Evidence-based
Health Practice

Evidence-based Health Practice

Edited by
Valerie A. Wright-St Clair
Duncan Reid
Susan Shaw
Joanne Ramsbotham

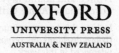

OXFORD
UNIVERSITY PRESS
AUSTRALIA & NEW ZEALAND

OXFORD
UNIVERSITY PRESS

Oxford University Press is a department of the University of Oxford.

It furthers the University's objective of excellence in research, scholarship, and education by publishing worldwide. Oxford is a registered trademark of Oxford University Press in the UK and in certain other countries.

Published in Australia by
Oxford University Press
8/737 Bourke Street, Docklands, Victoria 3008, Australia

National Library of Australia Cataloguing-in-Publication entry

    Author: Wright-St Clair, Valerie, author.

    Title: Evidence-based health practice / Valerie Wright-St Clair, Duncan Reid, Susan Shaw,
        Joanne Ramsbotham.

    ISBN: 9780195585230 (paperback)

    Notes: Includes index.

    Subjects: Medicine—Research—Australia.
        Research—Methodology.

    Other Authors/Contributors: Reid, Duncan, author.
                  Shaw, Susan, author.
                  Ramsbotham, Joanne, author.

Dewey Number: 610.72

Reproduction and communication for educational purposes

Edited by Joy Window
Text design by Sardine Design
Typeset by diacriTech, Chennai, India
Proofread by Bette Moore
Indexed by Jeanne Rudd
Printed and bound in Australia by Ligare Book Printers Pty Ltd
Cover image: Annie Griffiths/National Geographic Society/Corbis

FOREWORD

I suspect everybody reads a book like this a bit differently. I confess that I seldom ever read the foreword of a book. The times I read it is when the book has been so good that I want to savour every last drop. That is when I remember there is a bit as yet unread; it's a gift to have one last taste. The other time I read the foreword is when it is a book that I am struggling to understand, like when I am trying to read some of the philosophers. That's when I think 'Maybe whoever wrote the foreword can help me here'. And often they do; they simplify some of the complexities and point out the handholds.

So the question is, at what point in your book-experience are you reading this, and how might I be of any help? If you are fairly new to research, chances are this book initially felt a bit overwhelming. I doubt you have sat down to read it chapter by chapter from start to finish; life is too busy for that. You will have had an assignment, an exam—something that has prompted your reading. The great thing about this book is how clearly the information you might need has been laid out. It starts with overviews of research concepts. The 'me' who likes to get things done quickly might be tempted to bypass these chapters, but the 'wise' me would say 'slow down; get a grasp of the foundations, learn the language, understand how it all fits together. That will get me there quicker in the end'. Then there is the section on how to do research. Maybe it will be years before that's what you do, but to be able to critique any research you have to be able to understand if they did it 'right'. And tucked in the midst are gems, like Chapter 14 (identifying and evaluating multiple sources of information) and 15 (presenting and publishing research), which will be relevant for all your scholarly endeavours. They are both chapters to consult time and again.

Part 2 makes this book uniquely 'ours'. It acknowledges the indigenous communities of New Zealand and Australia, drawing our attention to both the cultural underpinnings of research and the cultural imperatives. Again, the insights from these authors go way beyond the subject of research itself. Remember they are here; they will be valuable resources in all sorts of ways.

My guess is that many of you will have headed straight for home base! You will have found the chapter about your chosen discipline and read it eagerly. This is the door that opens you to understanding the knowledge base that will underpin your practice. I encourage you, however, to make friends with other chapters. The world of health-care practice is becoming increasingly interprofessional. That means we need to get to know each other. In doing that, time and again we find we have more in common than we have differences.

So, is there any point to all of this? Maybe your grandmother was a nurse, or your uncle was a physiotherapist in an era when you just got on and did your best. There was no fuss about research back then. It was good basic care that mattered. David Nicholls, in Chapter 16, has us standing in a quandary by the bed of a patient with complex health and social issues, wondering what we should do. In those moments, you will be glad you have equipped yourself with the knowledge that research has gifted to your basket. At the same time you will know that, in itself, research will never be enough. Part 4 provides you with skills that will ensure you arrive at the practice encounter as ready as you can be to provide 'best care', yet you will always be called to respond to each unique situation. The thinking skills we encounter in research are great training for the dilemmas of practice.

Do not forget the index! Many of the notions within this book are threaded through chapter after chapter, like the melody of a song. You may not get it on the first read, but once you have heard the same melody represented in slightly different ways, it will stay with you. You will find yourself humming it without even having tried to commit it to memory.

None of us knows everything there is to know about research. There are several chapters in this book that I want to go back to because I know there are important insights within them 'as yet unlearnt' in my own long research journey. Therefore, this is not a book to sell at the end of the year. Keep it with you; return to it whenever you come up against something 'new'.

One imagines research books to be written by serious minded, scholarly people who either wear white coats or hide away at their computers wearing very thick glasses. Let me assure you the authors of this book are dynamic, enthusiastic and passionate about their subject. Like you they were once new to all of this, in an era when research itself was fairly new to the health disciplines. Many of us had to learn from teachers who were reading the text book one chapter ahead of us. In contrast, the authors of this book have all been involved in doing research, in teaching research to students and in supervising research projects. They have learnt what matters and what does not. Heidegger, the philosopher I try to read, once said that the only way to learn to ski is on skis. I had my own experience of trying to learn to ski from the book. It was only as I flew down the mountain that I realised I hadn't covered the chapter that told me how to stop! These authors will make sure they pass on the crucial information; at the same time they share a hope that one day you too will become a researcher inspired by their stories.

Knowledge is always socially constructed and privileged (or not). At the other end of the research journey when one's PhD goes out for examination, 'who' the examiners are can make a huge difference. It is not uncommon for two examiners to praise a thesis and a third to be very critical. This reminds us that life is complex; nothing is ever simple and straightforward. The good thing about drawing from a book written by local experts is that their expectations of what the 'right' answer is will be included in their writing. When I was first at university I came to recognise that the first assignment for every new teacher involved testing the waters, getting a feel for what they wanted. I might quote from international authors not knowing that 'my' teacher had quite a different view on things. This book keeps you within safe territory. Not only has the local author laid out their way of seeing things, but the local editors have nodded in agreement. The insights from this book are congruent with the ways of thinking about research within this community.

My advice is to treat this book as a trusted friend, the sort of friend who makes no demands upon you but is always there when you need them. Do not be frightened or shy of this book. Understanding 'comes'. Sometimes slowly, but that's okay. Just keep reading. Talk to your fellow students about the bits that interest you, or confuse you. Note the bits that you really enjoy; maybe they are pointing to a road you might one day follow in your postgraduate research. Delight in meeting the authors and engaging them in conversation about what they have written.

After my first read of this book I rang up Valerie, one of the editors, to congratulate her and her team on a splendid book. She was excited that I liked it. Having been privy to conversations with many of the authors over recent months as they found the time to write their pieces, and hearing how the editors often spent their weekends polishing this book into its readiness for you, I am very aware that every page is a labour of love. This is a gift from one generation of scholars to the next. Its purpose is not so you can pass your assignments (although that's definitely a plus!) but so that you can take hold of the flaming torch that will lead your generation forward in the challenge of keeping health care as good as it can be amidst the possibilities and challenges that lie ahead. This book is to grow you and strengthen you in your quest to become a health professional. May you delight in the learning, thinking and equipping that it offers. One day, you will look back and say, 'Look how far I have come'.

Dr Elizabeth Smythe
Associate Professor School of Health Care Practice
Faculty of Health and Environmental Sciences
AUT University

BRIEF CONTENTS

EXPANDED CONTENTS

LIST OF FIGURES AND TABLES

FIGURES

TABLES

LIST OF CASE STUDIES

LIST OF CLINICAL REFLECTIONS

LIST OF RESEARCH ALIVE BOXES

PREFACE

Research is one of the subjects that students in the health professions often find challenging and yet the process of finding, critiquing, using and evaluating information is essential to professional development and practice. This book has been designed to introduce fundamental research concepts that are relevant to the wider health-care and disability support sector while also making strong connections to the various areas of practice that students identify with.

The explanation of foundational concepts and illustrations from practice are designed to present research as relevant and useful to practitioners. Developing an understanding of research in a specific area of practice is enhanced by an appreciation of the work of other practitioners and disciplines. The increasing emphasis on interprofessional learning and collaborative practice means that students and practitioners need to understand concepts that are used by colleagues from other disciplines.

The research endeavour and practice go hand in hand as practitioners develop and reflect on their practice, explore current thinking, debate and contribute to analysis and critique, and suggest new or refined approaches to their work. It is essential that students develop the skills to explain, articulate and defend practice with relevant evidence.

This book presents an innovative approach to teaching research to students in the health sciences, linking research to practice, the identity of professions and the context of interprofessional learning and practice.

Valerie Wright-St Clair
Duncan Reid
Susan Shaw
Joanne Ramsbotham
Auckland, August 2013

STYLE GUIDE

The chapters in this book include features that are designed to support learning and provide a range of resources to consolidate and extend understanding. They are explained in the order you will find them in the book.

OVERVIEW

Each chapter begins with an overview in which the headings within the chapter are listed, providing a guide to the content.

KEY TERMS

At the beginning of each chapter a list of key terms is presented. These terms appear within that chapter in bold print and may be found in the glossary. Many of these words appear in more than one chapter, but they are only listed as key terms when they are essential to the flow and understanding of the content and presented in bold text when it does not interfere with the context within the text.

CASE STUDIES

Specific information is identified within chapters as case studies. These are situations, information or examples of interactions that illustrate links between research and practice. These provide a focus for class, tutorial or group discussion and debate.

RESEARCH ALIVE

These sections in each chapter showcase key research concepts or illustrate major research studies relevant to the chapter.

CLINICAL REFLECTIONS

Clinical reflections are provided to illustrate links between research and practice. They present real questions or issues that need to be considered by practitioners and encourage reflection on learning and practice.

SUMMARIES

Summary information is presented at the end of chapters to provide a brief overview of the information presented.

REFLECTION POINTS

Each chapter includes a list of reflection points, which are designed to assist with appreciating the communication process.

STUDY QUESTIONS

Key points from content of each chapter can be explored in more detail by responding to the study questions at the end of each chapter.

WEBSITES

The references at the end of chapters also include relevant websites to enable easy links to current debates and information. Some information about specific websites is also provided within the chapters.

GLOSSARY

A comprehensive glossary of terms is included at the end of the book and directly reflects the key terms from the chapters.

ABOUT THE AUTHORS

EDITORS

Valerie A. Wright-St Clair MPH, PhD, DipProfEthics, DipBusStudies, DipOccTherapy

Valerie is a registered occupational therapist with over 20 years' experience as an educator and researcher at Auckland University of Technology, with previous practice experience in gerontology, rehabilitation and neurology. She is currently Co-Director of the Active Ageing Research cluster, Person Centred Research Centre, and Associate Professor within the School of Rehabilitation and Occupation Studies. Valerie's teaching includes research for evidence-based practice, older adult health and wellness, ethical reasoning, and practice philosophies across undergraduate and postgraduate health professional programmes. Her current research projects span the fields of gerontology, occupational science, cross-cultural research and interpretive phenomenology. She holds a particular interest in how indigenous, non-indigenous and migrant seniors' participation in everyday activities influences longevity, health and wellness; seniors' integration and participation within communities; and understanding the meaning of what people do.

Duncan Reid BSc, MHSc, DHSc, PGDipHSc(Manipulative Physiotherapy), DipMT, DipPhys

Duncan is an Associate Professor of Physiotherapy and Associate Dean of Health in the Faculty of Health and Environmental Sciences, Auckland University of Technology. His areas of interest are teaching musculoskeletal physiotherapy at undergraduate and postgraduate level. In particular he has expertise in manual and manipulative therapy, especially manipulation to the cervical spine, a topic he has taught both nationally and internationally for over 25 years. Duncan's research interests are in the areas of muscle viscoelasticity, the management of osteoarthritis and sports injury prevention and screening. He is currently Vice President of the International Federation of Orthopaedic Manipulative Physical Therapists Association (IFOMPT). He is a Fellow of the New Zealand College of Physiotherapy and a life member of NZ Manipulative Physiotherapists Association.

Susan Shaw BN, MEdAdmin(Hons), EdD, DipTchg(Primary), NZRGON

Susan has a background in education and health care, having originally qualified as a primary school teacher and then a nurse. She holds professional registrations in teaching and nursing. Susan has worked at the Auckland University of Technology (AUT) since 1992 in several roles including teaching, academic leadership and staff development. During this time she has maintained her clinical practice in surgical, medical and palliative care settings. She is currently Associate Dean (Undergraduate), a director of the National Centre for Interprofessional Education and Collaborative Practice (NCIPECP) and Head of Nursing within the Faculty of Health and Environmental Sciences at AUT. Her research interests include quality education and clinical practice along with the responses of patients and health professionals towards experiences of chronic illness and disability. Her doctorate investigated nursing education in relation to chronic pain.

Joanne Ramsbotham BN, M(ClinicalNursing), PhD, RN, EM

Jo has coordinated and taught in nursing and midwifery programmes, and has expertise and a range of experience in employing and evaluating the impact of learning and teaching approaches in this area. Jo's research interests include how nursing students transfer prior learning from theoretical contexts into the practice environment, how past theoretical experiences inform students' development of dimensions of competence and factors that influence this dynamic process. Jo has a nursing clinical background in a variety of rural and metropolitan settings, most recently in paediatric acute services. She is based at the Queensland University of Technology.

CONTRIBUTORS

Anita Bamford-Wade MA, DNurs, DipBus (PMER), RN

Anita has wide experience in leadership and governance within New Zealand Health Care. Anita has been a senior lecturer at Auckland University of Technology (AUT) since 2005, after completing 15 years as Director of Nursing in both the public and private sectors. Her governance experience has been within district health boards and the secondary education sector. Anita was Joint Head of Nursing at AUT 2006–2012. Her doctoral thesis was action research entitled: *Leadership for culture change: generating new growth from old*. Anita teaches in the Doctor of Health Science programme at AUT. She also supervises both master's and doctoral students and is a regular peer reviewer for the *Journal of Nursing Management, Nurse Education Today, Nurse Leader: Journal for the International Council of Nurses, Journal of Clinical Nursing* and the *International Nursing Review*.

Felicity Bright BSLT(Hons), MHSc(Hons), MNZSTA

Felicity is a speech-language therapist and doctoral candidate at AUT University in Auckland. She is employed at Auckland University of Technology to lecture on speech-language therapy-related issues to allied health students, and provides clinical education to physiotherapy students focusing on communication skills and integrating a client-centred approach to rehabilitation. She works clinically with patients with a variety of acquired neurological conditions at both AUT and in private practice. Felicity's PhD is about exploring how rehabilitation providers engage with their patients who have communication difficulties in stroke rehabilitation. Her research interests centre on therapeutic skills and ways of working in rehabilitation.

Heather Came BA, MA(Hons), PhD, PGDipSE, CertHP

Heather is a seventh generation Pākeha New Zealander. She has spent the last 20 years working in a range of grassroots and strategic health promotion/public health roles across Aotearoa. She is an activist scholar with a passion for working with Te Tiriti o Waitangi and the pursuit of social justice across a range of issue areas. She currently teaches health promotion and community development within the Department of Community Health and Development at Auckland University of Technology.

Susan Cartwright BDS, MEd (Hons), DipClinDent

Susan graduated from Otago University Dental School in 1983 with a BDS and completed a Diploma in Clinical Dentistry in Periodontology with Distinction in 1998. She has worked in private dental practice in Hamilton, London and Auckland. Susan completed a master's degree in Education in 2010 while working as the Head of the Oral Health Department at Auckland University of Technology. In September 2010 Susan took up the role of Scientific Affairs Manager for Colgate Oral Care in the South Pacific region and is now based in Sydney.

Brenda Costa-Scorse BHSc (Nursing), RGON

Brenda has been involved in emergency medicine and paramedic education for the larger part of her professional life. She is a senior lecturer in Paramedicine and Emergency Management at Auckland University of Technology. Her clinical background is predominantly in emergency medicine; both in hospital, and out of hospital in the ambulance and commercial ski-areas. Brenda is presently undertaking a PhD on injury preventions strategies in alpine skiing and snowboarding. She has a strong belief in strengthening the chain of survival by advancing collaborative research and educational opportunities for all people involved in out-of-hospital care and emergency management responses. In 2009 Brenda established the National Paramedic Research Forum, an annual one-day conference that informs, inspires and creates debate by showcasing student and emerging researchers work. At the heart of Brenda's research philosophy is working with people, for people, to harness the potential of research to affect positive change. Brenda is a member of Paramedics Australasia.

Caroline Day BSocP(Counselling), CertCommWk, PGCert Counselling, MNZAC

Caroline Day is the programme leader for the Bachelor of Health Science in Counselling at Auckland University of Technology. She has extensive experience in the field, working in various counselling agencies as a family therapist and counsellor, and for the Auckland Family Court. She has a small private practice focused on supervision of counselling practitioners. Her practice is based on Narrative Therapy. She has an interest in social justice and conflict resolution.

Tagaloatele Peggy Fairbairn-Dunlop BA(Hons), MA, PhD, DipTchg

Tagaloatele Peggy is Professor of Pacific Studies at the Institute of Public Policy, Auckland University of Technology (AUT). She has been researching and publishing Pacific development issues for over 30 years and has been prominent in critiquing global models for their appropriateness to Pacific people's experiences—including issues of sustainable development, gender equity, family security and family-based violence. Peggy has worked with most national planning offices in the Pacific and has been active in women's and youth NGO advocacy and community education programmes. Peggy returned with her family to New Zealand from Samoa in 2006 to be Director of the Vaaomanu Pacifica Programme at Victoria University of Wellington, and then moved to AUT at the end of 2009. Documenting our stories 'before these are lost' is another research focus as seen in the publications *Tamaitai Samoa: Their stories* (1996) and *Making our place; Growing up PI in New Zealand* (2006). Her priority to grow a vibrant and robust Pacific postgraduate community is seen in her coordination of the national Pacific Post Graduate Talanoa by access grid. Peggy is Sa Petaia (Te'o) and Sa Atoa.

Panteá Farvid BA(Hons), MA(Hons), PhD

Panteá Farvid is a lecturer in psychology at Auckland University of Technology and the Head of Postgraduate Studies in the School of Public Health and Psychosocial Studies. Her research focuses on the intersection of gender, sexuality, identity, culture and power. Panteá is an experienced qualitative researcher and uses a variety of discursive methods in her work. A few years ago she completed her PhD research, which examined the social construction of heterosexual casual sex, from a critical and feminist perspective. She is currently working on projects examining the sex industry within New Zealand and Iranian codes of gender and sexuality. She has previously worked on projects examining online dating, sugar dating, *Fifty Shades of Grey*, and teen girls' engagement with Tumblr.

Brenda Flood MSc(OT), DipOT, NZROT

Brenda is a senior lecturer within the School of Interprofessional Health Studies at Auckland University of Technology (AUT) and the National Centre for Interprofessional Education and Collaborative Practice (NCIPECP). Her role involves developing, implementing and evaluating interprofessional education and collaborative practice opportunities for students across the Faculty of Health and Environmental Sciences. Brenda has a keen interest in and commitment to interprofessional practice, completing her master's degree in Interprofessional Health & Community Studies, at Canterbury Christchurch College (UK) and is currently undertaking doctoral studies at AUT with a focus on interprofessional education development. Her clinical background focused on interprofessional collaboration in the areas of forensic and acute mental health care. Brenda is committed to ensuring that students develop the knowledge, skills, attitudes and values required to work collaboratively in teams and are able to transfer these competencies into practice environments with the aim of improving health outcomes.

Dawn Forman MBA, PhD, PGDip(Executive Coaching), PGDip(Research Methodology), TDCR, MDCR

Dawn is a consultant and executive coach currently working in the UK, having recently spent 15 months working in Australia. She is an adjunct professor at Curtin University and Auckland University of Technology, and visiting professor at Chichester University. Dawn is involved in a number of national and international consultancy and research projects primarily in interprofessional education, governance and leadership development, and provides executive coaching to senior professionals both in Australia and the UK. Dawn was an executive faculty dean for 12 years at two universities in the UK and has published widely including five books and over 50 chapters and peer-reviewed articles.

Sue Fyfe BAppSc(Speech and Hearing)(Hons), BEd(Hons), BSc, PhD

Sue is a Professor of Medical Education and Chair of the Programme of Research into Higher Education in the Faculty of Health Sciences at Curtin University. She is an epidemiologist, anatomist and speech pathologist with research interests in disability and educational research in tertiary health sciences. Sue was the inaugural dean of teaching and learning in the Faculty of Health Sciences in 2004, before taking up the role of head of school of Public Health from 2005 to 2011. Her research interests and educational publications include the development and evaluation of courseware for teaching and learning in human biology; the role, use and value of automated feedback for students; and curriculum change and development. She has a particular interest in integrating interprofessional education into the proposed Curtin medical course, building on the strengths and focus on interprofessional education in the Faculty of Health Sciences at Curtin.

Ray Gates BPhty, GradDip(Pain Management)

Ray Gates is an Aboriginal physiotherapist descended from the Bundjalung people of north-eastern New South Wales, Australia. He has been professionally involved in Aboriginal and Torres Strait Islander health issues in various capacities for over 16 years. He was a founding member and inaugural president of the National Association of Aboriginal and Torres Strait Islander Physiotherapists, Inc. (NAATSIP). He is an advocate for the use of physiotherapy in primary health care to address the poor health status of Aboriginal and Torres Strait Islander peoples, and is a strong supporter for the provision of culturally safe health care by non-indigenous services.

Rosemary Godbold PhD, RN

Until recently Rosemary was a senior lecturer in health-care ethics and executive manager of the Auckland University of Technology's ethics committee. She is a registered nurse and her research interests include ethics education, research ethics and the convergence of health law, health ethics and clinical practice.

Naomi Heap DipDPM, GradDipTertTchg

Naomi is a qualified institutional and clinical services manager with over 20 years of experience in health-care management ranging across both the private sector and educational settings. Currently the Clinical Services Manager of the Akoranga Integrated Health Clinic at Auckland University of Technology, she holds the Graduate Diploma in Tertiary Teaching and has special interest in the fields of quality health services management, infection control, and interprofessional education (IPE) and collaborative practice. Current research activities are in the fields of sustainability, students' response to IPE, and IPE clinic management. Naomi is presently engaged in a Master of Health Science in Leadership and Management.

Colleen Higgins BSc(Hons), PhD

Colleen has over 30 years' experience using the techniques of molecular genetics to research a range of topics in plant and human biology. She has worked in university, government and private biotechnology laboratories in Australia, New Zealand and the UK understanding gene/disease associations, developing genetically modified plants with improved characteristics, studying gene structure and function, and examining pathogen evolution and host responses. In 2004 she joined Auckland University of Technology where she is now a senior lecturer teaching molecular genetics at undergraduate and postgraduate levels to Science and Medical Laboratory Science students. She has an active research programme using molecular tools to study plant virus evolution and host responses to infection.

Graham J. Howie BA, MSc, PhD

Graham Howie first joined the Ambulance Service in 1975, in the days of single-crewed vehicles. It was a great time to enter pre-hospital emergency care—he surfed that wave of new skills and advanced life support that transformed the ambulance world in New Zealand from the mid-1970s onwards. He has held positions as an on-road advanced paramedic, as a station officer in central Auckland, as a lecturer and coordinator of the advanced care programme with the National Ambulance Officers Training School, as a professional standards and development officer (a form of clinical coach) and as principal tutor within St John Clinical Education. Graham completed a BA in Psychology in 1999, an MSc in Neuroanatomy in 2003, and more recently a PhD in Physiology (in the developmental origins of the metabolic syndrome). He is currently a senior lecturer and researcher within the discipline of Paramedicine and Emergency Management at Auckland University of Technology.

Marion Hunter BA, MA(Hons), ADN, RGON, RM

Marion completed her midwifery education in 1982 with a keen interest in women's health and a sense that maternity care needed to change. Marion has worked in various roles including staff midwife in primary and tertiary settings, hospital educator, charge midwife of a tertiary birthing unit, consultant midwife overseeing the tertiary hospital and three primary units, midwifery lecturer at Auckland University of Technology (AUT) combined with a small caseload as a Lead Maternity Carer midwife in rural/remote rural area for eight years. Currently Marion continues her role as a Midwifery lecturer at AUT and is a doctor of health science candidate at AUT. Marion is a director of the PHARMAC Seminar Series, an advisory board member for NZ Formulary and member of the Midwifery Council of New Zealand. Her research interests include place of birth, prescribing, and most aspects of midwifery and women's health. Marion is a researcher in the NZ Birthplace collaborative group, which published New Zealand birth outcomes from home, primary and secondary or tertiary settings in the *Birth and NZCOM Journal* during 2011 and 2012.

Nicola Kayes BSc, MSc(Hons), PhD

Nicola graduated with her master's degree in health psychology from the University of Auckland in 2000 and her PhD from Auckland University of Technology (AUT) in 2011. She has been working in the Health and Rehabilitation Research Institute at AUT since 2005 as part of the Person Centred Research Centre where she contributes to both research and teaching in her role as senior lecturer. Nicola's research predominantly explores the intersection between health psychology and rehabilitation. Key research interests include the exploration of factors influencing engagement in rehabilitation (including the role that practitioners play), the development of novel strategies for engagement, and the development of outcome measures responsive to what matters most to patients undergoing rehabilitation. Since joining AUT in 2005, she has contributed to a range of projects resulting in publications in reputable international journals including *Clinical Rehabilitation*, *Archives of Physical Medicine and Rehabilitation*, *Neuropsychological Rehabilitation* and *Journal of Psychosomatic Research*.

Paula Kersten BSc, MSc, PhD, PGCert (Academic Practice), Member HPC

Paula qualified as a physiotherapist in the Netherlands in 1988. She completed both her MSc Rehabilitation and PhD in the UK. In 2011 she joined Auckland University of Technology as an Associate Professor in rehabilitation and Deputy Director of the Person Centred Research Centre (PCRC) where she leads the outcomes research cluster. Paula's research focuses on the evaluation of the rehabilitation process and outcome measurement. For example, she has completed projects on the management of fatigue in multiple sclerosis (MS), secondary prevention after transient ischemic attack (TIA), and implementation intentions as a supportive strategy for mobility enhancing activities in stroke and MS. Paula has also developed and delivered postgraduate programmes, supervised MSc and PhD students to completion and provided leadership to a wide range of nursing and allied health postgraduate programmes.

Chris Krägeloh BA(Hons), PhD

Chris is a senior lecturer in psychology at Auckland University of Technology and recently finished a term as head of postgraduate studies in the School of Public Health and Psychosocial Studies. Chris is a founding member of the New Zealand World Health Organisation Quality of Life (NZ WHOQOL) Group and conducts research about quality of life issues in a wide range of health and educational settings. He is an experimental psychologist by training and has expertise in psychometric testing of questionnaires. His other research interests include applied linguistics, as well as conceptual and philosophical issues in psychology, especially regarding the concept of mindfulness.

Jason Landon BSc, MSc, PhD

Jason has a PhD in psychology from the University of Auckland and the American Psychological Association (Div 25) awarded him the prize for an outstanding dissertation in behavioural psychology. He was one of the first postdoctoral scientists appointed to the National Research Centre for Growth and Development at the Liggins Institute of the University of Auckland where he was part of a multidisciplinary team investigating the effects of early-life nutrition on development. He was then a senior advisor with public health intelligence at the Ministry of Health. He is currently a senior lecturer in the Department of Psychology and the Gambling and Addictions Research Centre at Auckland University of Technology, and Programme Leader for the BHSc in Psychology degree. He is a named investigator on several large externally funded gambling research projects, and has research interests in gambling, addictions, behavioural psychology, health psychology, quality of life, and noise sensitivity.

Janet Larkman BA, MEd, RN

Janet is a senior lecturer in the Faculty of Health and Environmental Sciences at Auckland University of Technology, in the Nursing School. She is currently the program academic leader for Nursing. Janet worked as a nurse for 20 years, mainly in acute care. Her research experience started while she was nursing. She has extensive teaching experience in nursing and research. Her research interests are currently focused on integrating research into the nursing curriculum and educational research.

Peter Larmer MPH(Hons), DHSc, DipPhysio, DipMT, DipAcup, MNZSP, FNZCP

Peter is currently Head of the School of Rehabilitation and Occupation Studies at Auckland University of Technology. Peter has been teaching in the Department of Physiotherapy since 1995 and in the Master of Health Science programme since 1999. Peter's professional background is in private practice in musculoskeletal physiotherapy. Peter is a past member of the Physiotherapy Board of New Zealand. He has been involved on a number of committees of Physiotherapy New Zealand. He is currently a member of the Clinical Reference Group of the Accident Compensation Corporation and is also Vice President of Arthritis New Zealand. Peter has a specific interest in critical appraisal tools and has published a number of systematic reviews. He also has a research focus on outcome measures and his doctoral thesis investigated outcome measures in relation to ankle sprains.

Litiuingi Lose 'Ahio BSc, MPH, PGDip (Public Health)

Litiuingi Lose 'Ahio is Tongan-born, permanently residing in New Zealand. Over the last 10 years, she has been working as a Health Science Teacher and an Equity Team Coordinator for Māori and Pacific students at the Faculty of Health and Environmental Sciences, Auckland University of Technology (AUT). She completed her Master of Public Health (MPH) from AUT and is currently a part-time student of the Master of Educational Leadership programme. In her MPH thesis, she conducted research to explore the context and perception of food security for Tongans in South Auckland. She has just received a 10 weeks' summer studentship from the New Zealand Health Research Council to disseminate her MPH Vaevae manava (sharing of food and other resources) thesis findings to the Tongan community in Auckland.

Judith McAra-Couper BA, PhD, RGON, RM

Judith trained to be a midwife in Auckland in 1989 for the express purpose of going and working in Bangladesh. Her beginning midwifery was spent among the women and midwives of St Helens and Middlemore in Auckland, New Zealand, and this has had a lasting influence on her practice. Judith then spent many years in Bangladesh where the Bengali people and their lives touched her deeply and in terms of midwifery she experienced much that was challenging, tragic and amazing. Since her return to New Zealand in 1996 she has worked at Auckland University of Technology (AUT) as a midwifery lecturer. For 12 years she has held a joint appointment at Counties Manukau where she worked as a clinical midwife educator in the birthing unit. Judith has been involved in academic study for many years, and completed her PhD in 2007. In 2009, Judith returned for three months to Bangladesh where she worked for the World Health Organization and helped write a midwifery curriculum and syllabus for nurse midwives. This work has continued and Judith is now involved in the implementation of the programme and the curriculum development for Direct Entry Midwifery in Bangladesh. Judith received a STAR Post-Doctoral Scholarship in 2010, enabling her to develop as a researcher and to be involved in a number of research areas such as maternal mental health, sustainability of midwifery practice and place of birth. Judith is Co-Director of the Midwifery and Women's Health Research Centre at AUT and leads a number of research projects both at AUT and in collaboration with midwives and doctors from other institutions.

Antoinette McCallin BA, MA (Hons), PhD, RN

Antoinette McCallin is an Associate Professor in the Faculty of Health and Environmental Sciences and a director of the National Centre for Interprofessional Education and Collaborative Practice. Antoinette teaches postgraduate students in a variety of areas and supervises master's and doctoral research projects. The main emphasis of her research and writing has been on interdisciplinary teamwork, collaboration in professional–client relationships, and the development of interprofessional collaboration in health professional education. Antoinette is an internationally recognised, classic grounded theory researcher, a Fellow of the International Grounded Theory Institute in San Francisco, and a facilitator of international grounded theory workshops in the US and at Oxford in the UK. Her active involvement working with many students from wide-ranging disciplines and cultures over the years situates her well to work with professional practitioners seeking professional development through higher education.

Barbara McKenzie-Green MHSc (Hons), PhD, PGDip(Counselling), RN

Barbara has worked with older adults in acute care, community and long-term care settings. She has conducted research into residential life in long-term care, ageing with disability, oral health and older adults, relocation of older adults residing in long-term care, and registered nurses and supervisors' work in long-term care. Currently a senior lecturer at Auckland University of Technology, Barbara coordinates the older adult health and wellness postgraduate qualification. Her research methodology is grounded theory although she has taught and supervised thesis students in a range of qualitative methodologies. She co-facilitates a grounded theory group of thesis students with Shobah Nayar.

Sue McNaughton MBChB, MEd(Hons), GradDipTchg(Sec)

Sue has a background in medicine, clinical administration and science teaching. She currently lectures on interprofessional papers in the Faculty of Health and Environmental Science. Her academic interests include mapping, the development of beliefs and values, and the role of the body in clinical wisdom. She is currently doing her PhD around these interests using mixed phenomenological methods, and has also been involved in another project using mixed ethnographic methods.

Kathryn M. McPherson BA(Hons), PhD, DipHV, RN, RM

Kathryn is Professor of Rehabilitation (Laura Fergusson Chair) in the School of Rehabilitation and Occupation Studies and Director of the Person Centred Rehabilitation Centre at Auckland University of Technology. Previously, Kath was Associate Dean Postgraduate Studies at the University of Otago (Wellington) and Reader in Rehabilitation at the University of Southampton (UK). She has authored or co-authored more than 140 peer-reviewed publications. She also disseminates research and scholarship in training for organisations in New Zealand (the district health boards, the Accident Compensation Corporation, and other health and social services). She is a Visiting Professor at Kings College (University of London) and the University of Southampton. Kath's research has focused on person-centred rehabilitation—particularly in long-term neurological conditions, pain-related conditions, cancer survivorship and palliative care—including research measuring what matters, quality of care, informing rehabilitation by psychological approaches, quality of life, goal-setting, promoting engagement in rehabilitation, promoting participation, understanding the experience of disability, and theory in rehabilitation.

Russell B. Millar BSc(Hons), MSc, PhD

Russell is an Associate Professor at the University of Auckland. He obtained his PhD in Statistics from the University of Washington and has expertise in the development and application of statistical methodology for the modelling of real data, specialising in challenging problems such as those encountered in ecology and fisheries research. He has over 100 publications in the primary literature, and is currently Editor of the journal *Biometrics*.

C. Jane Morgan BA, MEd, RGON

Jane has an extensive background in tertiary teaching in health disciplines, and more recently in academic, information and research literacies. She is currently a lecturer in the School of Interprofessional Health Studies at Auckland University of Technology, teaching research methods within an enquiry-based learning framework. Jane takes a constructivist approach to teaching–learning activity, developing students' understanding of research in practice, processes inherent in research activity and the lenses that inform research methodologies. Jane's research focuses on interprofessional collaboration, specifically on the intersection of identity as a health professional and collaboration in graduate practice, and generally on notions of professionalism in health and allied health practices.

Juliet Boon-Nanai BA, MA, PhD

Juliet is an Equity Academic Pasifika leader within the Faculty of Health and Environmental Sciences. She is also a postgraduate supervisor in the Centre for Community Investment and Development within the Institute of Public Policy. Her research interests are in the general and holistic well-being of Pasifika people within New Zealand. Juliet has worked in academic institutions for 20 years, mainly with social science education and postgraduate students in the Samoan master's programme. Juliet's doctoral degree in geography from Ochanomizu University, Tokyo, Japan focused on sustainable development and examined community-based conservation activities within Iriomote Island and Samoa. Juliet obtained her master's degree from the University of the South Pacific, and her thesis examined the impact of socio-economic activities on mangrove degradation. The paper derived from this study was published in the *Geographical Review of Japan* and was nominated the best contribution to the journal's edition of 1991. Juliet also obtained her Bachelor of Arts degree in Geography from the University of Canterbury, Christchurch. Juliet is Samoan.

Shoba Nayar BHSc(OT), MHSc, PhD, NZROT

Shoba trained as an occupational therapist and is currently the Associate Director of the Centre for Migrant and Refugee Research and a senior lecturer in postgraduate public health at Auckland University of Technology. Her interest lies in developing understandings of Asian mental health, particularly the relationship between occupation and mental health and well-being, for immigrants and refugees living in New Zealand, and what health professionals and community organisations can do to support this population. Her doctoral work explored the occupational processes in which Indian immigrant women engage as they create a place for themselves and their families in New Zealand. This work has been the basis for current studies exploring the settlement experiences of immigrant communities in New Zealand and internationally.

David A. Nicholls MA, PhD, GradDip, MPNZ

David has a career as a practitioner, lecturer and researcher spanning three decades. In the 1980s he trained as a physiotherapist in England and became a physiotherapy practitioner. In the 1990s he moved into teaching, completed a master's degree in Research Methodology, and began researching using qualitative research approaches. In 2000 he emigrated to New Zealand to take up a teaching post at Auckland University of Technology and completed his PhD entitled *Body politics: A Foucauldian discourse analysis of physiotherapy practice*. David has taught on a range of undergraduate and postgraduate programmes for 20 years and is a passionate advocate for qualitative research, postmodern philosophy, pedagogy and critical theory.

Deborah Payne BA, MA, PhD, RN

Deborah's expertise is in qualitative research. She has a longstanding interest in women's health issues. Her PhD thesis was a Foucauldian discourse analysis of 'elderly primigravida', the term given to women who are pregnant for the first time at the age of 35 years or over. Her methodological expertise is in descriptive qualitative research and Foucauldian discourse analysis. Recent research projects have explored issues in relation to women and disability (for example, motherhood and disability, and sexuality and physical disability); assisted reproductive technologies (women's perceptions of short cycle IVF; IVF and work); and breastfeeding and work. Deborah is an experienced supervisor of master's and doctoral thesis students.

Holly Perry MAppSc(Hons), Registered Medical Laboratory Scientist, NZIMLS

Holly is a medical laboratory scientist with over 30 years' experience in transfusion science, both in clinical diagnostics and in tertiary education. In the clinical laboratory, Holly held a senior position in New Zealand, performing DNA-based typing and matching for transplant patients in the 1990s. Currently, Holly teaches undergraduate students of medical laboratory science, specialising in Transfusion Science at Auckland University of Technology in New Zealand. Holly's research areas are disease association studies, and designing new educational tools to teach Transfusion Science students. Holly also informs her teaching by attending conferences, such as the American Association of Blood Banks international meeting in 2012. She is a member of the New Zealand Institute of Medical Laboratory Science, and is the convenor of the NZIMLS Transfusion Science Special Interest Group. This group is responsible for promoting the profession through the provision of continuing education.

Kirk Reed MOccTherapy, DHSc, DipOccTherapy, Registered Occupational Therapist, MNZAOT

Kirk is Head of Occupational Science and Therapy at Auckland University of Technology. He is an occupational therapist with 22 years' experience in the mental health and tertiary education sectors. Kirk's doctoral thesis used a hermenutic phenomenological method and is entitled *Resituating the meaning of occupation in the context of living*. His research interests include the contribution that participation in meaningful occupation makes to health outcomes, interprofessional education and practice, and evidence for occupational therapy in primary health care. He teaches on undergraduate and postgraduate papers, supervises postgraduate thesis students, and is a director of the National Centre for Interprofessional Education and Collaborative Practice.

Heleen Reid (nee Blijlevens) BHSc(Occupational Therapy), MHSc

Heleen is Programme Leader for the Occupational Science and Therapy Department at Auckland University of Technology. She has a particular interest in evidence-based practice and occupation-focused practice through both her postgraduate research, and involvement with the *Journal of Occupational Science*. She has been involved in the review of a number of Australasian evidence-based practice textbooks. Teaching an evidence and practice paper for a number of years to both second and final year students has established her commitment to ensuring students develop their own skills in being critical consumers of research.

Keith Rome BSc(Hons), MSc, PhD, FCPodM SRCh

Keith is a Professor and Co-Director of the Health & Research Rehabilitation Institute, Auckland University of Technology with a clinical and academic background in podiatry. His research focuses on disorders affecting mobility in rheumatological conditions and incorporates studies of balance, falls risk factors, the effects of rheumatic disease on gait and foot function, and the effects of foot disorders and footwear. His research expertise extends from laboratory-based human movement studies through to the conduct of clinical trials. He has published four book chapters, 85 peer-reviewed journal articles, six editorials/letters/reviews and 75 conference abstracts. He has published in the most prestigious journals in the fields of rheumatology and biomechanics, including *Arthritis Care and Research*, *Rheumatology*, *Clinical Biomechanics* and *Gait & Posture*. Keith has a strong national and growing international reputation, as evidenced by 20 invited conference presentations, including presentations in the UK, the USA, Australia and Italy.

Sandy Rutherford BA(Soc Sci), MSc(Rehabilitation), DipOT, PGDip (Occ Practice), NZROT, MNZOTA

Sandy is an occupational therapist and doctoral candidate at Auckland University of Technology (AUT). She works in the Person Centred Research Centre as a research officer on a longitudinal qualitative study exploring the experience of recovery after Stroke. She is completing her PhD as a part of this study focusing on self-management. Sandy also works as a lecturer in the department of Occupational Science and Occupational Therapy. She coordinates the occupational therapy service based in the AUT clinic, which is part of the National Centre for Interprofessional Education & Collaborative Practice. Her research interests include the strategies people with health conditions use to participate in occupations and experience well-being and goal planning in rehabilitation.

Rhoda M. Scherman BA(Psychology), MA, PhD

Rhoda is a senior lecturer in the Department of Psychology, where she teaches Social Psychology and Critical Evaluation in Psychology within the undergraduate programme, and facilitates the postgraduate dissertation class for the BHSc(Hons) in Psychology. Rhoda is also the Head of Research for the School of Public Health and Psychosocial Studies, where she supports and assists academic staff to enhance their research activities. Originally from the US, she immigrated to New Zealand in 1997 in order to complete her master's degree and PhD at the University of Auckland, where she could specialise in adoption-related research owing to New Zealand's unique and progressive adoption practices. Rhoda continues to research and supervise in the broad field of adoption, as well as in areas of collaborative learning and teaching environments, the use of novel methods for assessing social attitudes, the influence of sporting outcomes on violence against women, and the experiences of refugee children settling in New Zealand.

Elizabeth Smythe BSocSc, PhD, RGON, RM

Elizabeth comes from a background of nursing and midwifery, but has developed a strong commitment to interprofessional learning at master's and doctoral levels. She is currently Programme Leader of the Doctor of Health Science, exploring approaches to changing practice from within the practice setting. Her research methodological expertise is phenomenological hermeneutics.

Deb Spence BA, PhD, DipTertiaryTeaching, PGDip(Soc Sci Dist), RN, RM, MCNANZ

Deb has a strong practice background in acute care nursing and teaches at bachelor, master's and doctoral levels. Interests and strengths in relation to her teaching and research include cross-cultural practice, advanced nursing practice, qualitative methodologies (particularly hermeneutic phenomenology), action research, appreciative inquiry and working collaboratively to advance clinical practice. She has a particular interest in making the less tangible dimensions of practice more visible. In her joint role as Head of Nursing, Deb has committed to implementing a culture of shared governance within nursing and the School of Health Care Practice. Current areas of research include curriculum development and the collaborative implementation of a student supervision model supporting the development of clinical practice.

Robin Sutcliffe MHSc(Hons), DipPsychotherapy, PGDip HSc

Robin Sutcliffe is a teacher on the Bachelor of Health Science in Counselling at Auckland University of Technology. She began her counselling training in 1987 with a course in person-centred counselling with Presbyterian Support Services and then went on to complete a Diploma in Psychodynamic Psychotherapy, a postgraduate Diploma of Health Science in Clinical Supervision and a Master of Health Science. She has also trained in psychodrama, Transactional Analysis, NLP and solution-focused counselling. Robin has many years experience working within a residential mental health service as a counsellor and therapist, and as a counsellor for a community women's centre. She also supervises mental health support workers and counsellors.

Alice Theadom BSc, MSc, PhD, MNZPsS, MIHP

Alice trained and worked as a psychologist in the UK, before moving to New Zealand in 2009. Alice is based within the National Institute for Stroke and Applied Neuroscience at Auckland University of Technology and leads the traumatic brain injury research programme. Alice has a key interest in the application of psychology in health care, with a particular emphasis on the role of sleep in neurological conditions, individual adjustment to illness and impact on family functioning, and trialling of novel interventions in neurorehabilitation. Alice has published many authored and co-authored journal articles in a range of medical and psychology journals including *The Lancet*

Neurology, *European Journal of Neurology*, *Sleep Medicine* and the *Journal of Psychosomatic Research*. Alice is Assistant Editor for the journal *Neuroepidemiology*, and a member of the Medical Advisory Board for Fibromyalgia Syndrome in the UK.

Keith Tudor BA(Hons), MA, MSc, PhD, DipPsychotherapy, CQSW, CTA(P), TSTA(P)

Keith has a background in probation, social work, counselling, mental health and psychotherapy. He is an Associate Professor at Auckland University of Technology where he is also Head of the Department of Psychotherapy. He is the author or editor of over 300 publications, including 11 books; the editor of a book series, *Advancing theory in therapy* (London: Routledge), of the journal *Psychotherapy and Politics International* (Wiley-Blackwell), and, with Alayne Hall, of the journal *Ata: Journal of Psychotherapy Aotearoa New Zealand*.

Wee-Leong Joe Chang BMLS MMLS, PGCert (Applied Sci), GradCert Bus, GradCert Information Tech

Joe is a senior laboratory scientist in clinical chemistry, with a background in research and development adept at distilling complex scientific and medical issues into easily understandable packets in both written and verbal formats, with 15 years' experience in laboratory medicine and eight years as a lecturer in the BMLS pathway. Currently he works part time at Auckland University of Technology as a clinical chemistry lecturer and a senior medical scientist at the Auckland District Health Board. His role includes providing medical education and training, regulatory compliance, and significant interaction with peers on issues in diagnostic testing. In addition he also provides support in the laboratory information system as an IT analyst.

Tineke Water PhD, GradDip, DipNsg, RCpN

Tineke has a background in child-health nursing and currently teaches on the postgraduate child-health pathway at Auckland University of Technology (AUT), as well as working at Starship Children's Hospital as a research fellow. Tineke's research interests include ethical issues around the provision of care for children and young people, ensuring that children and young people's voices are included in any decision-making around their health care, and promoting research with children rather than on children. She is currently the Head of Research for the School of Health Care Practice and Co-Director of the Child Health Research Centre, and is on the Auckland University of Technology's Ethics Committee. Her PhD was on the ethical dilemmas faced by health professionals and families when a child requires health care.

W. Lindsey White BSc, PhD

Lindsey completed his PhD at the University of Auckland in 2001. He was awarded a three-year Post-Doctoral Fellowship from the New Zealand Foundation for Research, Science and Technology and in 2004 took up a position as senior lecturer in the School of Applied Science at Auckland

University of Technology (AUT). He is currently Head of the School of Interprofessional Health Studies at AUT. Dr White's research interest is seaweed utilisation, both by humans and by marine herbivores. In terms of seaweed utilisation by humans, he is interested in seaweed farming—both understanding and limiting the environmental impacts of seaweed farming. To examine plant–herbivore interactions he has employed a nutritional ecology perspective, entailing a synthesis of information about both the algae (for example, their abundance and nutritional composition) and the herbivore (for example, diet choice and digestive physiology).

Denise Wilson BA(SocSc), MA(Hons), PhD, RN, FCNA(NZ), Fellow of Te Mata o te Tau

Denise is an Associate Professor of Māori Health and the Director of Taupua Waiora Centre for Māori Health Research at Auckland University of Technology. She has an extensive background in undergraduate and postgraduate nursing education, and currently teaches and researches in the area of Māori health. Her research and publication activities are focused on Māori and indigenous health, cultural safety, family violence and health (particularly Māori), and workforce development. She is a Fellow of the College of Nurses Aotearoa (NZ) and Te Mata o te Tau (Academy of Māori Research & Scholarship), the Editor-in-Chief of *Nursing Praxis in New Zealand*, and has been appointed to the Health Research Council's College of Experts, the Health Quality and Safety Commission's Family Violence Death Review Committee and Māori Roopu. She is also an elected member of the Nursing Network for Violence Against Women International, and a member of the national steering group for Ngā Manukura ō Āpōpō.

Grace Wong BA, MPH, RCpN

Grace's work is devoted to tobacco control, nurses and equity. She is a senior lecturer in Nursing at Auckland University of Technology. Grace was a public health nurse, researcher and policy analyst at Action on Smoking and Health New Zealand, and lecturer in research methods. She is the director of Smokefree Nurses Aotearoa/New Zealand.

PART 1

RESEARCH CONCEPTS

CHAPTER 1

WHAT, WHY AND HOW OF RESEARCH

VALERIE A. WRIGHT-ST CLAIR, DUNCAN REID AND SUSAN SHAW

CHAPTER OVERVIEW

This chapter covers the following topics:

- The interplay of research and practice
- The nature of knowledge
- What is evidence?
- Evidence grows and changes
- Evidence in the world of practice
- The impact of evidence on practice
- Thinking critically about research

KEY TERMS

Control	Paradigm shift
Data	Practitioner
Design	Qualitative evidence
Evidence-based practice	Quantitative evidence
Expertise	Research
Intuition	Science

Evidence-based practice
Practice that is informed by the careful consideration and evaluation of relevant information, and client/patient and practitioner experience and preference.

Research
The purposeful collection and consideration of information to investigate a defined question.

There are many reasons for choosing to study in the health sciences—some students are motivated by the opportunity to work alongside patients (the words 'patient', 'consumer', 'client' and 'service user' will be used interchangeably throughout this book) and others have a particular career plan in mind. All students will find themselves learning about evidence-based practice and research during their studies. These concepts are central to learning and practice in the health sciences and may initiate a range of responses in students from strong interest to the sense that this may one of those subjects that just has to be survived! Some students may have been involved with research projects at school or in other settings and therefore have an understanding of the processes and the work involved. For others this will be a new area, possibly creating a certain sense of trepidation about what lies ahead.

THE INTERPLAY OF RESEARCH AND PRACTICE

Practitioner
A person recognised by a professional group.

It is common for students to wonder about the relevance of research, especially if their aim is to be the best health practitioner that they can. However, most people interested in the area of health science already have questions about practice such as why things are done in certain ways, what way is best, or how current thinking or practice can be improved. Often these questions emerge from personal experience and play some role in students' choice of study. It is common for people in general and health practitioners in particular to form opinions about what they think is best. These opinions are informed by personal understandings and the views and opinions of others, including colleagues and patients. The processes of thinking, questioning, investigating and reflecting on information from a wide range of sources, people and contexts are at the heart of finding and using evidence to guide practice.

This is what a student (we will call her Lauren) said when reflecting back on how her undergraduate education had prepared her for getting her first job:

> I entered my degree thinking I probably wasn't going to change the world, but I intended to change the world for my clients, that's for sure. I wanted my clients to have every opportunity to engage in the life they wanted; not settle for a life they should be grateful for, or a life that would do. So how will my degree enable me to do this? I can see how my degree armed me with the skills and knowledge to understand people in different settings, to know what to assess and [how to] design interventions, to reason and make decisions. And let's not forget the dreaded research papers. How will we, as newly graduated practitioners, know how to achieve better health outcomes for our clients and promote our profession's credibility without evidence? And when better to plant that seed than when I'm first learning everything? (Lauren, September 2012)

It is not surprising that health science students want to become the best practitioners they can be. As a student it is easy to see how being a good communicator, learning practice techniques, and engaging in clinical and professional reasoning come together to help make good practitioners. This is the stuff of everyday practice. Evidence and research are threaded through practice and professional work and study in the health sciences.

THE NATURE OF KNOWLEDGE

One of the features of the modern world is the vast array of information that is generated and the access that people have to it; the world of student health practitioners is no different. One of the challenges is to know how to manage, understand and use this information. This requires having tools for finding, sorting and evaluating information as well as skills for interpreting and using it.

One of the expectations of students graduating from entry level degrees is that they will be critical consumers of research. In other words, health science students and graduates are expected to use research-generated knowledge, or evidence, to design, implement and evaluate the most effective interventions for the people and communities they serve. This expectation changes at the postgraduate level of study where students are expected to make a contribution to a field which may be described in terms of new knowledge; this involves actually doing research rather than just accessing and understanding it.

Design
The process of planning and creating a solution to a problem.

Gaining a bachelor's degree-level qualification in the health and disability sector requires becoming familiar with research in a way that informs practice decisions. The interplay of research evidence and practice therefore ensures that advancing knowledge contributes to the delivery of services and ultimately to enhancing outcomes for service users. This is what evidence-based health practice means; it involves questioning what to do, searching for relevant information, critically considering the information available, building new knowledge and reflecting on it in a way that develops effective practice.

WHAT IS EVIDENCE?

The statement 'not everything that counts can be counted, and not everything that can be counted counts' has been attributed to Einstein and Cameron (Cameron, 1963) and while the exact phrase and history of it are difficult to track, the principle that 'just because information exists does not mean it is useful' is important to consider. Evidence-based health practice has been described as 'the integration of best research evidence with clinical experience and client values' (Sackett, Straus, Richardson, Rosenberg, & Haynes, 2000, p. 1). As such, equal privilege is afforded to available knowledge arising from rigorous and trustworthy research (qualitative and quantitative evidence), practice wisdom, and the consumers' needs, goals and aspirations. The nature of the question asked determines the nature of the evidence that is most relevant and useful.

CASE STUDY 1.1

TYPES OF EVIDENCE—NUMBERS AND STATISTICS GIVE ONE VIEW WHILE NARRATIVE GIVES ANOTHER

Quantitative evidence
Information collected through rigorously conducted research processes with an emphasis on the quantity of data.

Qualitative evidence
Information collected through a rigorous research process that emphasised the quality and richness of data.

Control
A research cohort not treated in an active way to provide a point of comparison.

Quantitative evidence (such as numbers and statistics) and qualitative evidence (such as stories and narrative) combine to present a comprehensive picture—to tell the 'whole story'.

Drawing on trustworthy evidence from quantitative and qualitative research is valuable when designing effective interventions. To illustrate, unintentional falls are a major cause of injury and disability for older New Zealanders. In 2010 alone, over 3,100 serious, non-fatal falls were reported for those aged 75 and older, showing a pattern of increasing annual frequency (Statistics New Zealand, 2011). The personal, social and health care costs of serious and less serious falls are significant. Numerous studies in Aotearoa New Zealand, Australia and other countries have considered the efficacy and cost–benefits of falls prevention programmes that target modifiable risk factors. For example, a recent intervention study in the United Kingdom of 204 community-dwelling seniors who had fallen, but not been admitted to hospital, is fairly typical of the multi-factorial programmes being tested and implemented. As well as being more cost-effective, the structured falls-prevention programme led by nurses, occupational therapists and physiotherapists resulted in better participant outcomes, including fewer subsequent falls and higher quality of life, than the existing rehabilitation services (Sach et al., 2012). Yet, even though both programmes were making a difference, participants still withdrew from both the experimental and control groups. Qualitative research offers some suggestions as why older people do not participate in or complete community and clinic-based falls-prevention programmes (Child et al., 2012; Elskamp, Hartholt, Patka, van Beeck, & van der Cammen, et al., 2012).

When interviewed about their own and others' experiences of falling, as well as likelihood of falling in the near future, older people in South Australia wanted to be viewed by others as not the type of person who falls. In other words, participating in a falls-prevention programme threatened their sense of who they were (Dollard, Barton, Newbury, & Turnbull, 2012).

Similarly, older people in The Netherlands who were seen by emergency services following a fall thought of themselves as being too well to attend a falls-prevention programme (Elskamp et al., 2012). Such qualitative research adds depth to understanding what is going on and why. Making use of different forms of research evidence means richer understandings can be taken into account when designing effective health, disability or social services.

Thinking critically about evidence helps to broaden the range of information that a practitioner may bring to any situation. An appreciation of the notion of expertise can lead to seeing the client or patient as an expert, with knowledge that is based on lived experience and can contribute to understanding the situation and addressing it. Trusting human intuition and experience can also inform the planning and delivery of health-care and disability support services (Welsh & Lyons, 2001). Most experienced practitioners can tell stories of situations in which they 'knew' there was a problem before it was completely obvious and acting on their intuition and clinical judgment had a positive outcome whereas if they had waited for objective information to appear, it may have been too late to have made such a difference.

Expertise
Expert skills and knowledge.

Intuition
The process of knowing something as a result of personal and/or professional insight.

EVIDENCE GROWS AND CHANGES

In order for evidence to inform practice, research needs to be relevant and useful. However, what is known and its relevance change and develop over time. It is important to appreciate that the usefulness of research can be altered as a consequence of the development of a field of knowledge, or when the context in which the problem exists changes. Research activities include various processes designed to ensure the integrity of new information. The concepts of review and debate are highly valued within the research community. Practitioners and researchers alike need to be aware of new and emerging concepts and how such knowledge impacts on their understanding and approach to any given practice situation.

CASE STUDY 1.2

PREPARING PATIENTS FOR SURGERY

Aotearoa New Zealand has a particularly high incidence of bowel cancer and therefore is a nation in which much bowel surgery takes place every year. Practitioners working with these patients follow routine protocols to prepare

(continued next page)

VALERIE A. WRIGHT-ST CLAIR, DUNCAN REID AND SUSAN SHAW

them for this type of surgery. A surgeon working in Auckland (Mattias Soop) is part of an international team which has been investigating pre-surgery preparation for bowel surgery patients through extensive analysis of research and practice and has challenged a number of conventional parts of this preparation (Fearon et al., 2005; Lassen et al., 2009)—see Table 1.1.

TABLE 1.1 PROBLEMS AND RESEARCH-BASED SOLUTIONS

TRADITIONAL PRACTICE	PROBLEMS IDENTIFIED	RESEARCH-BASED PRACTICE
Extensive preoperative bowel preparation	Dehydration, fluid and electrolyte imbalance Risk of cardiac complications	Patients undergoing colonic resection should not receive routine oral bowel preparation.
Fasting from midnight on the day of surgery	Thirst and hunger anxiety Not a major risk factor	Patients should fast for liquids for two hours and solids for six hours preoperatively.

Changes in practice based on this information benefit patients not only in terms of outcomes but also positively influence their experience of this treatment.

It is tempting to think that any specific piece of evidence may be ultimately right and therefore indisputable but, in reality in the context of practice, the need to keep seeking a more detailed understanding and the advent of new technology means that new questions constantly can be asked and new perspectives sought. The continued consideration of problems and attempts to seek new answers lead to changes in practice even in what may appear to be very developed fields of knowledge.

EVIDENCE IN THE WORLD OF PRACTICE

Human existence and the contexts in which practitioners and those they serve involve many variables. One of the challenges when linking research to practice is that often the most precise and definitive research only answers a very small question which may be only partially helpful for the particular situation that the practitioner and the patient find themselves in. A large amount of research in the health and disability sector is undertaken in relation to medications. The specific research questions often relate to the effectiveness of the medication.

CASE STUDY 1.3

NEW PERSPECTIVES ON OLD INFORMATION—PHARMACOGENETICS

Despite extensive resources spent on researching medicines there is evidence that unless patients have a genetic code that equips them to fully metabolise the specific components within it they will not be able to fully benefit from it. Research from the UK by Brian Spear and his colleagues (2001) identifies the proportion of the world's population which have the genetic code to gain the most benefit from various types of medications.

TABLE 1.2   EXAMPLES OF FINDINGS ABOUT THE PROPORTION OF THE POPULATION ABLE TO BENEFIT FROM TYPES OF MEDICATIONS BASED ON GENETIC PROFILE

TYPE OF ISSUE	EFFICACY (%)
Alzheimer's disease	30
Asthma	60
Diabetes	57
Oncology	25
Rheumatoid arthritis	50
Schizophrenia	60

Source: Spear, Heath-Chiozzi, & Huff, 2001

This information could help explain why some patients do not seem to respond to or benefit from medications to the same extent as others.

The existence of research in relation to any specific issue or problem does not mean that all of the relevant questions have been asked or answered. Existing information may not be providing a comprehensive picture when there are questions about the sample or the relevance of the specific question in relation to the complex world of practice (Shaw, 2006).

THE IMPACT OF EVIDENCE ON PRACTICE

Paradigm shift
A change in the theoretical framework or perspective from which information and knowledge has been viewed.

Practice changes over time as evidence evolves, as do the approaches to asking questions and seeking answers. The concept of a paradigm shift refers to a situation in which there has been a significant change in thinking within a field of knowledge or practice. This usually involves commonly held assumptions about the things that are thought to be true in current practice being challenged and questioned. The concept of the paradigm shift was suggested by Kuhn (1970) and denotes a change from one way of thinking to another. Such journeys within groups of practitioners and fields of knowledge are often driven by people who act as agents of change. In the case of scientific endeavour this change agent is new research or evidence.

CASE STUDY 1.4

PARADIGM SHIFT

An example of a paradigm shift in the world of musculoskeletal practice is the treatment of tendinitis, in particular the Achilles tendon. Generally speaking when an anatomical structure is mentioned with the suffix 'itis', this implies an inflammatory process affecting the structure (for example, appendicitis can be defined as inflammation of the appendix). Therefore any patient presenting with a sore tendon was diagnosed with an inflamed tendon or tendinitis. Within this paradigm the methods of treatment to help resolve this problem revolved around reducing inflammation and swelling, rest, ice, compression, elevation, massage, ultrasound, stretches and anti-inflammatory medications.

However, not all patients who presented with this type of condition improved with this regimen; many of them had the condition for months well beyond the accepted time for normal inflammation to have resolved. Some patients also required surgery despite the best conservative care (Alfredson, Pietila, Jonsson, & Lorentzon, 1998; Maffulli, Sharma, & Luscombe, 2004). Research identified that these types of tendon problems were not inflammatory—in fact, tendon biopsy showed no inflammatory cells in the tendon, but there were instead great degeneration in the tendon and types of collagen that did not tolerate normal loads well (Khan, Cook, Taunton, & Bonar, 2000, Maffulli et al., 2004).

So the paradigm shift involved rethinking the concept of inflammation in the tissues; this in turn debunked the model of care that had been predicated on inflammation. It led to a change in treatment from emphasising rest and reduced loading to one of gradually increasing load via strengthening the muscles and tendon, and return to a sport or activity programme (over a 12-week period). The shift in treatment approach has now been demonstrated to be more effective than surgery in people with this type of condition (Alfredson, Pietila, Jonsson, & Lorentzon, 1998). This shift has been reflected in a change of name from tendinitis to tendinopathy, which more accurately reflects the pathological process in the tendon. There is also now a body of research that supports this approach in a wide range of tendon conditions (Svernlov & Adolfsson, 2001; Mafi, Lorentzon, & Alfredson, 2001; Norregaard, Larsen, Bieler, & Langberg, 2007; Ohberg, Lorentzon, & Alfredson, 2004).

There are many examples of practice within health science that have been considered standard for a long time and yet have been challenged by research. Research which investigates a real-life question and explores information from various perspectives (such as qualitative information from patients and practitioners, and quantitative information from mechanical analysis) is likely to be the most meaningful and useful. Understanding evidence and research is necessary to the provision of high-quality care within the health-care and disability support sector.

THINKING CRITICALLY ABOUT RESEARCH

Research, like most areas of human endeavour, has the potential to challenge territories, boundaries and interests. The pressure for industry to use research to produce and market products (such as pharmaceuticals) and the demands on practitioners and academic health professionals to describe and reflect on their practice requires that high standards are maintained and that critical questions are asked. The existence of research results does not mean that the new knowledge is useful or relevant. If the research did not pose a useful question or did not investigate it in a manner that represented real life or practice then it may demonstrate good science but not be of any use.

Engaging in research often means asking challenging questions or questioning the status quo. This is not always an easy place to be. Historically, there are examples of people having suffered for their new ideas which were deemed radical and foolish. In the 1780s Semmelweiss suggested that practitioners should wash their hands between patients and particularly between carrying out postmortems and delivering babies. He was ostracised for his views (Widmer, 2000) but today hand washing is considered by the World Health Organization to be of the greatest importance (Pittet, Allegranzi, & Boyce, 2009) for professionals and the general population.

Science
The body of processes used to develop and extend knowledge (often with an emphasis on empiricism and positivism).

VALERIE A. WRIGHT-ST CLAIR, DUNCAN REID AND SUSAN SHAW

RESEARCH ALIVE 1.1
RESEARCH AND PRACTICE

There are many developments underway interrogating the interface between research and practice. A particularly innovative approach is that of the REACT (randomised evaluations of accepted choices in treatment trials).

The traditional approach to medical (especially pharmaceutical) research has been to randomise patients into groups at the beginning of the study comparing two treatment approaches. This process is complex and time-consuming. The REACT trials involve links in the software and records that are routinely kept by general practitioners. At the point where a particular diagnosis is made and more than one accepted treatment is available the system asks specific questions and then links the patient's **data** into the system. This enables follow-up and analysis via the information kept in the health system and also provides long-term information about 'real life' outcomes (such as adverse health events that patients experience) rather than surrogate outcomes (such as changes in cholesterol or blood pressure) (van Staa et al., 2012).

Data
Information that is gathered for the purpose of analysis and research.

SUMMARY

Evidence and research are concepts that students need to understand. They are central to understanding and developing practice and necessary to keeping up to date with knowledge and innovations, ultimately contributing to the delivery and evaluation of the best possible care and support. A foundation knowledge of these concepts gained during undergraduate education will also equip practitioners well to further develop their careers in practice, teaching or research.

REFLECTION POINTS

- Thinking back on this chapter, what are the main messages that you draw from it?
- How has your thinking about the relevance of research to your learning changed?
- How has this chapter challenged and/or affirmed your understandings and beliefs about research?

STUDY QUESTIONS

1 How would you describe the concept of evidence?
2 Why would evidence be relevant to an undergraduate student in the health sciences?
3 What are the differences between quantitative and qualitative evidence?
4 Why is research important for practitioners and patients?

ADDITIONAL READING

Goldacre, B. (2012). *Bad pharma*. London: Fourth Estate.

Salsburg, D. (2001). *The lady tasting tea: How statistics revolutionized science in the twentieth century*. New York: Henry Holt.

REFERENCES

Alfredson, H., Pietila, T., Jonsson, P., & Lorentzon, R. (1998). Heavy-load eccentric calf muscle training for the treatment of chronic Achilles tendinosis. *American Journal of Sports Medicine, 26*(3), 360–366.

Cameron, W. B. (1963). *Informal sociology: A casual introduction to social thinking*. NewYork: Random House.

Child, S., Goodwin, V., Garside, R., Jones-Hughes, T., Boddy, K., & Stein, K. (2012). Factors influencing the implementation of fall prevention programmes: A systematic review and synthesis of qualitative studies. *Implementation Science, 7*, 91.

Dollard, J., Barton, C., Newbury, J., & Turnbull, D. (2012). Falls in old age: A threat to identity. *Journal of Clinical Nursing, 21*, 2617–2625.

Elskamp, A. B. M., Hartholt, K. A., Patka, P., van Beeck, E. F., & van der Cammen, T. J. M. (2012). Why older people refuse to participate in falls prevention trials: A qualitative study. *Experimental Gerontology, 47*, 342–345.

Fearon, K., Ljungqvist, O., Von Meyenfeldt, M., Revhaug, A., Dejong, C., Lassen, K., Nygren, J., et al. (2005). Enhanced recovery after surgery: A consensus review of clinical care for patients undergoing colonic resection. *Clinical Nutrition, 24*(3), 466–477.

Khan, K, M., Cook, J. L., Taunton, J. E., & Bonar, F. (2000). Overuse tendinosis, not tendinitis. Part 1: A new paradigm for a difficult clinical problem. *The Physician and Sports Medicine, 28*(5), 38–48.

Kuhn, T. S. (1970). *The structure of scientific revolutions*. Chicago: University of Chicago Press.

Lassen, K., Soop, M., Nygren, J., Cox, P., Hendry, P., Spies, C., et al. (2009). Consensus review of optimal perioperative care in colorectal surgery: Enhanced recovery after surgery (ERAS) group recommendations. *Archives of Surgery, 144*(10), 961–969.

Mafi, M., Lorentzon, R., & Alfredson, H. (2001). Superior short term results with eccentric calf muscle training compared to concentric training in a randomised prospective multicenter study on patients with chronic achilles tendinosis. *Knee Surgery, Sports Traumatology, Arthroscopy, 9*(1), 42–27.

Maffulli, N., Sharma, P., & Luscombe, K. (2004). Achilles tendinopathy: Aetiology and management. *Journal of the Royal Society of Medicine, 97*, 472–476.

Norregaard, J., Larsen, C., Bieler, T., & Langberg, H. (2007). Eccentric exercise in treatment of Achilles tendinopathy. *Scandinavian Journal of Medicine & Science in Sports, 17*, 133–138.

Ohberg, L., Lorentzon, R., & Alfredson, H. (2004). Good clinical results but persisting side-to-side differences in calf muscle strength after surgical treatment of chronic achilles tendinosis: A 5-year follow-up. *Scandinavian Journal of Medicine & Science in Sports, 11*(4), 207–212.

Pittet, D., Allegranzi, B., & Boyce, J. (2009). The World Health Organization guidelines on hand hygiene in health care and their consensus recommendations. World Health Organization World Alliance for Patient Safety First Global Patient Safety Challenge Core Group of Experts. *Infection Control and Hospital Epidemiology, 30*(7), 611–622.

Sach, T. H., Logan, P. A., Coupland, C. A. C., Gladman, J. R. F., Sahota, O., Stoner-Hobbs, Robertson, K., et al. (2012). Community falls prevention for people who call an emergency ambulance after a fall: An economic evaluation alongside a randomised controlled trial. *Age and Ageing, 41*, 635–641.

Sackett, D. L., Straus, S. E., Richardson, W. C., Rosenberg, W., & Haynes, R. M. (2000). *Evidence-based medicine: how to practice and teach EBM*. New York: Churchill Livingstone.

Shaw, S. M. (2006). A critical approach to evidence provided through clinical trials. *Nursing Times, 102*(36), 36–38.

Spear B. B., Heath-Chiozzi, M., & Huff, J. (2001) Clinical application of pharmacogenetics. *Trends in Molecular Medicine, 7*(5), 201–204.

Statistics New Zealand (2011). *Serious injury outcome indicators: 1994–2010.* Wellington: Author.

Svernlov, B., & Adolfsson, L. (2001). Non operative treatment regime including eccentric training for lateral humeral epicondylalgia. *Scandinavian Journal of Medical Science and Sports, 11*, 328–34.

van Staa, T-P., Goldacre, B., Gulliford, M., Cassell, J., Pirmohamed, M., Taweel, A., et al. (2012). Pragmatic randomised trials using routine electronic health records: Putting them to the test. *British Medical Journal, 344*, e55.

Welsh, L., & Lyons, C. M. (2001). Evidence-based care and the case for intuition and tacit in clinical assessment and decision making in mental health nursing practice: An empirical contribution to the debate. *Journal of Psychiatric and Mental Health Nursing, 8*, 299–305.

Widmer, A. F. (2000). Replace hand washing with use of a waterless alcohol hand rub? *Clinical Infectious Diseases, 31*, 136–143.

WEBSITES

Is the five-second rule true?
http://www.youtube.com/watch?v=rYXdsOEWBj0&feature=b-mv

Health Research Council of New Zealand:
http://www.hrc.govt.nz
http:// www.hrc.govt.nz/funding-opportunities/maori-development

New Zealand Social Science Data Service:
http://www.nzssds.org.nz/surveys_in_nz/nzsrda:

Te Pou—supporting and developing the mental health, addiction and disability workforce in New Zealand:
http://www.tepou.co.nz

Unite for Sight—why research matters:
http://www.uniteforsight.org/research-course/module2

CHAPTER 2

OVERVIEW OF RESEARCH APPROACHES

C. JANE MORGAN

CHAPTER OVERVIEW

This chapter covers the following topics:

- World views (paradigms)
- Reasoning
- Research approaches

KEY TERMS

Constructivist	Quantitative
Deductive reasoning	Realism
Engagement	Relationships
Epistemology	Relativist
Inductive reasoning	Reliability
Interpretation	Social
Interprofessional collaboration	Theory
Ontology	Validity
Positivist	World view
Qualitative	

Research, like any other organised activity, does not happen by chance. The approach taken to plan, resource and implement an investigation is dependent on a number of factors: the context (situation) in which answers are being sought, the focus of the enquiry, perceived or actual 'gaps' in current knowledge, and the questions.

CASE STUDY 2.1

KEY QUESTIONS TO ASK

Enquiry Context

Where is the enquiry situated? Are you asking questions related to a specified health discipline issue or are you focused on broader interdisciplinary concerns? Once you have established the context, you begin to focus on your specific area of interest.

Focus of Enquiry (Initial Area of Interest)

In the area of interest, what is the current literature telling you? What studies have previously been conducted and how were the studies designed? To answer these questions you read literature that is relevant and appropriate to your area of interest.

What are the similarities and differences noted between study findings? To answer this question you critique (compare, contrast, evaluate) specific research designs and findings.

What is currently known in the area of interest? To answer this question you synthesise (draw together) information and discuss commonalities and differences in relation to your area of interest.

'Gaps' in Knowledge

You will have some answers to your initial enquiry, but often you conclude with more questions due to the expanding knowledge base. Through your critique of relevant information and research designs you will come to realise there are 'gaps' that warrant further investigation. Arguing the need for further investigation requires sound reasoning, and provides justification for pursuing answers through one or more focused research questions.

Research Questions

A research question must be clear, directive and contain the essence of what you want to explore, investigate, examine, evaluate or test. Your research questions will guide what approach you take in designing a study that may produce answers to your questions.

C. JANE MORGAN

WORLD VIEWS (PARADIGMS)

Ontology
The view an individual holds about the nature of being or existence.

Epistemology
The study of the basis of knowledge.

Realism
A view that emphasises external sources of existence independent of human interpretation.

World view
A set of beliefs or concepts held by an individual informing how they interpret their environment and experience.

Positivist
An approach that emphasises natural phenomena, objectivity and empirical scientific approaches to knowledge.

Relativist
A view that information must be considered according to its relationship with other known facts.

Interpretation
Adapting or explaining information in a meaningful and relevant way.

Constructivist
A view that learning is not passively received, but actively constructed by individuals or groups.

Relationships
The similarities and connections between people or variables in any given situation.

Many answers to the above questions are logical and easily answered. However, the way the world is viewed (ontology) has implications for understandings of what knowledge is (for example, facts, thoughts, opinions and experiences) and how knowledge is obtained and constructed (epistemology). Realism is the term used to refer to the world as an objective reality that may only be accurately captured by humans through unbiased 'detached' discovery (Liamputtong, 2010). In this world view, reality is objective, residing separate to human awareness, and accessed through rigorous study and ability to 'tap into' what already exists outside human consciousness. From a realist perspective, knowledge is absolute and can only be challenged through discovering 'new' facts that contradict or negate what was previously obtained. A positivist lens refers to the ways realists view knowledge and how knowledge is obtained within their world views. Knowledge of human anatomy falls within a realist-positivist paradigm, with people generally consensual on the foundational aspects of the human body structures.

If, however, people believe that knowledge is constructed by individuals and in groups, with meaning and understanding varying between individuals, then this could be thought of as a relativist world view of reality (Denzin & Lincoln, 2011). Within this paradigm, humans create meaning through experiences, interactions and interpretation towards new understanding, and therefore knowledge is constructed, rather than obtained or discovered. A constructivist lens refers to the ways relativists view knowledge and how knowledge is created, either individually or through social interaction (Fosnot, 2005). From this perspective humans do not think in isolation of their social and cultural perspectives with individual history influencing how humans perceive, interpret and generate meaning from new experiences (Creswell, 2007). This is true also of groups, and influences cultural and socialisation processes. Table 2.1 summarises the different world views.

Within the continuum between strictly positivist and strongly constructivist stances on what constitutes knowledge (epistemology) are a number of hybrid lens that encompass aspects of both objective and subjective world views. Some terms are postpositivism, advocacy/participatory, pragmatism and postmodernism (Creswell, 2009). These terms also relate to ways of thinking about what constitutes knowledge and how knowledge is created. In reality there are few people who are solely positivist thinkers or purely constructivist because humans generally like to rely on certain knowledge as consistent and dependable (positivist), and most have interpersonal relationships where meanings can alter over time and through interaction (constructivist). In relation to research activity, people's ontological world view on what constitutes reality (realism or relativism) and associated epistemological view on what constitutes knowledge acquisition (positivist or constructivist) influence recognition and acceptance of knowledge in a specified field. How an individual views the nature of reality (ontology)

TABLE 2.1 OVERVIEW OF TERMINOLOGY RELATED TO WORLD VIEWS AND RESEARCH

WORLD VIEWS (PARADIGMS)		
Ontology *(nature of reality)*	Realism	Relativism
Epistemology *(nature of knowledge)*	Positivist	Constructivist
Axiology *(values)*	Objectivity	Subjectivity
Reasoning *(logical thinking)*	Deductive	Inductive
RESEARCH		
Aim	Explain, predict, confirm, test theory	Understand, create meaning, build theory
Approaches	Quantitative	Qualitative
Researcher	Detached	Integral
Methodology	Descriptive Experimental/manipulative	Descriptive, interpretive, naturalistic
Methods	Observation, measurement	Observation, dialogue, participation
Data (information collected)	Numerical	Written text, visual 'text'
Analysis (information examined)	Statistical	Thematic, discourse
Findings (communicated to audience)	Tables, graphs, charts, statistics	Descriptive text and/or interpretive text

and knowledge (epistemology) can also influence personal choice of research approach, design and implementation.

In summary a realist, through a predominately positivist lens, maintains detached objectivity towards knowledge—knowledge is waiting to be discovered through asking the right questions and continual scrutiny of current answers towards the 'ultimate truth' (Crotty, 1998). In contrast a relativist, through a predominately constructivist lens, views knowledge as fluid, malleable and open to interpretation. From this perspective, knowledge is not fixed and waiting to be discovered. Instead, knowledge is variable, interlinked with experiences and the meaning attributed to those experiences.

Realistically humans oscillate between objective and subjective thinking, depending on what they are doing and their aims at a designated time. This is important when considering research, which, as previously stated, is focused activity. Graziano and

Raulin (2013) use the term 'a prepared mind' to illustrate the methodical preparation required in developing a research design—aligning a focused question with a research approach that is likely to produce answers.

REASONING

Reasoning is the ability to think logically or rationally, towards decision-making on what constitutes knowledge. The ability to reason is strongly influenced by whether knowledge is viewed as waiting to be discovered (positivist lens), or constructed through social interaction (constructivist-interpretive lens). It is important to remember, as stated previously, that in reality humans are seldom only positivist or only constructivist. However, in research terms, inductive reasoning involves building knowledge from research data, progressing from information (data) produced directly during research activity to increasingly more complex ideas and concepts in the area of interest (Neuman, 2009). From this line of reasoning, a researcher uses research data to construct new knowledge, new understanding and new meaning, and for grounded theory approaches generation of theory is viewed as an outcome of research (Bryman, 2008). Conversely, deductive reasoning commences with an 'educated guess' on what may be found through research in a specified area of interest (Neuman, 2009). From this line of reasoning Bryman (2008) advocates the use of existing theory to guide research.

Inductive reasoning
An approach to thinking that involves developing general propositions from particular examples.

Theory
An explanation of a phenomenon.

Deductive reasoning
An approach to thinking that involves identifying common principles from which specific conclusions can be drawn.

RESEARCH APPROACHES

The approach taken to finding answers to focused questions is influenced by the researcher's world view, questions asked and the logical reasoning that aligns with the world view. A positivist world view aligns well with deductive reasoning, or logic. From this perspective knowledge is absolute and through research new discoveries confirm, add to or negate what is currently known (Bryman, 2008). Those who are interested in testing current knowledge, to determine validity (legitimacy) and reliability (dependability) of what is currently known in an area of interest are inclined towards a quantitative research approach to study designs. This implies that, following extensive review of relevant literature, the researcher uses deductive reasoning and quasi or experimental research designs for the purpose of adding to, negating or confirming knowledge in the area of interest. The use of quasi (pseudo) or experimental research designs sits within a quantitative research approach, aiming at discovery of knowledge.

Validity
Fitness for purpose.

Reliability
The extent to which the same results are elicited when an investigation is repeated.

Quantitative
Relating to analysis based on quantity of information.

Inductive reasoning aligns with a constructivist world view, whereby individuals and/or groups construct meaning to existing or new experiences, with the purpose of constructing 'meaning' that may be consistent with current knowledge, or may be entirely novel. This research approach is generally exploratory by nature, with research data from participants providing the basis for developing ideas, or new ways of viewing the world. Exploratory research designs sit within a qualitative research approach, aiming at construction of knowledge.

The approach to research can be polarised from purely qualitative (exploratory) through to purely quantitative (experimental), but may include design aspects of both qualitative and quantitative approaches based on what questions are being asked, in a specified interest area. Qualitative data (information) provide in-depth rich textual information from relatively small numbers of people or groups, and is often referred to as social research (Bryman, 2008). Collection of measurements and observations to determine correlations (linked associations) between naturally occurring factors or through manipulating one or several factors to determine causal relationships provides quantitative data. Table 2.1 provides a simplistic summary of terms associated with particular world views, namely realism-positivist and relativism-constructivist. Human thinking seldom fits neatly into either paradigm; however, familiarity with the terms and how they fit into research approaches assists with planning a relevant research journey.

Qualitative
Relating to analysis based on quality rather than the quantity of information and the value of human experience.

Social
Relating to people and the interactions between them.

CLINICAL REFLECTION 2.1: THINKING ABOUT STUDENT PLACEMENTS

During your undergraduate study as a health science student in a clinical programme, you are expected to undertake clinical placement requirements. This can cause anxiety and uncertainty as you negotiate your way into new and often complex interactive relationships with patients/clients, other health teams and allied health-care practitioners. Additionally you have academic study requirements that must be met while you are immersed in practice placements off-campus. If you wanted to know how other students respond to the expectations of practice, what research approach would be most appropriate if you were interested in knowing the following:

a   Does the timing of placements affect students' ability to study?
b   How do students 'juggle' the dual demands of academic study and learning in placements?
c   What challenges face students in practice settings?
d   What strategies students use to communicate effectively with placement staff.
e   How students interact with patients/clients.

ANSWERS
a & d Quantitative approach may be most appropriate
b, c & e Qualitative approach may be most appropriate

Curiosity, uncertainty or perplexity direct people towards the relevant enquiry questions to ask, and towards designing a research plan that will allow them to either discover or explore potential answers. The epistemological world view of an individual on what constitutes knowledge and whether knowledge is discovered or constructed will influence how research is viewed.

Aligned with the research approach for each of the questions, think about what type of knowledge would be gained through use of the approach. What is the world view that underpins the approach and what is the associated logic or reasoning that informs the world view? It is worthwhile asking, 'What does the person asking the question want to know'? Is the question asked to explore students' perceptions or experiences of placement interaction? If so, the question sits within a qualitative research approach and seeks to find answers from a constructivist-interpretive world view on what constitutes knowledge. If the question seeks answers on cause–effect relationships between observable factors, then it fits in a quantitative research approach that is underpinned by a positivist world view. The following chapters will enlarge on qualitative and quantitative research approaches in greater depth.

RESEARCH ALIVE 2.1
COLLABORATION

Interprofessional collaboration is viewed as a way forward in providing effective, efficient health-care services (World Health Organization, 2010). However, the ability to work with other health professions does not occur automatically. One reason is that students enter university with stereotypical expectations of their chosen profession, influencing how and whom they interact with. Pollard (2009) was interested in exploring how students who enrolled in health-related disciplines engaged with other health professions, and what their views on interprofessional engagement included. Interactive observations and interviews with a small number of students who had experienced interprofessional interaction provided data (information), which Pollard analysed thematically in order to understand the meaning students had attributed to their experiences of working collaboratively. Pollard's findings indicated a number of factors influencing successful student engagement, including students' confidence levels and the availability of support networks in the clinical context. Results from the study identified the need for senior clinical staff members to scaffold learning experiences of an interprofessional nature with undergraduate students. Earlier research by Perkins, Horsburgh and Coyle (2008) discovered stereotypical attitudes of senior practitioners as

Engagement
Meaningful interaction.

a contributing factor to maintenance of negativity towards **interprofessional collaboration** by undergraduate medical and nursing students. Perkins et al. surveyed both students and practising professionals from nursing, medicine and pharmacy disciplines on their attitudes, values and beliefs related to collaborative work. Statistical results indicated a strong correlation between practising professionals' attitudes, values and beliefs and those of emerging professionals. Although Pollard (2009) explored student perspectives only, and Perkins et al. (2008) surveyed both students and registered practitioners, findings from both studies indicate the influence that health-care practitioners have on student attitudes and willingness to engage in collaborative practice.

Interprofessional collaboration
The process of practitioners from different professionals working together in a meaningful way.

SUMMARY

Research requires an understanding of world views (paradigms) on what constitutes reality and knowledge. This involves appreciating the concepts of ontology (the nature of reality) and epistemology (the nature of knowledge); then research approaches and aligned designs become clearer. A primary consideration in research design is what the researcher is seeking to find in the context and the initial enquiry and to identify gaps in the literature leading to research questions. The research approach taken in designing a study will depend on the type of answers being sought: exploration into …, investigation into …, examination of … and/ or experimentation with …

This chapter provides an overview of qualitative and quantitative research approaches, and the philosophical underpinnings that inform each approach. It is important to remember that this is just the beginning, with expansion and elaboration through the research continuum provided in further chapters.

REFLECTION POINTS

- As you delve into further chapters, think about the philosophical concepts of ontology and epistemology that expand research approaches.
- Do you have a clear understanding of the alignment between your perspectives on the nature of reality, on what constitutes knowledge, and how these perspectives inform and influence the types of questions you seek answers to?
- How does your world view on reality and knowledge affect the types of research literature you read and are informed by?

STUDY QUESTIONS

1 'Mind map' or graphically display your world-view perspectives on the nature or reality and knowledge. Link the two with the types of knowledge you rely on to inform your clinical practice.

2 What research approaches align with your world view?

3 What aspects of clinical practice are you interested in researching? What research considerations are required in designing a study that may provide answers?

ADDITIONAL READING

Crookes, P., & Davies, S. (2004). *Research into practice* (2nd ed.). Toronto: Elsevier.

DePoy, E., & Gitlin, L. N. (2011). *Introduction to research: Understanding and applying multiple strategies* (4th ed.). St Louis: Mosby.

Polgar, S., & Thomas, S. A. (2008). *Introduction to research in the health sciences* (5th ed.). Toronto: Churchill Livingstone Elsevier.

REFERENCES

Bryman, A. (2008). *Social research methods.* (3rd ed.). New York, NY: Oxford.

Creswell, J. W. (2007). *Qualitative inquiry & research design* (2nd ed.). Thousand Oaks, CA: Sage Publications.

Creswell, J. W. (2009). *Research design: Qualitative, quantitative, and mixed methods approaches* (3rd ed.). Thousand Oaks, CA: Sage Publications.

Crotty, M. (1998). *The foundations of social research: Meaning and perspective in the research process.* Sydney: Allen & Unwin.

Denzin, N. K., & Lincoln, Y. S. (Eds.). (2011). *The Sage handbook of qualitative research.* Thousand Oaks, CA: Sage.

Fosnot, C. T. (Ed.). (2005). *Constructivism: Theory, perspectives, and practice* (2nd ed.). New York, NY: Teachers College Press.

Graziano, A. M., & Raulin, M. L. (2013). *Research methods: A process of inquiry* (8th ed.). Upper Saddle River, NJ: Pearson.

Liamputtong, P. (2010). *Performing qualitative cross-cultural research.* Cambridge: Cambridge University Press.

Neuman, W. L. (2009). *Understanding research.* Boston, MA: Pearson Education.

Perkins, R. J., Horsburgh, M., & Coyle, B. (2008). Attitudes, beliefs and values of students in undergraduate medical, nursing and pharmacy programs. *Australian Health Review, 32*(2), 252–255.

Pollard, K. (2009). Student engagement in interprofessional working in practice placement settings. *Journal of Clinical Nursing, 18*, 2846–2856.

World Health Organization. (2010). *Framework for action on interprofessional education and collaborative practice.* Retrieved from http://www.who.int/hrh/nursing-midwifery/en

WEBSITES

Health Research Council of New Zealand:
http://www.hrc.govt.nz

Centre of Asian and Ethnic Minority Health Research:
http://www.fmhs.auckland.ac.nz/soph/centres/cahre

Tōmaiora Māori Health Research Centre:
http://www.fmhs.auckland.ac.nz/faculty/tomaiora

Centre for Mental Health Research:
http://www.fmhs.auckland.ac.nz/son/cmhr

CHAPTER 3

QUALITATIVE APPROACHES

SUE McNAUGHTON

CHAPTER OVERVIEW

This chapter covers the following topics:

- What is qualitative research and why do it?
- Qualitative research dimensions
- Qualitative research methods

KEY TERMS

Behaviour	Mental
Community	Methods
Critical	Naturalistic
Critical theory	Objective
Cultural	Participants
Data	Phenomenology
Ethnography	Qualitative research
Evaluation	Social
Holistic	Theoretical
Interviews	

The way in which any research is planned and undertaken should reflect the question that is being asked and the best way of getting quality information. Qualitative research approaches provide opportunities for exploring complex questions in their context. The experience of pain is a good example of a complex concept that lends itself to qualitative research.

Qualitative research
Research carried out in a qualitative manner.

WHAT IS QUALITATIVE RESEARCH AND WHY DO IT?

'What is the pain like?' 'How much does the pain impact on life?' These common health-care questions may be explored using measurable and scientific methods of investigating what is at least in part a physical problem. Yet a report using a World Health Organization quality of life assessment by Skevington, Lotfy and O'Connell (2004) noted that, compared with other factors such as energy or work, pain was quite poorly correlated with the physical domain of quality of life. What does this mean? Is pain something other than physical, or is bodily experience only one aspect of pain? How does pain affect a person's evaluation of quality of life? These are questions that a statistical examination, even one using rigorous quantitative methods and large global samples, cannot answer. The qualities of things, people and events cannot be fully expressed in numbers.

Methods
Systematic procedures for undertaking an inquiry.

Evaluation
The process of determining value.

Rather, there are multiple individual and collective qualitative ways to go about attempting to answer questions such as 'What is the pain like?' Pain is used in this chapter to explore some of these ways and the sorts of answers they might give to questions about the nature of the phenomenon. The examples presented here are based on real patients and pain research.

QUALITATIVE RESEARCH DIMENSIONS

To investigate the nature of pain qualitatively, researching practitioners must decide whose pain to explore, what sort of information to collect, and what theoretical position to take. Figure 3.1 illustrates these three dimensions of qualitative research using common qualitative terms. The participants (who), the kind of information (data) to collect and the research approach are all influenced by the theoretical positions and world views.

Theoretical
Relating to theory.

Participants
People who choose to take part in research.

Data
Information that is gathered for the purpose of analysis and research.

FIGURE 3.1 QUALITATIVE DIMENSIONS

The diagram shows a spectrum of qualitative research ranging from quite structured, 'outsider-looking-in' approaches where a detached researcher determines how the research is conducted and what data are collected, right through to an unstructured, 'insider-looking-in' view where the participants and an involved researcher together determine how the data are collected and sometimes the whole research process (Bryman, 2008). Narratives (stories), experiences, social and environmental interactions, cultural documents and artefacts (human-made objects) and naturally occurring events are common sources of data for qualitative research.

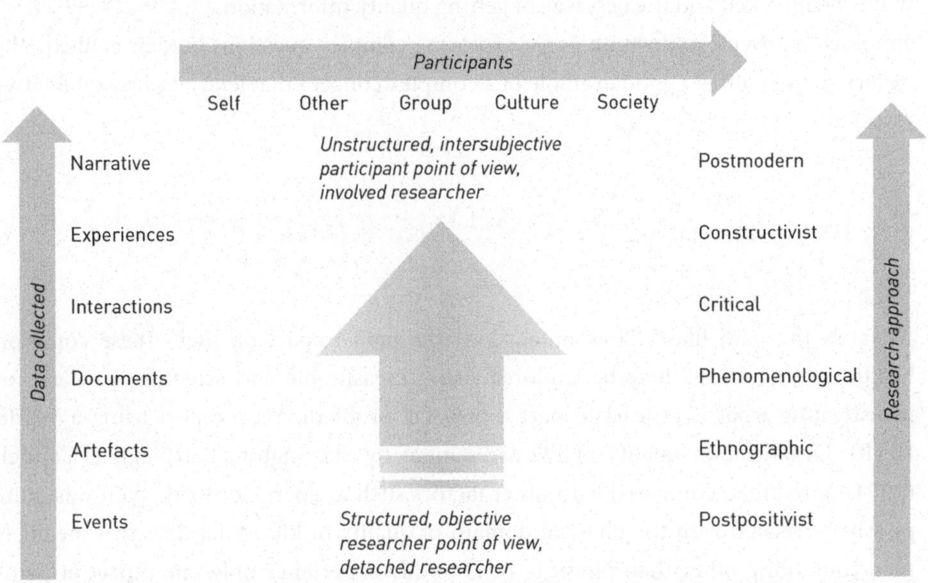

Social
Relating to people and the interactions between them.

Cultural
Relating to beliefs, traditions, practices and rituals originating within the family and community into which a person is born and raised, and transmitted from one generation to the next through a common language.

Interviews
Conversations held for the purpose of gathering information.

QUALITATIVE RESEARCH METHODS

Qualitative research provides a lot of scope for choosing methods (ways of doing research). Embarking on qualitative research requires carefully considering what methods will best fit the research question, the theoretical approach and the participants' particular characteristics. Reading published qualitative research articles is a good way to find descriptions of what and why the particular methods were used. Figure 3.2 shows some data collection methods and where they tend to sit within the qualitative dimensions. Some, for example interviews, are used with many different approaches and participants, but this does not always mean that they are the most appropriate.

FIGURE 3.2   POSSIBLE QUALITATIVE DATA COLLECTION METHODS

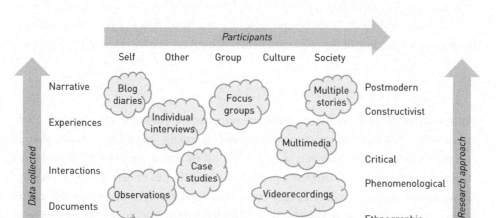

CASE STUDY 3.1

RESEARCHING EFFECTIVE TREATMENT

Allan is 49 years old, lives in a small New Zealand town, and has had rheumatoid arthritis for 15 years. Different medications have reduced the pain he experiences in his ankles and elbows, but he has progressively lost the movement and strength in these joints. A friend suggested he try a special diet which excluded all processed foods, flour, sugar and meat. Allan has been on the diet for six months and recently stopped taking his prescribed medications because he felt the pain had reduced to a manageable level and his joint function was unchanged. If you were interested in conducting qualitative research on the effects of dietary changes on rheumatoid arthritis pain:

- What sorts of participants would you want to include?
- What kinds of qualitative data could be collected?
- What data collection methods could be used?

SUE McNAUGHTON

Considering these questions would ideally highlight a fundamental qualitative research problem: the topics are usually complex and deciding how to recruit participants or collect data is difficult. Some compromises are usually needed, so it is important to have a basic understanding of the important beliefs behind qualitative research approaches.

POSTPOSITIVIST APPROACHES

Postpositivist research applies experimental principles to qualitative research; this might seem contradictory since experimental research is usually quantitative. While sharing the positivist view that research is an objective process aimed at explaining or predicting through valid and reliable methods, postpositivism differs in understanding knowledge as never complete, and nature as only ever understandable in terms of probable causes rather than laws (Denzin & Lincoln, 2011). This has led to criticism of post-positivism as a thinly disguised positivist, scientific view of the world, lacking in the acknowledgment that the researcher interprets the process and the product of research (Giddings & Grant, 2007). Nevertheless, for researchers with a realist world view who want to investigate topics qualitatively but retain some quantitative principles, the postpositivist approach allows the researcher to be more distanced from the participants, use scientific methods, define criteria to analyse the data and search for correlations between factors.

Objective
An approach that implies a completely external or detached view of an object or phenomenon.

RESEARCH ALIVE 3.1
PAIN AND UNBORN CHILDREN

Chin's (2011) discussion of foetal pain illustrates how researchers' models of the foetus differ between positivist and post-positivist approaches. One group of researchers view the foetus as an 'incomplete adult' while the other group views the foetus as an 'unborn patient' (2011, p. 307). The 'incomplete adult' model researchers base their view on research into the foetal brain, which does not develop the cortical structures and functions that adults require to subjectively experience pain until the third trimester of pregnancy. These researchers believe foetuses prior to this stage cannot feel pain since they do not have the necessary structures. The 'unborn patient' model researchers base their view on experimental studies detecting stress hormone levels in preterm neonates and in-utero surgery. They suggest that the foetus may experience pain in unique ways, perhaps via subcortical structures and processes. In their view, the foetus is a unique kind of patient, not an incomplete adult (Chin, 2011).

Although based on two different understandings of the foetus, both research groups use similar scientific methods. The more positivist researchers see the foetus as subject to the same knowable developmental and physiological laws as the adult human, while the postpositivist researchers see the foetus as a unique and partly unknowable entity that cannot be subjectively experienced.

ETHNOGRAPHIC APPROACHES

Ethnography is literally the writing or drawing of culture, which usually means the close observation of a group of people or society going about its usual activities (Murchison, 2010). Ethnography has a history in detailed field studies by researchers taking a naturalistic approach, which means observing and describing the culture and world from the participants' perspective in a non-interventionist and respectful way (Hammersley & Atkinson, 1995). This naturalistic focus has produced other ethnographic approaches such as ethnomethodology, in which researchers study the way that conversation and activity create and produce social structures and functions (Bryman, 2008). It has also produced a lot of overlap between ethnography and other types of qualitative research, especially critical research which is concerned with social structures. Ethnography today is frequently less interested in describing activities and events and more interested in patterns of behaviour and the shared symbols and meanings of groups and cultures (Murchison, 2010). As an approach to studying cultural practices, including workplace interactions, ethnography is very useful for researching both health-care practitioners' and patients' daily lives, practices and cultures, and for investigating the meanings of health-care activities. In response to criticisms of ethnography as too detached and objective, participant-observer or insider research, where the researcher is a member of the culture being studied, has become increasingly popular (Denzin & Lincoln, 2011). Being a participant-observer may improve the researcher's authentic understanding of the culture, but it does not completely eliminate the distinction between researcher and participant and must still be appropriate and ethical (Murchison, 2010).

Ethnography
The process of recording and describing human behaviour.

Naturalistic
An approach that emphasises viewing and exploring things in their natural environment.

Critical
Of significance or a deliberate attempt to bring about social change.

Behaviour
The response of a living thing (including people) to stimulation.

CASE STUDY 3.2

THINKING ABOUT HOW TO INVESTIGATE

Kate is a physiotherapist on an orthopaedic ward in a large hospital and David is a nurse on the same ward. Their daily workplace interactions involve relating to patients who are often heavily medicated in order to control the pain from

[continued next page]

SUE McNAUGHTON

their injuries. Kate has observed that pain perception in these patients varies greatly on a day-to-day basis and this affects the interventions she uses. David has noticed that the patients respond well to Kate and that his interactions are better with the patients she assists, particularly in conversations about their pain.

- How might an ethnographic approach be used to study the management of pain in a hospital setting?
- What potential problems might occur in studying health-care culture in the hospital setting?

PHENOMENOLOGICAL APPROACHES

Phenomenology
The study of human experience and consciousness.

Mental
Relating to the mind.

Holistic
An emphasis on the whole, rather than separate parts.

Phenomenology is primarily interested in people's lived experiences of the world and how they make sense of them (Bryman, 2008). Meaning can be explored through the interpretation of texts (hermeneutics), through stories and events (Heideggarian phenomenology), social interaction, or through perception—what messages human senses convey through bodily and mental subjectivity (Husserlian phenomenology). In all phenomenological research, it is the experience of the participants that is central, yet the presence of the researcher is acknowledged as influential. The intertwining of the body and the world in some phenomenological approaches has made them popular as a more holistic way to investigate people's experiences of health and health care. Finlay (2011) describes her own long-term experience of pain from a complex head of humerus fracture. She explains how the pain became not simply sensation and reaction to movement, but a mental negotiation filled with fear and anxiety, leading to a new meaning for pain and '… a new way of moving in my world …' (Finlay, 2011, p. 154). Rich descriptions of experience and interpretation of what living and being mean may be presented as themes, categories or variations in phenomenological studies, but these are always recognised as partial views of a bigger integrated whole (Merleau-Ponty, 2002).

CASE STUDY 3.3

FINDING THE RIGHT RESEARCH APPROACH

Christine is 56 years old and has chronic back pain from a car accident 10 years ago; the accident resulted in three crushed vertebrae and a fractured ankle, now held together by metal screws. She has found it hard to exercise and has recently become overweight. Her general practitioner has increased her pain medication, but she often feels tired and depressed. A psychologist suggested joining a group activity but Christine feels too embarrassed. A friend has suggested she see a podiatrist so that she could learn to walk more comfortably, but Christine is worried this will cost too much.

- What are some of the experiences of chronic pain that this case illustrates?
- How might a phenomenological approach be used to investigate these?

CRITICAL APPROACHES

Critical approaches are not a single entity and 'critical' may be used to qualify other approaches, as in 'critical ethnography'. These approaches share a common ancestry in critical theory, which insists that all human activity takes place in societies with histories, structures and values that favour some people, viewpoints and interpretations and ignore or suppress others (Denzin & Lincoln, 2011). Power relations are assumed to be present in all forms of society, with formal and informal community rules and conventions allowing or restricting all social practices, including writing, speaking and research (Hyland, 2009). Critical approaches seek to analyse the social, political, cultural, ethnic, gender and economic influences that shape the practices and identities of communities (Hyland, 2009) to produce social change or emancipation (Denzin & Lincoln, 2011). Critical approaches emphasise honestly representing the community in question, which often includes initial consultation and ongoing feedback opportunities for the participants (Murchison, 2010). Health-care research uses critical approaches to examine the power relationships that exist between and within communities of health-care practice, and between patients and health-care providers or society. One example of this is the work of occupational therapists Nilsson and Townsend (2010) on the exclusion of older people from leisure activities and everyday technology opportunities. They argue for an occupational justice framework for health practitioners to reduce alienation, marginalisation and discrimination in occupational activities for older people.

Critical theory
An approach that examines hidden imbalances of power and knowledge in society and involves an in-depth analysis of social constructs in order to effect change.

Community
A group of people with defined commonality. This may include geographical location, belief systems or any other social construct.

CONSTRUCTIVIST APPROACHES

Constructivist approaches to qualitative research take the view that people actively create their own reality and make their own meaning of things, primarily through social interaction and language (Denzin & Lincoln, 2011). Constructivist approaches, of which discourse analysis is probably the best known, are concerned with both participant and researcher views of the research topic. Discourse is usually described as all the interconnected texts, images and social processes through which people bring things into existence and make them meaningful (Gee, 2011). Meaning arises from the connections between what people are, say and do, so discourse analysis can include looking at how language and context work to create meaning at many different levels, including the personal, social and political (Gee, 2011). In health care there are strong connections between language, context and practice, but Smythe (2005) suggested that there is a lack of reflection on researchers' constructions because of the focus on practical results rather than the thinking behind outcomes in health-care research. Constructivist research approaches have been used effectively to investigate health-care discourses such as socially determined representations of the body, and conflicting discourses of patient and practitioner identities (MacLeod, 2011). Interpersonal interaction is central to constructivist approaches, making them useful for research in social or collaborative settings.

RESEARCH ALIVE 3.2
THE PAIN OF BURNS

In their review of the management of pain for burns patients, Richardson and Mustard (2009) noted that the experience of pain is very complex and affected by many different factors, including expectations and anxiety associated with treatment. Interestingly however, they found that while patient factors were very significant, there was also inadequate management of pain by health-care staff. Good prescribing knowledge was not matched by pharmacological understanding or positive attitudes towards pain medication among junior medical and nursing staff in particular. These findings might be seen as somewhat surprising when one considers that pain is something all health-care practitioners deal with. Other research has suggested that negative perceptions of illness are well-established in clinical students before they reach practice settings (Ross, von Fragstein, & Cleland, 2011). It appears that there are conflicting constructions and discourses of pain and illness among patients and practitioners.

POSTMODERN APPROACHES

Postmodern (or poststructural or deconstructive) research has its origins in the work of philosophers such as Derrida. Postmodernism suggests that social activity is time- and setting-dependent, and that meaning is always an intersubjective, shifting and unstable interpretation of a constructed reality that emerges through language

(Hammersley & Atkinson, 1995). In health-care research this often translates into studies that challenge the investigators' understandings of the setting and search for hidden perspectives to capture the multiple aspects of the inquiry and the shifting perspectives of the participants and the researcher (Ironside, 2005). This may produce ongoing reshaping of the research process and multiple readings of the data. Narrative or story is often used in postmodern research because the partial and incomplete identities of people can be explored without a defined end-point and because single or generalisable truths are not sought since these do not exist for the postmodernist (McEldowney, 2005). Postmodern research can appear difficult to understand or apply to concrete situations, but it is useful in health-care research when there are multiple criss-crossing threads or where conflicting concepts exist, because it pushes the researcher to examine their own frameworks and consider all voices and interpretations as equally relevant.

RESEARCH ALIVE 3.3
END-OF-LIFE QUESTIONS

Palliative or end-of-life care is a special pain context. Zimmermann and Wennberg (2006) conducted a deconstructive analysis of some conflicting end-of-life palliative care concepts. They considered how natural and medicalised death, and acceptance and denial, have become polarised opposites rather than points on continuums along which patients' and health professionals' understandings move. Pain relief is an important part of palliative care, but, as Zimmermann and Wennberg note, polarised opposites 'may encourage the view among patients, health care providers, and policy-makers alike that a choice must be made between two counterpoised alternatives: a peaceful, pain-free death and a painful, heroic fight to the end' (p. 256). The authors argue for an integrated, individualised approach to palliative care that disputes these polarisations and balances patient needs and wishes with medical perspectives.

SUMMARY

Qualitative research can be thought of as the interplay between research approach, participants and data collected, within which various methods can be used. There is a range from more objective, structured, researcher-distant qualitative approaches that have some similarities to quantitative research, through to more intersubjective, unstructured, researcher-immersed approaches. The six approaches briefly outlined in this chapter represent some points along this continuum. Examples of the uniquely useful contributions of each approach have been provided to illustrate their value in health-care research. Qualitative researchers should weigh the fit of the research methods chosen with their approach, and with participant needs, potential pitfalls and ethical issues.

REFLECTION POINTS

- Revisit chapters 1 and 2 on research approaches and methods and consider your own ontological and epistemological positions.
- Does this help you to understand why you are more or less attracted to particular qualitative approaches?
- What are the potential biases associated with this position?

STUDY QUESTIONS

1 In what ways might the approach, participants or data collection constrain qualitative health-care research and why?
2 Western societies are often portrayed as obsessively individualistic. How might some of these qualitative research approaches enhance collaborative research?

ADDITIONAL READING

Pope, C., & Mays, N. (Eds.). (2008). *Qualitative research in health care*. (3rd ed.). London: BMJ Books.

REFERENCES

Bryman, A. (2008). *Social research methods* (3rd ed.). Oxford: Oxford University Press.

Chin, C. (2011). Models as interpreters (with a case study from pain science). *Studies in History and Philosophy of Science, 42,* 303–312.

Denzin, N. K., & Lincoln, Y. S. (2011). *The Sage handbook of qualitative research* (4th ed.). Los Angeles, CA: Sage Publications.

Finlay, L. (2011). *Phenomenology for therapists. Researching the lived world.* Chichester, United Kingdom: Wiley-Blackwell.

Gee, J. P. (2011). *An introduction to discourse analysis. Theory and method* (3rd ed.). New York, NY: Routledge.

Giddings, L., & Grant, B. (2007). A Trojan horse for positivism? A critique of mixed methods research. *Advances in Nursing Science, 30,* 52–60.

Hammersley, M., & Atkinson, P. (1995). *Ethnography: principles in practice.* London: Routledge.

Hyland, K. (2009). *Academic discourse: English in a global context.* London: Continuum International Publishing Group.

Ironside, P. M. (2005). Introduction. In P. M. Ironside (Ed.), *Beyond method: Philosophical conversations in healthcare research and scholarship* (pp. ix–xix). Madison, WN: University of Wisconsin Press.

Macleod, A. (2011). Caring, competence and professional identities in medical education. *Advances in Health Sciences Education, 16,* 375–394.

McEldowney, R. (2005). Combining interpretive methodologies: Maximizing the richness of findings. In P. M. Ironside (Ed.), *Beyond method: Philosophical conversations in healthcare research and scholarship* (pp. 148–190). Madison, WN: University of Wisconsin Press.

Merleau-Ponty, M. (2002). *Phenomenology of perception.* (C. Smith, Trans.). London: Routledge. (Original work published 1945.)

Murchison, J. M. (2010). *Ethnography essentials.* San Francisco, CA: Jossey-Bass.

Nilsson, I., & Townsend, E. (2010). Occupational justice—bridging theory and practice. *Scandinavian Journal of Occupational Therapy, 17,* 57–63.

Richardson, P., & Mustard, L. (2009). The management of pain in the burns unit. *Burns, 35,* 921–936. doi:10.1016/j.burns.2009.03.003

Ross, S., von Fragstein, M., & Cleland, J. (2011). Medical students' illness-related cognitions. *Medical Education, 45,* 1241–1250.

Skevington, S. M., Lotfy, M., & O'Connell, K. A. (2004). The World Health Organization's WHOQOL-BREF quality of life assessment: Psychometric properties and results of the international field trial. A report from the WHOQOL group. *Quality of Life Research, 13*(2), 299–310.

Smythe, E. (2005). The thinking of research. In P. M. Ironside (Ed.), *Beyond method: Philosophical conversations in healthcare research and scholarship* (pp. 223–258). Madison, WN: University of Wisconsin Press.

Zimmermann, C., & Wennberg, R. (2006). Integrating palliative care: A postmodern perspective. *American Journal of Hospice and Palliative Medicine, 23,* 255–258.

WEBSITES

National Collaborating Centre for Methods and Tools:
http://www.nccmt.ca/index-eng.html

Qualitative research and Cochrane reviews:
http://www.igh.org/Cochrane/tools/Ch20_Qualitative.pdf

Centre for Health Evidence:
http://www.cche.net/text/usersguides/qualitative.asp

CHAPTER 4

QUANTITATIVE APPROACHES

W. LINDSEY WHITE AND RUSSELL B. MILLAR

CHAPTER OVERVIEW

This chapter covers the following topics:

- What is quantitative research and why do it?
- Key statistics: the mean and standard deviation
- How important is the normal distribution?
- Experimental design

KEY TERMS

Average	Measurement	Random
Bias	Normal distribution	Replicate
Confidence interval	Null hypothesis	Sampling
Empirical	Probability	Standard deviation
Hypothesis	*P*-value	Treatment
Mean	Quantitative research	Variability

The quantitative approach to research is, in essence, about taking measurements of something and using statistical analysis to quantify the strength of evidence for there being a difference, or no difference, between different groups. It's a bit like being a detective, with the data you measure being used as evidence in order to come to the right verdict. It stems from a positivist perspective in which the only way to know things about the world is to investigate it in an empirical, scientific sense.

WHAT IS QUANTITATIVE RESEARCH AND WHY DO IT?

Often research is seeking to determine whether there are differences or similarities between things or groups. This can be as diverse as trying out different medicines or other treatments on groups of patients and observing if there are any benefits, or applied to ecology, seeking to identify the factors involved in the spatial distribution and abundance of organisms.

Quantitative research is about gaining information from sensory experiences, aided by logical or mathematical arguments. Sensory experience refers to empirical data that can be gathered by instruments or counted physically. The main difference between quantitative and qualitative research is that quantitative research uses measurements or counts that do not rely on subjective measurements. For example, measuring levels of fatigue following hard exercise in a qualitative way might involve interview questions about how participants were feeling. In a quantitative investigation we would use a more objective measurement, perhaps taking blood and measuring physiological parameters. To carry out quantitative research a hypothesis is formulated, an experiment to test the hypothesis is designed and carried out, and the data analysed to see if the hypothesis can be rejected.

In order to gain an appreciation of quantitative research a few basic statistical terms need to be understood, along with how they determine whether two treatments or samples differ in some way.

KEY STATISTICS: THE MEAN AND STANDARD DEVIATION

The first concept is the mean and it is a simple concept. This is just fancy terminology for the average, which is something that you probably have an intuitive feel for. It is calculated by adding up the numbers to be averaged and dividing by the number of items in the data set. As an example, the mean age of the Smith sisters (aged 34, 35 and 36 years) is 35 years old.

Empirical
Relating to a scientific approach to defining knowledge based on objective information and processes.

Quantitative research
Research carried out in a quantitative manner.

Measurement
The process of measuring the size or amount of something; also, the size or amount itself.

Hypothesis
A speculative explanation for a problem that can be tested by further research.

Mean
A particular type of average value calculated by the addition of all values in a data set, divided by the number of data points.

Average
A measure that represents the middle point in a set of data (mean, median or mode are all types of average).

It is useful in research to be able to talk about the mean, as it provides a useful summary of the data collected. Another useful concept is about how variable the data set is. Think about this: compare the mean age of the Smith sisters with the mean age of the Brown sisters (aged 15, 35 and 55 years). The Browns' average age is also 35 years. But the two families seem fundamentally different, don't they? The Smiths were all born within just a few years while the Browns were born at least a decade apart—so the Browns' ages are more variable. Using the mean to summarise the ages of the two families does not really capture enough information about them.

This is where the standard deviation (SD) comes in. It is also a very simple concept. This involves figuring how much variation there is around the mean value. In the Smith family the mean is 35, so how much does each sister's age deviate from the mean? Well, sister 1 deviates by one year, sister 2 by zero and sister three by one year. Using a basic formula for SD (which you can find in most calculators, in Excel or even in Wikipedia), these deviations give us an SD of 1. In the Brown family the deviations are 20, 0 and 20 years respectively, giving an SD of 20. The SD of the Browns is larger and thus the data are more variable.

Standard deviation
A description of how widely data points are spread around a mean value.

The mean and the standard deviation are two statistics that form a basis for understanding the way quantitative research is used to determine differences and similarities between groups in research.

HOW IMPORTANT IS THE NORMAL DISTRIBUTION?

Figure 4.1 shows the size frequency distribution of some surf clams (*Dosinia anus*). Specifically, 936 clams were collected and the shell measured across the longest dimension (more details about these clams later). In the graph the *x*-axis (horizontal axis) is the size classes of clams while the *y*-axis (vertical axis) shows how many clams were found in each of these size classes. So there were five clams that were 10 mm long, and 30 clams that were 24 mm, and so on.

When a smoothed curve is placed over these data, a bell-shaped curve can be seen (see Figure 4.2). This curve is known as the normal distribution, commonly called the bell curve. Many things in this world are distributed in a similar fashion. Think about any parameter about humans that can be measured—height for example. In any random group of people there will be few very tall people, few very short people, with the vast majority somewhat closer to the average. If this pattern was plotted on a graph, it would create the same pattern as for the clams—that is, the normal distribution. Indeed, this is why it is called 'normal' (Kruskal & Stigler, 1997), because it is.

Normal distribution
A statistical concept that describes the expected symmetrical distribution of a set of data around the mean.

Random
Without plan or pattern.

FIGURE 4.1   LENGTH FREQUENCY OF CLAMS (*DOSINIA ANUS*) FOUND IN
SHALLOW WATER

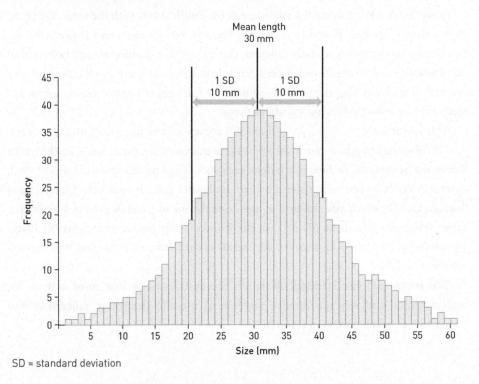

SD = standard deviation

FIGURE 4.2   NORMAL DISTRIBUTION OF CLAM LENGTHS SHOWING
PERCENTAGE OF CLAMS THAT ARE 1 AND 2 STANDARD DEVIATION
UNITS FROM THE MEAN

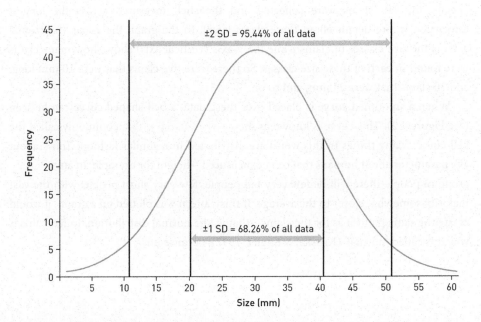

In a data set that is distributed normally, the standard deviation shows how much of the population is contained within a certain part of the curve. Drawing a line down from 1 standard deviation either side of the mean (as in Figure 4.2), 68% of the samples in the data set will be in that group (see Figure 4.2), so for the shallow-water clams 68% of them will be between 20 and 40 mm long. If this is extended out to 2 SDs either side of the mean (30 mm ± 20 mm), then 95% of all clams fall in this range. So a clam that is larger than 50 mm can be considered to be uncommonly large, since such clams occur only 2.5% of the time. If you came across lots of these big clams on the beach, you might start to wonder whether they really were from the shallow-water population. This is precisely the kind of evidence that needs to be judged when trying to compare this shallow-water data set with data from other locations, or from deeper water on the same beach.

Continuing the clam example above, suppose now that you knew that the SD of clam sizes was 10 mm, but you did not know what the mean size was. If you measure a single clam, then you know that its size is within 20 mm of the mean size with probability 0.95. So if the measured clam was 43 mm, you could say that the mean size is between 23 and 63 mm with high confidence. In statistical lingo, the interval 23–63 mm is called a 95% confidence interval. In practice, we never know what the SD of the population is, but we can calculate it from a sample taken from the population.

Probability
The likelihood of a particular outcome.

Confidence interval
A range of values within which a parameter is expected to lie.

A last point about normal distribution curves: they are not all exactly the same shape as the one in Figure 4.2. Some are taller, some shorter, some wider and some thinner (Figure 4.3). What is key is that the shape of the curve is determined by only two statistics: the mean and the standard deviation of the data. The position of the curve is determined by the mean while the width of the curve is determined by the standard deviation (how variable the data are—remember the Smith and Brown sisters). This is clear in Figure 4.3, which shows two different normal curve shapes, with different means and standard deviations determining the shapes.

In Case Study 4.1 it was of interest to know whether the shallow and deep clams had the same size distribution. This is an example of a hypothesis test. To do a hypothesis test, you have to determine whether the observed data are plausible under the hypothesis that there is no difference between the groups. The hypothesis of no difference is called the null hypothesis, and in the clam example (Case Study 4.1) the null hypothesis would be that there is no difference in size between the shallow clams and deep clams. That is, the two depths have the same size distribution of clams.

Null hypothesis
The position that states there is no relationship between defined variables.

Statisticians use p-values to quantify how plausible the data are under the null hypothesis. A p-value is a probability, and must be between 0 and 1. A small p-value indicates that the data are very unlikely under the null hypothesis. If the p-value is below 0.05, it is said to be 'statistically significant', and the null hypothesis is rejected. For the clam data in Figure 4.4, statistical calculations based on the normal curve produce a p-value less than 0.000001. We can be very sure that the two depths have different size distributions of clams.

P-value
The statistical probability that the result is arrived at by chance.

FIGURE 4.3 TWO DIFFERENT NORMAL DISTRIBUTIONS

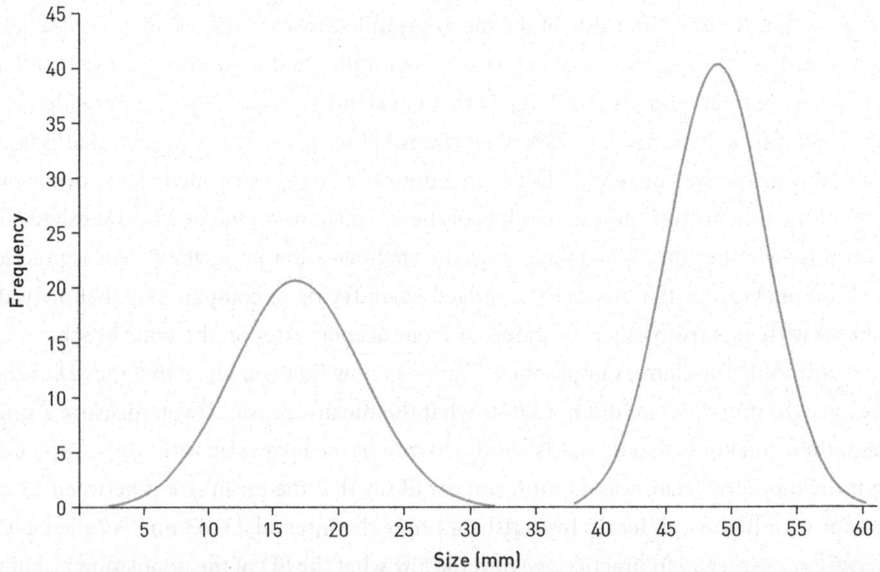

CASE STUDY 4.1

THE SIZE OF SURF CLAMS (DOSINIA ANUS)

I am interested in finding out if the surf clams (*Dosinia anus*) are different sizes depending on where they grow. Figures 4.1 and 4.2 were graphs about 936 clams that were collected from shallow water. Following this, a further 616 clams of the same species were collected from deeper water, and all of them had their shells measured along the longest dimension. It was found that the mean of the shallow clams was 30 mm and the mean of the deep clams was 65 mm. Is this difference big enough to say that there are two different populations, or is this difference just pure chance? Did we just happen to measure more large ones from the deep water? What of the standard deviation in the two data sets?

From the information above, you now have a good grasp on what the mean is, and how this and the standard deviation helps us determine the shape of the normal curve. You also know that in every single normal curve (no matter what shape it happens to be) that less than 2.5% of the data set under the curve lays outside a line taken 2 standard deviations from either side of the mean. So you now have the tools to compare two samples (shallow vs. deep) and see if they are different sizes and (importantly) exactly how sure are we of that.

Take a look at Figure 4.4. On this graph are plotted the data from both the shallow water (the left-hand curve) and the deep-water clams (curve on the right). Remember that the standard deviation of the shallow-water data set was 10 mm and the mean was 30 mm. So two SDs above the mean is 50 mm. There is only a 2.5% chance of a shallow-water clam being this big. Given that virtually all of the clams from the deep water are larger than 50 mm, a sample of clams that contained a lot of big clams would provide evidence that the clams were from deep rather than shallow water. We need to know if the evidence is strong enough to say that the clams were definitely from deep water. A statistical test uses the properties of the normal distribution to answer this question.

What could explain the different size distributions of the two populations of clam?

FIGURE 4.4 LENGTH FREQUENCY DATA FOR BOTH THE SHALLOW- AND DEEP-WATER CLAMS (*DOSINIA ANUS*)

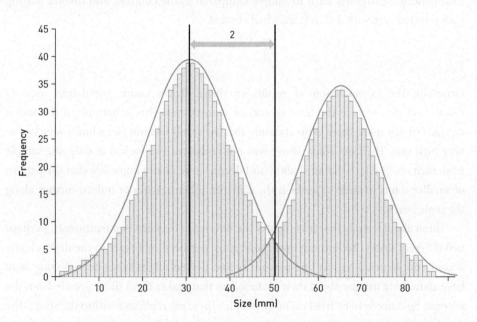

EXPERIMENTAL DESIGN
SAMPLE VERSUS POPULATION MEANS

When comparing two treatments or groups to determine if they are different (or similar), it is usually impossible to measure or assess the entire population, so it is necessary to take a sample instead. For example, in the clam study above, there is no way to collect every clam along a beach, so a sample of the clams (from both shallow and deep water) is taken and the results are extrapolated to the entire population. Since we cannot measure the true population means of the clams, we have to use the means of the sampled clams instead. Similarly, we cannot measure the true standard deviation of the entire population, and must instead work with the standard deviation from the sample.

The key is to select an appropriate sample so that it is truly representative of the population because it is only then that the average measurement can represent the whole population. Ensuring that the sample actually represents the population usually requires taking a random sample. This helps to avoid bias towards any particular subgroup within the population. However, there can be situations where a random sample is very inefficient, and then it may be better to have a more active role in determining how the sampling is conducted. For example, case-control designs are used when the case treatments are extremely hard to sample compared to the controls, and involve pairing each selected case with a closely matched control.

Bias
The preference of one particular response over another one.

Sampling
The process of identifying participants for a study.

REPLICATION

Generally, the extrapolation of results to those of the entire population requires researchers to replicate the tests several or many times. This is because, if the test is carried out just once, there is no certainty that the result was not just a lucky very low or very high one. The clam study above was not replicated (we looked at only one sample from each treatment—that is, shallow and deep), so we do not know whether the pattern of smaller clams in shallow water is the same on other beaches or indeed further along the same beach.

Think about a study that investigates the difference between two treatments, perhaps two different drugs. To find out how the average person might react to the drug, clearly it could not be tried on just one person, as that person might be an outlier—they may have something unique about their metabolism that makes them differ greatly from the average. So it needs to be tried on more people. These are replicates within the study. The number of replicates needed to be able to extrapolate findings to the entire population depends directly on the variability of the results among the replicates.

Replicate
The process of repeating an investigation.

Treatment
The act of carrying out an intervention for the purpose of alleviating or curing a problem.

Variability
An indication of the spread of data values.

CONTROLS AND CONFOUNDING VARIABLES

When experiments are designed to test a particular treatment, it is important to consider variables in addition to the one being tested. For example, imagine wanting to test a new fertiliser on a species of plant to see if it will make the plants grow taller. The experiment could be designed with several replicate plants (20 plants total), and 10 will get the treatment and 10 will not. The ones that do not get the treatment are called the 'control' plants. But more than this, knowing there are other factors that could influence growth of the plants requires ensuring that these factors do not bias the results. It is important that the other factors are 'balanced' between the treatment and control groups. Light and temperature are known to influence plant growth, so making sure that both groups of plants receive equal amounts of light and temperature is essential. One sensible approach would be to randomly assign the 20 plants to places in the greenhouse or garden to ensure there was no bias in these factors, thus achieving a rough balance for variation in light and temperature in the two groups. Another option would be to use an experimental design in which the treatment and control plants were planted alternately (for example, treatment-control-treatment-control …) in each row. This is a form of balanced design. It is not a fully random design, but is guaranteed to give very good balance of light and temperature.

RESEARCH ALIVE 4.1
IS EDUCATION LEVEL A CONFOUNDING VARIABLE
IN A RANDOMISED CONTROLLED TRIAL?

Kiser et al. (2011) tested a new patient education technique for self-management of inhaled medications with patients who had chronic pulmonary disease. Patients were randomly assigned to two groups: the new education technique (the group where the variable of interest was being tested) or usual care (the control group). Data was collected on all patients' medication use, health behaviours and measures of disease to determine if the new education technique made a difference to these variables. In the initial analysis the two groups were compared to see if they had similar characteristics at baseline, so any difference in results could be attributed to the new patient education technique. Education level was significantly different between the groups, with a higher percentage of patients in the control group not having completed high school. This was a potential confounding variable as low education levels are associated with poor health outcomes and low health literacy (health literacy is the 'cognitive and social skills which determine [a person's] motivation and

[continued next page]

ability ... to gain access to, understand and use information in ways which promote and maintain good health' (World Health Organization, 2013)). The difference in education levels between the two groups, rather than the new patient education technique, may have caused the differences in the trial results in the areas of medication use or health behaviours. The researchers therefore had to consider whether this difference between groups would bias their appraisal of the results.

CASE STUDY 4.2

PREDICTORS OF MENTAL HEALTH: A COMPLEX INTERACTION OF VARIABLES

Humans are very complex, so research designs that are used to investigate human health outcomes need to be complex too. In quantitative contexts, sophisticated statistical modelling can be used to account for person-to-person variables in a sample; it can also be used to analyse data and investigate research questions. This case study illustrates the complex nature of quantitative health research and of determining significant relationships in a sample.

Seib, Anderson, Lee and Humphreys (2013) hypothesised that there was a relationship between three groups of variables affecting the mental health of 340 Australian women aged 60–70 years. These were:

1 socio-demographics (age, marital status, income, employment);
2 modifiable lifestyle factors (BMI, diet, exercise, alcohol, smoking, sleep);
3 health status and quality of life indicators (clinical biomarkers, physical health, chronic illness).

Multiple data collection strategies were used to obtain a very large data set and a complex analysis was undertaken. Results from this sample demonstrated that current mental health status was predicted by sleep disturbance and past mental health problems, while socio-demographics and lifestyle variables had little impact on mental health status.

CLINICAL REFLECTION 4.1: PEOPLE ARE UNPREDICTABLE

Real people in real health care situations don't behave predictably: one person might be similar to, but isn't the same as, the next. The studies above highlight how complex quantitative health research can be and the challenges researchers face when they use scientific methods to investigate how factors such as education level or sleep quality interact and affect health outcomes.

SUMMARY

Quantitative research uses empirical measurements to test for differences and similarities between groups. Proper experimental design requires planning in terms of correct replication and controls. If this is done correctly it then allows for accurate statistical analysis of the resulting data and extrapolation of those results to the wider population.

This method of research underpins all scientific advances. It informs the way the world works. Without it we would not be able to address and answer the questions about the world, human health and medicine that are so important to human development.

REFLECTION POINTS

- Why would a quantitative design be chosen over other options?
- What are the strengths of quantitative research in the health-care sector?

STUDY QUESTIONS

1   If you were designing a test of a new drug for weight loss, how would you choose your study participants to avoid bias and ensure that the results could be extrapolated to the general population? How would you take into account differences in how the drug might work on different ages, ethnicities and genders?
2   In a study to test the effects of a new formulated feed for salmon, how would you design the study? What factors need to be controlled for?

ADDITIONAL READING

Burns, N., & Grove, S. K. (2005). *Understanding nursing research: Building an evidence based practice* (5th ed.). St Louis: Elsevier/Saunders.

Creswell, J. W. (2013). *Research design: Qualitative, quantitative, and mixed methods approaches*. Thousand Oaks, CA: Sage Publications Incorporated.

Polgar, S., & Thomas, S. A. (2008). *Introduction to research in the health sciences*. Edinburgh: Churchill Livingstone.

REFERENCES

Bailey, R. A. (2008). *Design of comparative experiments*. Cambridge: Cambridge University Press.

Giddens, A. (1974). *Positivism and sociology*. London: Heinemann.

Hinkelmann, K., & Kempthorne, O. (2008). *Design and analysis of experiments. Volume I: Introduction to experimental design* (2nd ed.). New York: John Wiley & Sons.

Kiser, K., Jonas, D., Warner, Z., Scanlon, K., Shilliday, B., & DeWalt, D. (2011). A randomised controlled trial of a literacy-sensitive self-management intervention for chronic obstructive pulmonary disease patients. *Journal of General Internal Medicine, 27,* 190–195.

Kruskal, W. H., & Stigler, S. M. (1997). Normative terminology: 'Normal' in statistics and elsewhere. In B. D. Spencer, (Ed.), *Statistics and public policy*. Oxford: Oxford University Press.

Mann, P. S. (1995) *Introductory statistics* (2nd ed.). Canada: John Wiley & Sons.

Marsaglia, G., & Tsang, Wai Wan (2000). The ziggurat method for generating random variables. *Journal of Statistical Software, 5,* 1–7.

Seib, C., Anderson, D., Lee, K., & Humphreys, J. (2013). Predictors of mental health in post-menopausal women: Results from the Australian healthy aging of women study. *Maturitas, 76*(4), 377–383.

Stigler, S. M. (1986). *The history of statistics: The measurement of uncertainty before 1900*. Cambridge, MA: Harvard University Press.

World Health Organization. (2013). *The WHO health promotion glossary*. Retrieved from www.who.int/healthpromotion/about/HPG/en

WEBSITES

An example of a quantitative research proposal:
http://www-distance.syr.edu/quantproposal.html

Quantitative research design:
http://www.sportsci.org/jour/0001/wghdesign.html

CHAPTER 5

MIXED METHODS APPROACHES

VALERIE A. WRIGHT-ST CLAIR AND KATHRYN M. McPHERSON

CHAPTER OVERVIEW

This chapter covers the following topics:

- Combining diverse research methods
- Reasons for using mixed methods
- Doing mixed methods research
- 'Quality' in mixed methods research

KEY TERMS

Clinical trial
Mixed methods
Participation
Rigour
Triangulation
Variance

Mixed methods
An approach to research that encompasses multiple elements—commonly both qualitative and quantitative approaches.

Just as the name implies, mixed methods research brings together methodologically diverse, yet complementary, ways of doing research within a single study. It is an approach that uses the strengths of each methodology to enrich the results. This can be thought of as being a bit like building a new house; the design and the construction process itself will determine whether it results in a quality home that is fit for purpose. A home's overall quality is highly dependent upon working to plan, and using quality materials, as well as each tradesman coming to the job with the right skill-set and doing things in the right way at the right time. The carpenter's construction of a robust frame lays the foundation for the electrician to fit the wiring, for the plumber to lay the pipework, and so on. In the same way, good mixed methods research relies on researchers being skilled in the different methodologies. Doing so will yield stronger and more complex understandings about the phenomenon of interest. This chapter sets out to show how mixed methods approaches in health and social research have the potential to produce deep knowledge that can enhance practice outcomes.

COMBINING DIVERSE RESEARCH METHODS

Triangulation
The process of linking more than two pieces of information to improve the trustworthiness of findings.

Mixed methods research typically includes quantitative and qualitative approaches to study a practice concern or health issue. It is one way of providing triangulation of the data as each method yields different forms of evidence to help answer the research question. Carroll and Rothe (2010) make a case for using mixed methods designs based on the complementary nature of subjective and objective knowledge, gained by both '"looking in" [and] "looking at"' (p. 3482) something. Corresponding to qualitative and quantitative research approaches, each view effectively complements the other to result in a fuller understanding of what is being studied.

Rigour
The degree to which research process and findings stand up to challenge.

Without a doubt, mixed methods research is gaining popularity in health science and social research. What seems most evident with the recent methodological advancement of mixed methods studies is a move away from a long-standing, futile debate opposing the merits and rigour of quantitative and qualitative research approaches, to an accepted position of valuing what each brings to the applied research field (McPherson & Kayes, 2012; Sackett & Wennberg, 1997). So, when the two dominant approaches to research (qualitative and quantitative) can and do stand alone across many research fields, why apply mixed methods? An answer to this question may be best illustrated by possibly the first randomised, controlled drug trial using mixed methods research in the early phase of the study (Berk et al., 2011). The qualitative component uncovered the participants' experiences of diminished or persistent symptoms not revealed by the quantitative measures. The investigators concluded that 'the integration of qualitative methods into rigorous, placebo-controlled randomized designs provides additional insight … and broadens the scope of the trial process' (Berk et al., p. 913).

Further examples of the diverse range of topics where researchers have used mixed methods include:

- exploring whether participation in 'adapted dynamic cycling' enhanced activity engagement and quality of life for children with cerebral palsy (Pickering, Horrocks, Visser, & Todd, 2013);
- identifying how effective Talking Mats (a communication tool for people with disabilities) are in aiding communication for people with Huntington's disease (Hallberg, Mellgren, Hartelius, & Ferm, 2013);
- enhancing understanding of older people's everyday experiences, functional abilities and fear of falling during community-based recovery following hip fracture (Jellesmark, Forsyth Herling, Egerod, & Beyer, 2012) (see Case Study 5.1);
- investigating how occupational perspectives of transitioning into assisted living are experienced by older Americans (Mulry, 2012);
- unpicking physiotherapists' experiences and views of implementing differing client interventions as part of a randomised controlled trial (Bampton et al., 2012); and
- developing and evaluating the validity of a skin care beliefs scale for people who live with spinal cord injury (King et al., 2012).

Case Study 5.1 illustrates how the investigators in one project brought together quantitative and qualitative methods to strengthen and deepen the research findings.

CASE STUDY 5.1

OLDER PEOPLE'S FEAR OF FALLING AND FUNCTIONAL ABILITY DURING RECOVERY FROM A HIP FRACTURE

Jellesmark, Forsyth Herling, Egerod, and Beyer (2012) conducted what they believe is the first mixed methods study exploring fear of falling. Responding to the research evidence that experiencing falls in later life commonly results in a reduced quality of life and a fear of falling, the investigators set out to explore a gap in current knowledge: the associations between fear of falling, functional changes and activity avoidance for community-dwelling seniors, three to six months after discharge following hip fracture. They designed a 'sequential explanatory mixed method study' (Jellesmark et al., p. 2125).

[continued next page]

Thirty-three people (26 women and seven men) aged 65 years and older who met the inclusion and exclusion criteria were recruited from two hospital orthopaedic departments. Beginning with an interview-based quantitative research phase, participants completed four different outcome measures: the Fall Efficacy Scale-International (FES-I) assessing the person's level of worry about falling; the Modified Survey of Activities and Fear of Fall in the Elderly (mSAFFE) measuring the extent of activity avoidance due to fear of falling; the Functional Recovery Score (FRS) evaluating participation in everyday activities; and the New Mobility Score (NMS) designed to measure post–hip fracture mobility in different indoor and outdoor environments (Jellesmark et al., 2012)

Those who scored highly for fear of falling (FOF) had varying functional ability levels, and were able to engage in a conversation about their situation (19 participants), were purposively selected for an in-depth individual interview. This qualitative phase was designed to explore the person's subjective experiences of everyday functioning and fears about falling. It enabled the investigators to understand how participants thought about their abilities as well as their fears and to understand why they avoided usual activities. As the study was a cross-sectional design, they could not infer causation, but found 'a significant association between FOF and functional ability 3–6 months after discharge from hospital. In addition, participants with a high degree of FOF avoided more activities, needed assistance in ADL [activities of daily living] and were less mobile' (Jellesmark et al., 2012, p. 2129). The qualitative data revealed participants' lessened quality of life and their sense of being protected from further falls by avoiding certain activities even though they were capable of doing the activity.

In this example, equal explanatory weight was given to the initial quantitative and subsequent qualitative phases; the mix of two different types of evidence extended the knowledge gained.

Participation
The process of being involved.

Interestingly, Austin and Williams-Mozley (2012) propose a different interpretation on mixed methods research and develop a novel methodological approach. Rather than bringing together quantitative and qualitative approaches, they mix 'indigenous and non-indigenous research paradigms or methods' (p. 102) in a study aimed at developing an 'indigenised' research process [see Research Alive 5.1].

RESEARCH ALIVE 5.1
AN 'INDIGENISED' RESEARCH DEVELOPMENT PROGRAMME

Disappointment with the outcomes of a research development project engaging Australian Aboriginal and non-indigenous researchers in the reciprocal sharing of research expertise led to the investigators, Austin and Williams-Mozley (2012), conducting a further study to design qualitative research methods inclusive of indigenous perspectives.

> The current project is an attempt to contribute to the legitimising of currently subaltern knowledge systems, and to provide those students from whose cultures such alternatives have been derived with a sense of belonging and pride in the cultural contributions made to research methods generally. (Austin & Williams-Mozley, 2012, p. 105)

What is emerging so far is how indigenous ways of communicating such as 'yarning' together might be formalised as a method of gathering narrative data with Aboriginal participants, rather than using Westernised focus group methods with semi-structured or unstructured interviewing.

REASONS FOR USING MIXED METHODS

Various conceptual frameworks illustrate when mixed methods designs are amenable to meeting the aim of a study. McPherson and Kayes (2012) propose applications including:

- when one method *informs* the other, such as doing a qualitative study to focus topics for a subsequent quantitative project;
- where one method *complements or extends* the other, such as when a qualitative approach is used to augment evidence gained through a quantitative study as in Jellesmark et al.'s (2012) fear of falling study described in Case Study 5.1 or to pursue interesting quantitative findings (in clinical trials or epidemiological studies); or
- to *develop or choose outcome measures*, when, for example, understanding that what is important to people is a significant factor in developing a new measure (for example, King et al. (2012) in their development of a new measure of behaviour as noted above).

McPherson and Kayes (2012) argue that a mixed methods research design is particularly suitable for practice-based questions, suggesting the following as key examples:

1 'How can the novel interventions we wish to evaluate be delivered in a way that is most acceptable to the patient population it will be tested in?' (p. 384).

VALERIE A. WRIGHT-ST CLAIR AND KATHRYN M. McPHERSON

To answer this question, an initial qualitative phase exploring how a representative sample of the relevant patient population experiences different aspects of their intervention programme and therapists' communication with them, by engaging them in focus group interviews, could be conducted in order to *inform* the development of a treatment manual to facilitate a standardised (and acceptable) clinical approach to delivering treatment.

2   'Can we extend understanding of the factors that explain why Group A appeared to benefit from the intervention more than Group B (beyond the variance accounted for by our measures)?' (p. 384).

This question might best be asked by first conducting a clinical trial comparing treatment outcomes for participants receiving the standard treatment (the control group) with those receiving a new treatment method (the experimental group), then purposely selecting participants from each group to engage in in-depth individual interviews to *extend* the understanding of why the different interventions are effective or not.

3   'Do our selected measures map onto issues of importance to our participants?' (p. 384).

With an increased focus on standardised assessment tools and outcome measures, this is a fundamentally important question in health care and practice. This question may be best answered by first engaging participants in in-depth individual interviews using open-ended questions to encourage stories about their experiences and/or needs in relation to the phenomenon of interest. An interpretation of the narrative data would reveal the emergent themes in relation to what matters to them for getting on with life. In the next research phase, one or more standardised measures aimed at examining the phenomenon of interest would be implemented, the results analysed, and the highly rated factors then compared with what people said was important to them. The standardised, quantitative measure that most closely mapped the qualitative evidence would help the practice team *choose* the best instrument for use within the service.

An initial understanding of how two different methodologies will *inform, complement or extend one another*, or enable the *development or choice of outcome measures* is the cornerstone of designing a good mixed methods study. It will determine the actual design for the study, such as whether it is a concurrent/triangulation mixed methods, embedded experimental before-intervention mixed methods, or sequential exploratory or sequential explanatory mixed methods design (Plano Clark & Creswell, 2008). When reading a mixed methods research article, it is a good idea to look for the authors' justification of why they used the approach they did.

DOING MIXED METHODS RESEARCH

Finally, two different studies, one recently published and one in progress, are outlined to further illustrate how mixed methods research can be done with rigour.

Variance
A measure of how far each value in a data set is from the mean.

Clinical trial
A formally structured approach to research which includes standards and processes for identifying the problem and investigating it.

CASE STUDY 5.2

BARRIERS TO TREATMENT IN AN ETHNICALLY DIVERSE SAMPLE OF FAMILIES ENROLLED IN A COMMUNITY-BASED DOMESTIC VIOLENCE INTERVENTION

Finding no evidence in the literature for family exposure to violence and the associated treatment attendances, barriers to attendance and treatment outcomes, Becker et al. (2012) designed a mixed methods study exploring the 'barriers to participation in a community-based domestic violence program' (p. 833) with a sample of 63 mothers, aged between 24 and 54 years old, who identified as Asian or Pacific Islander, and with up to six children, aged three to 18 years, also enrolled in the family domestic violence exposure programme.

The intervention entailed separate 90-minute 'psychoeducational,' 12-week programmes for mothers and their children. Pre- and post-intervention, the mothers and children were measured for their domestic violence coping skills using a 16-item scale. Mothers also answered a 25-item questionnaire measuring the emotional supportiveness of their parenting behaviours, and at their last attendance completed the Barriers to Treatment Participation measure. Last, mothers participated in an individual qualitative interview exploring two questions: 'Please tell us about any other situations related to domestic violence that made it hard to come to [the] group' and 'In your own words, please describe how you were able to overcome the difficulties of getting to [the] group' (Becker et al., 2012, p. 836).

The qualitative data *complemented*, and thereby strengthened, the quantitative findings; most often obstacles to attending the programme were pragmatic, such as everyday stressors like having car troubles, or children's sports; treatment-related, such as mothers being too upset to attend; or programme-related, such as the group being too early in the day. The qualitative data were particularly salient for illuminating what motivated mothers to attend; when their children were positive about the programme and when they experienced positive changes in the family.

As a consequence, effective evidence-based changes were made to the family violence programme.

VALERIE A. WRIGHT-ST CLAIR AND KATHRYN M. McPHERSON

RESEARCH ALIVE 5.2
COMMUNITY INTEGRATION OUTCOMES FOLLOWING TRAUMATIC BRAIN INJURY

Traumatic brain injury (TBI) is recognised as a major concern for older adults, with accidental falls being the main cause, yet little evidence from within Aotearoa New Zealand exists to guide people's reintegration into the community after a TBI. A summer studentship at AUT University funded by the Waitemata District Health Board (DHB) was undertaken by a third-year physiotherapy student, who explored older people's experiences of community integration following a mild or moderate TBI, and to test the appropriateness of two commonly used standardised instruments, the Community Integration Questionnaire (CIQ) and the Community Integration Measure (CIM). It was a small study to assist Waitemata DHB staff in the assessment and rehabilitation services select the best standardised measure of their clients' community integration after at least three months of living back home.

Participants—men and women, Māori aged 55 years or older or non-Māori aged 65 years or older, who had sustained a mild or moderate traumatic brain injury in the last year, had lived in their own home for at least three months following discharge from the Waitemata DHB, and lived within the DHB catchment area—were recruited through community advertisements.

Initially, qualitative descriptive data were gathered using a semi-structured interview guide to explore participants' community integration experiences and needs. Interviews of approximately 60–90 minutes duration were conducted in participants' own homes, or other venue of choice, with primary carers present if preferred. At the end of the interview, participants completed the interview-based CIQ (taking approximately 15 minutes) and the CIM (taking approximately 10 minutes). Separate interview times were arranged for participants that tired during the interview time.

Data analysis showed that issues identified as important by the participants in the qualitative interviews sometimes differed from the results derived from the standardised outcome measures. Results were shared with Waitemata DHB staff to inform the rehabilitation focus for community integration for older adults recovering from mild or moderate TBI, and outcome measures for older people, the CIQ or the CIM.

A summer studentship is a great way for an undergraduate student to gain experience as a novice researcher; they must conduct a rigorous, systematic literature review, establish partnerships with research partners, recruit participants, learn how to gather and analyse qualitative and quantitative data consistent with the underpinning philosophies, and work respectfully with research participants.

'QUALITY' IN MIXED METHODS RESEARCH

As the introductory metaphor of building a house suggested, researcher confidence in the results is the fundamental promise that a good mixed methods study offers (Plano Clark & Creswell, 2008). In turn, strong results from a quality mixed methods study means practitioners can be more confident in any decisions to change practice methods based on a study's findings. This is where 'the rubber hits the road'—practitioner confidence in research results lies at the heart of designing and delivering evidence-based health practice. Yet quality in mixed methods research is more than just in the design itself; it is necessarily dependent upon the researcher, or more likely the group of researchers, having the right set of knowledge about the different methodologies as well as being skilled in carrying out the research methods that are congruent with the design of each research component. The group requires an even greater range of skills to maintain quality than for a single strata research design. For example, if the qualitative component is exploring people's lived experiences of things, and is stated as being phenomenological in design, then all the methods used, from the research question up, to gather and analyse the qualitative data ought to be congruent, or fit together. Likewise, if the quantitative component is stated as being a clinical trial, then all the steps in the research process for this part of the study must be done with rigour, following accepted methods and processes.

The old adage holds true: quality in = quality out. Mixed methods research done well, using methods that are congruent with each of the underpinning philosophies, promises trustworthy results. Look for sound descriptions of research methods that fit with the named methodology and design when reading mixed methods research articles.

SUMMARY

Mixed methods research brings together methodologically diverse research approaches within a single study, and is a way of triangulating data. It can be used when one approach aims to *inform, complement or extend* the other, or to *develop or choose outcome measures*. Typically, mixed methods researchers use a carefully designed mix of qualitative and quantitative approaches. Alternatively, the term 'mixed methods' would apply to any study combining philosophically different approaches such as from indigenous and non-indigenous paradigms. Most importantly, researchers ought to make their reasons for using mixed methods research clear, and show how each different component is designed and carried out to bring about the most trustworthy results possible. The promise of good mixed methods research is more confidence in the results than a single methodology could offer, leading to practitioners being more confident when translating the results into evidence-based health practice.

REFLECTION POINTS

- What stands out for you after reading this chapter?
- How confident are you with knowledge gained from quantitative research? Why?
- How confident are you with knowledge gained from qualitative research? Why?
- What about your confidence in knowledge gained from a good mixed methods study? Why?
- What do you need to think about when critically reviewing a mixed methods research article?

STUDY QUESTIONS

1 Define mixed methods research in your own terms.
2 Write a question from your field of practice suitable for mixed methods research.
3 State three reasons for using mixed methods research.
4 State at least three things that influence the quality of mixed methods research. Justify your answer.

ADDITIONAL READING

Creswell, J. W., & Plano Clark, V. L. (2011). *Designing and conducting mixed methods research* (2nd ed). Los Angeles, CA: Sage Publications.

Johnson, R. B., & Onwuegbuzie, A. J. (2004). Mixed methods research: A research paradigm whose time has come. *Educational Researcher, 33*(7), 14–26.

Teddlie, C., & Tashakkori, A. (2009). *Foundations of mixed methods research: Integrating quantitative and qualitative approaches in the social and behavioral sciences.* Thousand Oaks, CA: Sage Publications.

REFERENCES

Austin, J., & Williams-Mozley, J. (2012). *An alternative view of mixed methods research.* Paper presented at the meeting of the 5th biennial International Indigenous Development Research Conference, Auckland, New Zealand. Retrieved from http://www.indigenousdevelopment2012.ac.nz

Bampton, J., Vargas, J., Wu, R., Potts, S., Lance, A., Scrivener, K., et al. (2012). Clinical physiotherapists had both positive and negative perceptions about delivering two different interventions in a clinical trial: a mixed methods study. *Journal of Physiotherapy, 58*, 255–260.

Becker, K. D., Mathis, G., Mueller, C. W., Issari, K., Atta, S. S., & Okado, I. (2012). Barriers to treatment in an ethnically diverse sample of families enrolled in a community-based domestic violence intervention. *Journal of Aggression, Maltreatment & Trauma, 21*, 829–850.

Berk, M., Munib, A., Dean, O., Malhi, G. S., Kohlmann, K., Schapkaitz, I., et al. (2011). Qualitative methods in early-phase drug trials: Broadening the scope of data and methods from an RCT of N-acetylcysteine in schizophrenia. *Journal of Clinical Psychiatry, 72*(7), 909–913.

Carroll, L. J., & Rothe, J. P. (2010). Levels of reconstruction as complementarity in mixed methods research: A social theory-based conceptual framework for integrating qualitative and quantitative research. *International Journal of Environmental Research and Public Health, 7*, 3478–3488.

Hallberg, L., Mellgren, E., Hartelius, L., & Ferm, U. (2013). Talking Mats in a discussion group for people with Huntington's disease. *Disability and Rehabilitation: Assistive Technology, 8*(1), 67–76.

Jellesmark, A., Forsyth Herling, S., Egerod, I., & Beyer, N. (2012). Fear of falling and changed functional ability following hip fracture among community-dwelling elderly people: An explanatory sequential mixed method study. *Disability & Rehabilitation, 34*(25), 2124–2131.

King, R. B., Champion, V. L., Chen, D., Gittler, M. S., Heinemann, A. W., Bode, R. K., & Semik, P. (2012). Development of a measure of Skin Care Belief Scales for persons with spinal cord injury. *Archives of Physical Medicine and Rehabilitation, 93*, 1814–1821.

McPherson, K. M., & Kayes, N. M. (2012). Qualitative research: Its practical contribution to physiotherapy. *Physical Therapy Reviews, 17*(6), 382–389.

Mulry, C. M. (2012). Transitions to assisted living: A pilot study of residents' occupational perspectives. *Physical and Occupational Therapy in Geriatrics, 30*(4), 328–343.

Pickering, D. M., Horrocks, L., Visser, K., & Todd, G. (2013). Adapted bikes: What children and young people with cerebral palsy told us about their participation in adapted dynamic cycling. *Disability and Rehabilitation: Assistive Technology, 8*(1), 30–37.

Plano Clark, V. L., & Creswell, J. W. (2008). *The mixed methods reader*. Thousand Oaks, CA: Sage Publications.

Sackett, D. L., & Wennberg, J. E. (1997). Choosing the best research design for each question: It's time to stop sqabbling over the 'best' methods. *British Medical Journal, 315*, 1636.

WEBSITES

United States Department of Health and Human Services, Office of Behavioral and Social Sciences Research:

   obssr.od.nih.gov/scientific_areas/methodology/mixed_methods_research/
   section2.aspx

Journal of Mixed Methods Research:

   mmr.sagepub.com

PART 2

CONTEXT

CHAPTER 6

MĀORI RESEARCH

DENISE WILSON

CHAPTER OVERVIEW

This chapter covers the following topics:

- Socio-historical context of Māori
- Māori and research
- Selecting evidence for use with Māori

KEY TERMS

Biomedical	Kaumātua	Tapu
Consensus	Kaupapa Māori	Te āo Māori
Determinants	Mana	Te reo Māori
Equity	Māori-centred	Tikanga
Guidelines	Mātauranga Māori	Tinana
Hapū	Noa	Treaty of Waitangi
Hauora	Participation	Wairua
Hinengaro	Partnership	Whānau
Iwi	Protection	

Whānau
Family.

Hapu
A subtribe.

Iwi
Main tribe.

Hauora
Philosophy of health.

Wairua
Spiritual well-being.

Tinana
Physical well-being.

Hinengaro
Mental well-being.

Concepts of health are constructed and practised within the socio-cultural reality of individuals, whānau (extended family), hapū (subtribe), iwi (tribal group), and communities (Wilson, 2008). The Māori (indigenous people of Aotearoa) concept of health, hauora ('the breath of the spirit of life' (Marsden, cited in Royal, 2003, p. 44), is broader than common understandings of health that occurs in the absence of illness or disease. Hauora, however, focuses on health and well-being (rather than ill-health) and encompasses a holistic understanding of health whereby the wairua (spiritual), whānau (extended family), tinana (physical) and hinengaro (psychological) dimensions function interdependently and are all important to Māori health and well-being (Durie, 2011). Despite the diversity among contemporary Māori in terms of the degree of traditional cultural beliefs and practises held by individuals and their whānau, biomedically constructed health practice and service delivery, for many, does not align to their world views and their health beliefs and practises.

The effective grounding of health practice in evidence for use with Māori must be accompanied by a critical analysis of the acceptability and appropriateness of its sources and outcomes, the unique understandings Māori have about health, and the socio-historical context which has resulted in the health inequities that burden Māori (Reid & Robson, 2006, 2007). It is important to note that while some health inequalities may be acceptable (such as gendered health conditions), Whitehead (1992) explains inequities as the 'differences which are unnecessary and avoidable, but in addition are considered unfair and unjust' (p. 431). In this chapter, a brief socio-historical background of contemporary Māori will be explored, along with the relevance of the Treaty of Waitangi to establish a context for considering evidence-based health practice. This will be followed by a discussion on Māori knowledge and the development of Māori-relevant research approaches for the production of evidence. Considerations for reviewing evidence to inform health practice involving Māori will then be discussed.

Treaty of Waitangi
The founding document of Aotearoa New Zealand signed between indigenous Māori and the British Crown in 1840.

SOCIO-HISTORICAL CONTEXT OF MĀORI

Māori have a complex but unique historical, social and cultural milieu that detrimentally influenced their health and well-being, as well as their ways of knowing and knowledge production (Durie, 1998). Any examination of the socio-historical context of contemporary Māori should be cognisant of the diversity in their cultural beliefs and practices—that is, there is no one Māori culture, although similarities across Māori do exist. Diversity exists within the contexts of iwi differences (also evident prior to colonisation), the dynamic nature of culture, and the effects of colonisation that resulted in many Māori being disconnected from their identity and cultural traditions and practices (Ihimaera, 1998; Webber, 2008). Nevertheless, similar to other indigenous peoples globally, Māori world views are holistic: steeped in spiritual, cosmological and environmental connections, relationships, connectedness, and a collective orientation (Chilisa, 2012; Durie, 1998). Marsden (cited in Royal, 2003) claims:

> Cultures pattern perceptions [sic] of reality into conceptualisations ['worldview of a culture'] of what they perceive reality to be; of what is to be regarded as actual, probable, possible or impossible. … The worldview lies at the very heart of the culture, touching, interacting with and strongly influencing every aspect of the culture. (p. 56)

Māori world views are often at odds with the biomedical world-view of health systems that focus on individuals and their illness or disease process. In Aotearoa New Zealand, it is the biomedical world view that informs the development of health service policy, planning and delivery, and consequently the dominant practice of those working within the arena of health.

Prior to the settlement of Aotearoa New Zealand, Māori possessed a legitimate, sophisticated knowledge system that guided communal living and traditional healing practices, aimed to keep everyone well and healthy. For example, daily life was dictated by concepts such as tapu (meaning restriction, sacred, protection) or levels of privilege or restriction applied to people, places, living creatures and events, for safety and protection from known risks. Noa (free from tapu, ordinary, unrestricted), on the other hand, provided a balance by providing situations without the protections and restrictions imposed by tapu. These two concepts guided members of Māori whānau and hapū about the protections and restrictions related to body parts (like the head, genitalia and heart), people, and food, for example (Durie, 1998).

It is beyond the scope of this chapter to provide an in-depth overview of the settlement and colonisation of Māori in Aotearoa, except to say the arrival of the British Crown, missionaries and settlers from Britain and Europe brought social and economic disruption for Māori, depopulation as a result of introduced diseases and warfare, and the loss of land, language, and cultural practices. Despite having a robust knowledge system, the colonising processes Māori were subjected to eroded their cultural traditions and invalidated mātauranga Māori and its acquisition (Tuhiwai Smith, 2012). Western and British cultural traditions and research practices dominated, invalidating Māori forms of knowledge and learning, denying, marginalising and silencing Māori as bearers of indigenous knowledge (Bishop, 2008; Chilisa, 2012; Denzin, Lincoln, & Smith, 2008; Tuhiwai Smith, 2012).

The Treaty of Waitangi ('the Treaty'), signed in 1840, established a bicultural relationship between Māori and the Crown and affirmed the status and right of Māori

Biomedical
Relating to a way of thinking about health and illness with a focus on diseases as physical entities that affect physical bodies. This is the dominant Western model of health care.

Tapu
A restricted or protected state, to be treated with the appropriate respect to ensure people are safe.

Noa
Normal (not sacred).

Mātauranga Māori
Māori knowledge and wisdom.

Te reo Māori
Māori language (voice).

Guidelines
Information providing
advice on how to
interpret policy or
procedure.

Partnership
Genuine and respectful
relationship between
people.

Participation
The process of being
involved.

Protection
The act of looking after
or taking care of.

Māori-centred
Focused on Māori
(by, for and about the
indigenous people of
Aotearoa New Zealand).

Kaupapa Māori
Philosophy or
agenda of the Māori
community.

to live their ways as the indigenous people of Aotearoa. In addition, it also guaranteed Māori protection and the equal rights others living in Aotearoa enjoyed (State Services Commission, 2005). Numerous breaches of the Treaty have occurred since its signing, in part because of the confusion about its meaning because two versions exist (one in te reo Māori (Māori language) and one in English), and also due to government legislation and policies enacted over time that have ignored the terms of this agreement. Nevertheless, it remains relevant today and its inclusion within the New Zealand *Health and Disability Act 2000* requires district health boards to be responsive to Māori health, and to recognise the Treaty obligations in decision-making and service delivery in order to reduce Māori health inequities and improve health outcomes (Durie, 2011). Te Ara Tika (Hudson, Milne, Reynolds, Russell, & Smith, 2010) provides guidelines for researchers to design and conduct ethical research with Māori and incorporates the Treaty principles, partnership, participation and protection, which can be used to understand the expectations of undertaking different types of research—mainstream, Māori-centred and kaupapa Māori ('by Māori, for Māori, with Māori').

MĀORI AND RESEARCH

Western science was imposed on Māori as the legitimate way of producing knowledge. Over time it dominated research with Māori and invalidated mātauranga Māori as a method of knowledge and knowledge development. This colonisation of Māori knowledge resulted in Māori becoming objects of investigation by researchers with little comprehension of the cultural relevance of the data they were collecting and their interpretion through a Western world view.

The marginalisation and invalidation of mātauranga Māori has led to research that has persisted over time and nullified information about Māori health beliefs and practices. But as Jahnke and Taiapa (1999) rightly claimed, 'Knowledge which makes sense in one particular cultural context cannot always be understood through the tools which govern the understanding of other belief systems and world views' (p. 41). Nonetheless, historically Māori have been over-researched in ways that systematically disempowered them, were disrespectful of their cultural traditions, and objectified their experiences with little regard to their social reality, important cultural interpretations and nuances. Without doubt Māori were subjected by non-Māori to research that was of little or no benefit, and frequently used to their disadvantage and to reinforce negative stereotypes. Tuhiwai Smith (2012) summed this simply: 'They came, they saw, they named, they claimed' (p. 83).

CASE STUDY 6.1

HEALTH DISPARITIES

Harwood and Tipene-Leach (2007) present research in Hauora IV that identifies morbidity, co-morbidity, and mortality disparities for Māori with type 2 diabetes. The statistical picture they present highlights the overwhelming nature of type 2 diabetes affecting many Māori. While these researchers acknowledge the many explanations for the high mortality and complication rates Māori experience, they also address issues related to unequal access to, and quality of, diabetes care for Māori rather than current policy and practice that focuses on individual behavioural change. For example, they position prevention within the structural changes, such as advertising, food regulation, and taxation incentives, that need to occur to help curb the diabetes epidemic affecting Māori.

The dominating agendas of Western scientific research endeavours disrupted any notion of social justice and the attainment of fairness and equity for all living in Aotearoa, and instead of producing evidence that would benefit Māori health outcomes Western scientific research reinforced unhelpful conclusions and interventions that lacked alignment with Māori constructions of health and well-being. This colonial construction of Māori knowledge and culture that often lacks relevance has contributed to a general sense of distrust in researchers and in the notion of research for many Māori. Tuhiwai Smith (2012) contends that past experiences are kept alive by the voices of elders, driven by the practices of researchers that disregarded tikanga (Māori cultural customs—the 'correct' way of doing things) and 'trampled' on their mana (status and authority). When Māori have minimal or no input into the planning, design, conduct of research and the interpretation of data, there is a high risk that the findings will not be beneficial for Māori and their communities (Tuhiwai Smith, 2012). At a minimum, it is important that Māori feel they have a voice in research they consider is important, and that the process is culturally safe (Chilisa, 2012; Tuhiwai Smith, 2012; Wilson & Neville, 2009).

Over the last four decades, Māori academics and communities have been engaged in recovering their research capacity, reclaiming mātauranga Māori, and asserting their right to undertake research in a culturally acceptable and appropriate manner. In the next section, an overview of things to look for when examining research-based evidence is presented.

Equity
Equal rights for all people in any situation.

Tikanga
Māori way of doing things; Māori protocol.

Mana
Pride or sense of esteem.

SELECTING EVIDENCE FOR USE WITH MĀORI

Chilisa (2012) provides important advice that is relevant for those using evidence to inform their health practice. She states: 'You will have a responsibility to critically assess the research process and procedures [of the evidence being reviewed] to see if they allow the researched to communicate their experiences from their frames of reference' (p. 39). There is a general consensus that research should benefit Māori, and Hudson et al. (2010) have gone so far as to say that, 'All research in Aotearoa New Zealand is of interest to Māori, and research which includes Māori is of paramount importance to Māori' (p. 1).

A variety of indigenous research approaches located within te āo Māori (the Māori world) has emerged—for example, Bishop (1996), Chilisa (2012), Durie (1996), and Tuhiwai Smith (2012). Research can be grouped depending upon the degree of control and involvement Māori have, and categorised into either mainstream, Māori-centred, or kaupapa Māori research (Cunningham, 2000). Kaupapa Māori research is based within an indigenous Māori world view, arises from the epistemological and metaphysical foundations of Māori culture and results in the production of Māori knowledge (Bishop, 2008; Nepe, 1991). Importantly, it rejects subjugation by dominant Western research traditions (Bishop, 2008).

A consequence of these developments is an advent of Māori aspirations driving research agendas, and Māori participation in research involving Māori from its inception to the dissemination of the findings and beyond. Readers of evidence should expect to see researchers critically locating their findings within a framework that critiques factors, such as structural, institutional, health system responsiveness, and determinants of health (Reid & Robson, 2006). Tuhiwai Smith (2012) provides a useful list of questions to guide reviewing evidence within a cross-cultural context:

> Who defined the research problem?
> For whom is this study worthy and relevant? Who says so?
> What knowledge will the community gain from this study?
> What knowledge will the researcher gain from this study?
> What are some likely positive outcomes from this study?
> What are some possible negative outcomes?
> How can the negative outcomes be eliminated?
> To whom is the researcher accountable?
> What processes are in place to support the research, the researched and the researcher? (pp. 175–176)

Therefore, when reading evidence it is important to scrutinise the purpose of any research and establish whether Māori participants are involved. Examine whether the study (1) does not involve Māori, or (2) involves Māori, (3) is Māori-centred, or (4) is a kaupapa Māori study. Table 6.1 shows a framework for the types of research with Māori outlined by Cunningham (2000). Defining features to explore include the research team

Consensus
A general agreement on any given issue.

Te āo Māori
Māori world.

Determinants
Factors that lead to a particular outcome.

composition, the participants, research methods used, the type of data collected, the data analysis methods, the standards against which the research is measured and the type of knowledge produced. Table 6.1 provides the key characteristics to assist in identifying each type of research.

TABLE 6.1 TYPES OF RESEARCH WITH MĀORI

	RESEARCH NOT INVOLVING MĀORI	RESEARCH INVOLVING MĀORI	MĀORI-CENTRED RESEARCH	KAUPAPA MĀORI RESEARCH
Description	Māori not participants or participation not sought Research will not have impact on Māori	Māori are participants	Māori are key participants	Māori are key participants
Research Team	May include Māori	Māori junior members	Māori senior members	Mainly Māori
Control	Mainstream	Mainstream	Mainstream	Māori
Māori participation	None	Minor	Major	Major
Research methods	Contemporary-mainstream	Contemporary-mainstream	Contemporary-mainstream and Māori	Contemporary-Māori and mainstream
Data collected	Mainstream	Māori	Māori	Māori
Analysis	Mainstream	Mainstream	Māori	Māori
Standards measured against	Western research	Western research	Western research–Māori	Māori
Knowledge produced	Mainstream	Mainstream	Māori	Māori

Source: Adapted from Cunningham, 2000

The principles of partnership, participation and protection can also be a useful guide to make judgments about the involvement of, and relevance of evidence to, Māori (Hudson et al., 2010). Thus, it could be expected that Māori have been involved in the formation of the research—a process enabling the building of relationships, identifying any potential impediments to the research progressing, and highlighting the benefits that can assist with Māori involvement in the research (Durie, 2011). The use of **kaumātua**

Kaumātua
Esteemed, wise members of the Māori community.

(respected elders), an advisory group, or Māori research assistants, for example, is an indicator of Māori participation in the research. The presence of kaumātua and advisory groups can also be an indicator that cultural values, beliefs and practices are respected and upheld by the research team. It is also important to look at how the findings are interpreted. The evolution of research has seen a rise in Māori centred qualitative research approaches, such as whānau and Māori communities using participatory action research that enable participants' research aspirations to drive the research project (see, for example, Cram & Kennedy, 2010; Eruera, 2010; Pipi, 2010).

It is useful to note that quantitative mainstream research, like epidemiological studies, often provides a 'big picture' of Māori health, although it can often portray Māori health negatively (Ministry of Health, 2010). Such research approaches, while helpful in providing information on health status and health gains, do little to generate information to inform health practice about local contexts that explain statistics or the strengths and health practices that Māori and their whānau possess and that are working well. Equal explanatory power has also been promoted for use in quantitative studies involving Māori in order to provide better powered studies to generate information for increased understanding, and enables addressing Māori health inequalities and health needs. This is achieved by purposely over-sampling Māori in sufficient numbers or equal to non-Māori—something to consider when reviewing evidence (Fink, Paine, Gander, Harris, & Purdie, 2011; Te Rōpū Rangahau e Eru Pōmare, 2002).

RESEARCH ALIVE 6.1
TOOLS IN CONTEXT

Pipi (2010) presents an analysis of the Planning Alternative Tomorrows with Hope (PATH) planning tool using a kaupapa Māori framework. The PATH planning tool is presented by Pipi as a person-centred approach to planning with individuals, whānau and communities. The PATH is presented as a way of moving people from one way of thinking to one that focuses on the future, current goals and aspirations. In addition, it assists people to identify strengths and other attributes they possess. The PATH is underpinned by self-efficacy (the belief that can undertake necessary actions to achieve success) and creativity (reflective of each unique person or group). This research is presented within a Māori context, and provides examples of its application in practice at various levels. The value of Pipi's evidence is the presentation of a tool that could be used with Māori and their whānau to focus on future aspirations and goals.

Undoubtedly, basing health practice on evidence is important. Equally important is that the evidence must be appropriate for use with Māori and inform interactions that are relevant. The above suggestions are simply an introduction into some of the things that should be considered when working with Māori.

SUMMARY

This chapter has given an overview of fundamental issues relating to Māori and evidence-based health practice, and has introduced some key issues for beginning readers to consider when reviewing evidence to inform their practice. The health of contemporary Māori is not simply the result of poor management by a collective of individuals, but rather it reflects the detrimental effects of colonisation and its ongoing effects, access to the necessary determinants of health, and the access to and quality of health services. Evidence to inform health practice with Māori should not be simply adopted, but carefully critiqued and ideally derived from research with Māori, interpreted by Māori.

REFLECTION POINTS

Think about whom you would seek assistance from to apply evidence to your health practice in the situations where you will work with Māori.

This chapter has focused on Māori, research and researchers and the potential for biases within the evidence. Equally important is recognising our own personal world views and biases when we select, interpret and use evidence based on research. A useful exercise is to divide a piece of paper into quarters, and then in each quarter write the following:

- What I think about Māori and evidence is …
- What I feel about Māori and evidence is …
- What I know about Māori and evidence is …
- What I need to know about Māori and evidence is …

Reflect on the answers you have written and develop strategies for any areas of development.

STUDY QUESTIONS

1   Why is it important to consider the socio-historical context for Māori health and how this may affect the use of evidence?
2   How can you ensure that evidence that informs health practice is relevant for working with Māori?

3   Using a piece of evidence you intend to draw on to inform your health practice, identify if the researchers created an opportunity to 'dialogue and negotiate' with Māori communities and participants, as suggested by Wilson and Neville (2009). What is the potential impact on the quality of the evidence?

ADDITIONAL READING

Durie, M. (1998). *Whaiora: Maori health development* (2nd ed.). Auckland, New Zealand: Oxford University Press.

Reid, P., & Robson, B. (2007). Understanding health inequities. In B. Robson, & R. Harris (Eds.), *Hauora: Maori health standards IV. A study of the years 2000–2005* (pp. 3–10). Wellington, NZ: Te Ropu Rangahau Hauora a Eru Pomare. Retrieved from http://www.hauora.maori.nz

Shaw, S., White, W. L., & Deed, B. (Eds.). (2013). *Health, wellbeing and environment in Aotearoa New Zealand.* Melbourne: Oxford University Press.

Tuhiwai Smith, L. (2012). *Decolonizing methodologies: Research and indigenous peoples* (2nd ed.). London: Zed Books.

REFERENCES

Bishop, R. (1996). *Collaborative research stories: Whakawhanaungatanga.* Palmerston North: Dunmore Press.

Bishop, R. (2008). Freeing ourselves from neo-colonial domination in research: A Maori approach to creating knowledge. In N. L. Denzin, & Y. S. Lincoln (Eds.), *The Sage handbook of qualitative research* (3rd ed., pp. 109–138). Thousand Oaks, CA: Sage Publications.

Chilisa, B. (2012). *Indigenous research methodologies.* Thousand Oaks, CA: Sage Publications.

Cram, F., & Kennedy, V. (2010). Researching whānau collectives. *MAI Review, 3,* 1–12. Retrieved from www.review.mai.ac.nz/index.php/MR/article/view/382/561

Cunningham, C. (2000). A framework for addressing Maori knowledge in research, science and technology. *Pacific Health Dialog, 7*(1), 62–69.

Denzin, N. L., Lincoln, Y. S., & Smith, L. T. (2008). *Handbook of critical and indigenous methodologies.* Thousand Oaks, CA: Sage Publications.

Durie, M. (1996, 1 February). *Characteristics of Maori health research.* Paper presented at the meeting of the Hui Whakapiripiri, Hongoeka Marae, Wellington, New Zealand.

Durie, M. (1998). *Whaiora: Maori health development* (2nd ed.). Auckland: Oxford University Press.

Durie, M. (2011). *Ngā tini whetū: Navigating Māori futures*. Wellington: Huia.

Eruera, M. (2010). Ma te whānau te huarahi motuhake: Whānau participatory action research groups. *MAI Review, 3*, 1–9.

Fink, J. W., Paine, S.-J., Gander, P. H., Harris, R. B., & Purdie, G. (2011). Changing response rates from Maori and non-Maori in national sleep health surveys. *New Zealand Medical Journal, 124*(1328), 52–63.

Harwood, M., Tipene-Leach, D. (2007). Diabetes. In B. Robson, & R. Harris, *Hauora: Maori health standards IV. A study of the years 2000–2005* (pp. 160–167). Wellington: Te Ropu Rangahau a Eru Pomare.

Hudson, M., Milne, M., Reynolds, P., Russell, K., & Smith, B. (2010). *Te ara tika Guidelines for Maori research ethics: A framework for researchers and ethics committee members*. Auckland: Health Research Council.

Ihimaera, W. (Ed.). (1998). *Growing up Māori*. Auckland: Tandem Press.

Jahnke, H. T., & Taiapa, J. (1999). Maori research. In C. Davidson, & M. Tolich (Eds.), *Social science research in New Zealand: Many paths to understanding* (pp. 39–50). Auckland: Longman Pearson Education.

Ministry of Health. (2010). *Tatau kahukura: Maori health chart book 2010* (2nd ed.). Wellington: Author.

Nepe, T. M. (1991). *Te toi huarewa tipuna: Kaupapa Māori an educational intervention system*. Unpublished master's thesis, University of Auckland, Auckland, New Zealand. Retrieved from http://hdl.handle.net/2292/3066

Pipi, K. (2010). The PATH planning tool and its potential for whānau research. *MAI Review, 3*, 1–10.

Reid, P., & Robson, B. (2006). The state of Maori health. In M. Mulholland (Ed.), *State of the Maori nation: Twenty first-century issues in Aotearoa* (pp. 17–32). Auckland: Reed Publishing.

Reid, P., & Robson, B. (2007). Understanding health inequities. In B. Robson & R. Harris (Eds.), *Hauora: Maori health standards IV. A study of the years 2000–2005* (pp. 3–10). Wellington, NZ: Te Ropu Rangahau Hauora a Eru Pomare. Retrieved from http://www.hauora.maori.nz

Royal, T. A. C. (2003). *The woven universe: Selected writings of Rev. Māori Marsden*. Ōtaki: Te Wānanga-o-Raukawa.

State Services Commission. (2005). *The story of the Treaty*. Wellington: Author.

Te Rōpū Rangahau e Eru Pōmare. (2002). *Mana Whakamārama—Equal explanatory power: Mäori and non-Mäori sample size in national health surveys.* Retrieved from www.fmhs.auckland.ac.nz/faculty/tkhm/tumuaki/_docs/Equal_explanatory_power.pdf

Tuhiwai Smith, L. (2012). *Decolonizing methodologies: Research and indigenous peoples* (2nd ed.). London: Zed Books.

Webber, M. (2008). *Walking the space between: Identity and Māori/Pākehā.* Wellington: NZCER Press.

Whitehead, M. (1992). The concepts and principles of equity and health. *International Journal of Health Services, 22,* 429–445.

Wilson, D. (2008). The significance of a culturally appropriate health service for indigenous Maori women. *Contemporary Nurse, 28*(1–2), 173–188.

Wilson, D., & Neville, S. (2009). Culturally safe research with vulnerable populations. *Contemporary Nurse, 33*(1), 69–79.

WEBSITES

Hauora: Māori Standards of Health:
http://www.hauora.maori.nz/hauora

Health Research Council—Te Ara Tika:
http://www.hrc.govt.nz/news-and-publications/publications/te-ara-tika-guidelines-m%C4%81ori-research-ethics-framework-researcher

Ministry of Health—Tatau Kahukura Māori Health Chart Book:
http://www.health.govt.nz/publication/tatau-kahukura-maori-health-chart-book-2010-2nd-editionRangahau:
http://www.rangahau.co.nz

CHAPTER 7

PACIFIC RESEARCH

PEGGY FAIRBAIRN-DUNLOP, JULIET NANAI
AND LITIUINGI AHIO

CHAPTER OVERVIEW

This chapter covers the following topics:

- Why Pacific health research?
- A Pacific world view
- Pacific health research models
- Guidelines on Pacific health research
- Applying a Pacific world view to research

KEY TERMS

Community	Holistic
Complexity	Model
Consensus	Pacific world view
Cultural	Power
Empowerment	Relationships
Equity	

Good health is fundamental for the well-being of individuals, families and communities and for national development. Good health enables people to engage in sports and recreation, for example, and in education and employment activities so as to achieve their life goals and contribute to the economic and social well-being of their communities. In line with its goals of equity, justice and aspirations as a culturally diverse nation, Aotearoa New Zealand directs considerable amounts to health research to support planning aimed at ensuring the good health of all citizens. Despite this investment, the health of Pacific peoples has been described as worse than other New Zealanders' health from childhood through to later stages of life (Statistics New Zealand and Ministry of Pacific Island Affairs, 2011).

Equity
Equal rights for all people in any situation.

WHY PACIFIC HEALTH RESEARCH?

Many factors influence good health, including socio-economic status. For example, because Pacific peoples are disproportionately represented in lower socio-economic groups and have lower incomes, it is likely that their food choices may be adversely affected by the affordability of food (Statistics New Zealand and Ministry of Pacific Island Affairs, 2011), they may live in over-crowded housing, and decisions about whether and when to go to a doctor will take place within a context of competing needs.

CASE STUDY 7.1

A SNAPSHOT OF DATA

- In 2006, the estimated life expectancy for Pacific men was 73.9 years and 78.9 years for Pacific women, more than four years less than for the total population.
- Between 2002 and 2006, Pacific children were 1.5 times as likely to be admitted to hospital for gastroenteritis and 4.5 times as likely as European children to be admitted to hospital for serious skin infections.
- Pacific children and young people (aged 0–24 years) are nearly 50 times more likely than European children (and twice as likely as Māori) to be admitted to hospital with acute rheumatic fever (ARF).
- Pacific young people are approximately twice as likely to have depression and anxiety issues, or to make suicide attempts, as the rest of the population.

- From 2006 to 2007, 10 per cent of Pacific peoples aged over 15 years were diagnosed with diabetes—approximately three times the diagnosis rate for the total New Zealand population.
- Between 2002 and 2004, the rate for new cases of stroke in Pacific adults was 318 per 100,000 compared with 179 per 100,000 for the total population.

Source: Statistics New Zealand and Ministry of Pacific Island Affairs, 2011, p. 13

Addressing Pacific health status has urgency for the quality of life of Pacific peoples but also because of the rapidly increasing Pacific population in Aotearoa New Zealand. Pacific peoples make up 7 per cent of New Zealand's total population and this is projected to rise to 9 per cent within the next few years. The diversity of the communities grouped together as 'Pacific' adds complexity. For example, Pacific peoples comprise over 22 ethnic groups, each with their own culture and language; 60 per cent are New Zealand born, and multi-ethnicity is increasing. 'Pacific peoples' is an umbrella term used to encompass the variety of Pacific Island nations and communities who are linguistically, culturally and geographically distinct from each other (Health Research Council of New Zealand, 2005).

Complexity
The result of interaction between entities that results in effects whose sum is greater than the effects produced by the component parts.

RESEARCH ALIVE 7.1
DEFINITIONS

PACIFIC COMMUNITY

There is no generic 'Pacific community' but rather Pacific peoples who align themselves variously and at different times along ethnic geographic church groups .... therefore it is important that these various contexts of Pacific communities are clearly defined and demarcated in the research process.

Anae, Coxon, Mara, Wendt-Samu, & Finau, 2001, p. 7

ETHNICITY

The ethnic group or groups that people identity with or feel they belong to. Ethnicity is a measure of cultural affiliation, as opposed to race, ancestry, nationality or citizenship. Thus ethnicity is self-perceived and people can affiliate with more than one ethnic group.

Gray, 2001

[continued next page]

PACIFIC OR ETHNIC SPECIFIC RESEARCH?
For a discussion of this point see Finau (2006) on cultural democracy.

PASIFIKA
'Pasifika' is commonly used in Aotearoa New Zealand to indicate that the Pacific community comprises a number of ethnic groups. Pacific health research must be 'informed first and foremost from within the continuum of the Pacific worldview'.

Health Research Council of New Zealand, 2005, p. 1

The use of generic research models cannot capture the realities of Pacific people's health experiences, challenges and enablers:

> Generic research models targeting the wider New Zealand population do not seem to be working as well for Pacific peoples. To increase understanding and knowledge and to build health literacy within Pacific communities, public health information needs to be tailored to the needs of specific community groups.

Statistics New Zealand and Ministry of Pacific Island Affairs, 2011, p. 43

Power
The exercise of strength or control.

Closely related to this is the fact that the assumptions and power relations underpinning the use of generic models has effectively ignored or devalued the understandings, beliefs and practices which Pacific peoples bring to the research process and which could have added to the pool of knowledge from which creative solutions could be made (Finau, 2006; Smith, 2004). As a result, research which could have been a mutually enriching, knowledge-sharing experience has proved to be disempowering. Evidence suggests that in many areas of health Pacific people have not had access to good information (Ministry of Health, 2008, 2011, 2012) and this has affected their ability to make informed decisions about their health or that of family members (Statistics New Zealand and Ministry of Pacific Affairs, 2011). It is likely that Pacific health interventions have been based on unverified assumptions of needs and what will work for Pacific peoples. Such outcomes represent a tremendous waste of resources that could have been used in other ways.

There is no such thing as value-free, neutral or strictly scientific research (Finau, 2006). Researchers (and participants) bring their own beliefs and understandings to the research process, and these influence how the research is framed, carried out and responded to, and the findings disseminated. Furthermore, research assumptions, concepts, language and terms used must be critically examined for their meaning to Pacific peoples. Otherwise it is questionable whether researchers and participants are talking about the same thing (Fairbairn-Dunlop, 2011).

RESEARCH ALIVE 7.2
DEFINING RESEARCH CONCEPTS: FOOD SECURITY

Here is an example of the different understandings of the term 'food security' (a term used in programme planning) held by the global community and members of a Tongan community in Aotearoa New Zealand.

Food security has been defined as the 'ability of individuals, households and communities to acquire appropriate and nutritious food on a regular and reliable basis by socially acceptable means' (McIntyre, cited in Rush, 2009, p. 9) and this definition is used in programmes to address food security. However, Ahio (2011) found that Tongan health workers and mothers in Aotearoa New Zealand conceptualised food security as having enough food available to feed the community rather than the family concept of day-by-day meals. Food security was connected to sharing and reciprocity, and to making sure there was enough food to fulfil cultural obligations. Having enough food for the family was a lower order requirement (Ahio, 2011).

Pacific researchers are increasingly using vernacular language to satisfy and claim the cultural nuances of meaning and value. Manu'atu's (2000) use of the Tongan terms 'mafana' and 'malie' to describe the tingling feelings of warmth which come from the heart when everything has been done in the culturally right way is a prime example.

Pacific peoples' health understandings and motivations are embedded in an intricate system of cultural beliefs and understandings which influence every facet of daily life. However, these are not static but have adapted to changing times and places (Health Research Council of New Zealand, 2005). Taufe'ulungaki (2000) expressed the responsibilities of Pacific research:

> The role of Pacific research is primarily not only to identify and promote a Pacific worldview, which should begin by identifying Pacific values in the way in which Pacific societies create meaning, structure and construct reality, but complementary to that is the need to also interrogate the assumptions that underpin western structures and institutions that we as Pacific peoples have adopted without much questioning. (p. 11)

Unfortunately there is little longitudinal data to plot the impact of changes over time in Pacific health status. AUT University's Pacific Island Family Study (PIFS) has pioneered this field and provides a veritable treasure chest of data for further research (see Case Study 7.2).

Cultural
Relating to beliefs, traditions, practices and rituals originating within the family and community into which a person is born and raised, and transmitted from one generation to the next through a common language.

CASE STUDY 7.2

THE PACIFIC ISLANDS FAMILIES STUDY (PIFS)

The Pacific Islands Families Study has been following a cohort of 1,400 Pacific children born (15 March to 17 December 2000) at Middlemore Hospital in South Auckland. Middlemore Hospital has the largest number of Pacific births in Aotearoa New Zealand, and includes the main Pacific Islands ethnic groups. PIFS aims to:

1   provide information on Pacific peoples' health, and the cultural, economic, environmental and psychosocial factors that are associated with child health and development outcomes and family functioning;

2   determine how such factors individually and interactively influence positive and negative child, parent and family outcomes over time; and

3   provide information that will help set quantifiable targets for Pacific peoples' health.

The study has followed individuals and families prospectively over time measurement points (at six weeks after the child's birth, at age 12 months, 24 months, at age 4 years and 6 years) with the present focus on the teenage years.

Source: AUT University, 2010

A PACIFIC WORLD VIEW

Pacific world view
A philosophical view that incorporates elements of Pacific culture and history.

Holistic
An emphasis on the whole, rather than separate parts.

A Pacific world view is described as being holistic in nature, encompassing three interconnected and interdependent elements. Tamasese Ta'isi (2007) describes a Pacific world view in this way:

> Imagine if you will, a worldview that understands the environment, humans, the animate and inanimate—all natural life—as having its sources in the same divine origin, imbued with the life force, interrelated and genealogically connected. (p. 13)

Pacific peoples see their place in the world as connected to the creator God (spiritual, sacred) and with natural environment and resources (material). Maintaining harmony and balance between these elements is fundamental to well-being. Tu'itahi (2005) proposes five interrelated dimensions as underpinning the health and well-being of Pacific people:

sino: physical

'*atamai*: mental and intellectual

laumalie: spiritual

kainga: community

'atakai: environment (both built and natural).

In every Pacific community behaviours and expectations aimed at ensuring a balance and harmony between these dimensions have developed over time.

The Pacific world view influences research in a number of ways. Overarching is the central place of the spiritual in every daily activity from planting, to travel, perceptions of what is good health, and what is required to achieve good health and healing processes. The interplay of the spiritual and the physical is a major consideration in Pacific health research. So too is the influence of the family and community. The extended family, under chiefly leadership systems (over 90 per cent of land in Pacific Island countries is still held in customary tenure under stewardship), is the main institution in Pacific communities, as sanctioned by the Gods which also allocated lands and sea resources to ensure family security. Because families are the main source of identity and social, political and economic participation, health is likely to be viewed as a communal rather than an individual responsibility and the role of leaders in promoting good health has additional importance. Maintaining the family good is paramount in all Pacific communities and this is achieved through acts such as sharing, reciprocity, and nurturing relationships through respectful behaviours, especially towards elders and seniors. The ideal of respectful behaviours is seen in the concept of va (the protected space) observed in many Pacific countries, and the feelings of health and well-being achieved when there is peace and harmony between people, nature and the Gods. While all knowledge was a gift from the Gods, there are distinctions between knowledge that is protected and sacred (as specialist knowledge) and knowledge that is communally owned and shared. For example, the specialist knowledge held by healers and midwives was closely guarded and shared within families such as the Samoan fofoa (massagers) and midwives while medicines and poultices were made from the available trees and crops. Communal knowledge, on the other hand, was constructed and validated in the many meetings which characterised life in these predominantly oral communities. Meetings were times when community members raised concerns and pooled their knowledge so as to identify solutions that would ensure the best community outcomes. Time was not a consideration—discussions continued until consensus was reached. The term 'talanoa' is now commonly used to signify these community knowledge construction processes (Vaioleti, 2006). This gathering of knowledge from multiple sources and the social engagement in critiquing these views together is a vastly different experience to the use of research surveys and questionnaires.

The place of the spiritual in health research and the importance of social engagement with communities of interest to reach solutions are noted as central. People's actions are underpinned by the belief in the spiritual and in a relationship between the spiritual and human actions.

Community
A group of people with defined commonality. This may include geographical location, belief systems or any other social construct.

Relationships
The similarities and connections between people or variables in any given situation.

Consensus
A general agreement on any given issue.

PACIFIC HEALTH RESEARCH MODELS

Model
A framework for
describing concepts.

A number of health research models have been devised aimed at drawing together
the multiple perspectives of the Pacific world view (see Figure 7.1). The Fonofale
health research model is regarded as both a Samoan and a pan-Pacific model (Pulotu-
Endemann, 2001).

In the Fonofale health research model the Samoan fale is used to symbolise the
holistic nature of the research process. The middle post of the fale represents the person,
individual or group. However, the individual does not stand alone but is grounded in
the family which in turn is sheltered by the cultural values and beliefs comprising the
spiritual, physical, mental and other dimensions. These values are symbolised by the
four posts (pou). In addition, the family sits and is influenced by the wider context of
environment (resources), concepts of time (the past, the present and the future) and
space (location).

FIGURE 7.1   THE FONOFALE MODEL

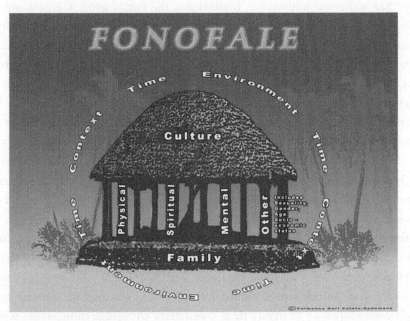

Source: Pulotu-Endemann, 2001, p. 3.

The relationship between each of these factors is integral to good health and
well-being. For research, this means not looking solely at the medical condition (the
physical manifestation) but taking account of the impact of other factors (such as socio-
economic, cultural and spiritual beliefs and aspirations) on the health issue, by applying

the holistic Pacific world view. Second, and related, the research process will feature face-to-face consultation and relationship-building with people and families at each stage of the research process, so as to gain an in-depth understanding of health challenges and enablers and ensure opportunities for the empowerment of Pacific peoples. Their participation in the production of knowledge will enhance their well-being and add to the global knowledge base. Finally, in the spirit of reciprocity, research findings must be shared with the participants as ongoing process.

Empowerment
Giving or receiving the power in a particular situation.

RESEARCH ALIVE 7.3
OTHER PACIFIC RESEARCH MODELS

The *kakala research model* by Helu-Thaman (1999), based on the traditional making of fragrant garlands, can be applied to identifying and selecting participants to collect information for a particular research topic. Making of the kakala garland involves three key processes: the 'toli'—the gathering of flowers for the garland (the information for research); the 'tui'—the weaving of the garland (design and collection and interpretation of data); and the luva or the presentation of the kakala after completion (the disseminating of the research findings back to the participants and other people so that findings can be used to improve health status).

Te Vaka Atafaga is a Tokelau assessment model for supporting holistic mental health practice with Tokelau people in Aotearoa, New Zealand (Kupa, 2009).

Other models are:

- *Tivaevae model*: a Cook Island model (Maua-Hodges, 2000);
- *Faafaletui model*: a Samoan model (Tamasese, Peteru, Waldegrave, & Bush, 2005);
- *Ta and Va model*: a Tongan model (Mahina, 1992);
- *Fonua model*: a Tongan model (Tu'itahi, 2005);
- *Fonofale model*: a pan-Pacific and Samoan model (Pulotu-Endemann, 2001).

GUIDELINES ON PACIFIC HEALTH RESEARCH

The Pacific health research guidelines (Health Research Council of New Zealand, 2005) outline 10 guiding principles for forming and maintaining ethical relationships with Pacific people. These are respect, cultural competency, meaningful engagement, reciprocity, utility, rights, balance, protection, capacity-building, and participation (see Health Research Council, 2005, pp. 12–43 for a full explanation of these).

CASE STUDY 7.3

THE GUIDELINES

The *Guidelines on Pacific Health Research* (Health Research Council of New Zealand, 2005) were developed through extensive community consultation. These ground-breaking guidelines reinforce the idea of the research process as being one of ethical engagement, and being a mutually empowering and beneficial knowledge exchange process in which developing, cultivating and maintaining principles and relationships is 'integral to all ethnical processes' (Health Research Council of New Zealand, 2005 p. 13). For ease, points drawn from page 11 of the guidelines have been re-grouped here under the headings of principles, Pacific research, process and responsiveness to changing contexts.

Principles: 'The primary role of Pacific health research is to gain knowledge and understanding that will improve the health of Pacific peoples.'

Pacific research 'will be informed first and foremost from within the continuum of Pacific world-views.'

'Pacific research will be underpinned by Pacific cultural values and beliefs and will be conducted in accordance with Pacific ethical standards values and aspirations.'

Process: 'Pacific health research requires the active involvement of Pacific peoples (as researchers, advisors and stakeholders) and demonstrates that Pacific peoples are more than just the subjects of research.'

'Pacific research will build the capacity and capability of Pacific peoples in research and contribute to the Pacific knowledge base.'

'The source material for Pacific health research will most likely be derived from Pacific peoples and from within Pacific realties—past, present and future.'

Response to change: 'Pacific approaches to research will aim to be responsive to changing Pacific contexts.'

Source: Health Research Council of New Zealand, 2005, p. 11

APPLYING A PACIFIC WORLD VIEW TO RESEARCH

There are a number of questions and actions to take account of when considering carrying out health research with Pacific peoples. The '*Ala Mo'ui Pathways to Pacific Health and Wellbeing 2010–2014* (Ministry of Health and Ministry of Pacific Island Affairs, 2010) report sets the current statement of health research needs.

RESEARCH ALIVE 7.4
STEPS AND QUESTIONS TO CONSIDER

STEP 1: QUESTIONS ARISING

- Are there differences by age, by gender, by ethnic group, by location (as New Zealand, homeland, those that travel between the homeland and Aotearoa New Zealand)?
- What could be potential influencing factors (economic, social and cultural), such as knowledge about strokes, access to information health services, and management?
- Is there a Pacific factor at play? For example, who is responsible for 'health'? Is health seen to be 'in the hands of the Gods'?
- Where is the best place to carry out this research, at this time?
- Should it be ethnic-specific? What does 'Pacific' mean? Which groups are in the sample (Polynesian, Melanesian, Micronesian groups)?
- Shall I focus on women?

STEP 2: DRAWING ON AVAILABLE KNOWLEDGE

- Consider the available reports and statistics.
- Tap community knowledge. At this stage it is wise to consult with members of the Pacific community. This will ensure people know about the study, add to the knowledge base of ideas and possibilities, encourage stakeholder buy-in and gain community support (and blessing) for the study. Community participation also supports a culturally safe entry into your research, provides an avenue for information sharing and increases the likelihood that findings will be shared and acted on. This is also the time to explore whether proposed definitions and terms are congruent with Pacific concepts and ideas (as illustrated in Research Alive 7.2); as is often said, 'community involvement will keep your research honest'. Church groups and women's groups are examples.

STEP 3: INTERVIEW SCHEDULE

Based on steps 1 and 2, prepare an interview schedule which is flexible and open to other ideas and suggestions. For the interviews themselves, it would be valuable to explore the use of the' talanoa' (see Vaioleti, 2006), which is the commonly used way of communicating in Pacific communities.

[continued next page]

STEP 4: RESEARCH METHODOLOGY AND DESIGN

Pacific research is likely to be qualitative because usually the data are already available and we are seeking people's perceptions of the data and what should be done.

Research design questions include:

- What approach will best answer my research question?
- Shall I use Pacific or Western methodology? (For example, phenomenology, case study or narratives)
- How are these research approaches the same or different?
- Is participatory action research useful?
- What data gathering methods shall I use?
- Shall I conduct interviews (talanoa), and will they be of individuals or groups?
- To whom shall I talk to ensure a comprehensive understanding of this issue?

The Samoan concept of fa'afaletui is often used to signify the weaving (tui) together of many different expressions of knowledge from within various community groupings. Concerns are expressed that researchers typically consult with Pacific Island-born elders, religious ministers and those in status positions (often male) and neglect to explore the views of grassroots groups, such as New Zealand-born youth.

STEP 5: DATA COLLECTION

- Will I need a translator?
- Can I create a culturally safe space for discussions (what are the protocols, courtesies and appropriate dress), allow enough time (pacing the interviews to ensure that customary communication protocols are observed and the views of participants are respected) and let participants lead our discussions?
- How much time should I allow?
- How should I show reciprocity?

STEP 6: DATA COLLECTION AND INTERPRETATION

- Consider using the community as a sounding board.

STEP 7: TAKING THE RESEARCH FINDINGS BACK TO THE PEOPLE

- Check to see if anything has been missed.
- Help inform community actions.

SUMMARY

Pacific health research must be informed first and foremost from within the continuum of the 'Pacific world view'. There are a number of key points underpinning a Pacific world view and suggestions about how they can be incorporated in Pacific health research guidelines and models. Using generic frameworks has not worked for Pacific people; in fact, the framing of health research from a Western perspective (with Western assumptions) has disadvantaged Pacific peoples by excluding their knowledge, expertise and experience. The foundational importance of spiritual beliefs to health and health practices must be acknowledged, along with the role of the family and family leaders in health education and the promoting of good health practices. Research with Pacific peoples must incorporate respect for their values, beliefs and the knowledge they bring to the process; otherwise the validity and credibility of any data collection will be questionable and of little use to forward planning.

REFLECTION POINTS

- How do your understandings of health compare to the Pasifika world view?
- Can the use of Pasifika research methods support Pacific peoples to have a voice in the Aotearoa New Zealand community?
- How might you go about conducting research that respects culturally appropriate and safe ways of data collection and analysis?
- How different are the Pacific research models from commonly used Western research models?

STUDY QUESTIONS

1 Why is there a need for Pasifika research?
2 What are the ethical principles that guide Pacific health research?
3 How do researchers know the research methodology they use is reliable and credible when carrying out research with Pacific peoples?

ADDITIONAL READING

Abel, S., Park, J., Tipene-Leach, D., Finau, S., & Lennan, M. (2001). Infant care practices in New Zealand: A cross-cultural qualitative study. *Social Science & Medicine, 53,* 1135–1148.

Ah Ching, P. L., Sapolu, M., Samifua, M., & Yamada, S. (2001). Attitudes regarding tuberculosis among Samoans. *Pacific Health Dialog, 8*(1), 15–19.

Blakely, T., Richardson, K., Young, J., Graham, P., Tobias, M., Callister, P., et al. (2009). Does mortality vary between Pacific groups? Estimating Samoan, Cook Island Māori, Tongan and Niuean mortality rates using hierarchical Bayesian modelling. *Official Statistics Research Series, 5*. Wellington: Statistics New Zealand. Retrieved from http://www.statisphere.govt.nz

Borrows, J., Williams, M., Schluter, P., Paterson, J., & Langitoto Helu, S. (2011). Pacific Island families study: The association of infant health risk indicators and acculturation of Pacific Island mothers living in New Zealand. *Journal of Cross Cultural Psychology, 42*(5), 699–724.

Craig, E., Jackson, C., Han, D. Y., & NZCYES Steering Committee. (2007). *Monitoring the health of New Zealand children and young people: Indicator handbook*. Auckland, New Zealand: Paediatric Society of New Zealand, New Zealand Child and Youth Epidemiology Service. Retrieved from http://www.paediatrics.org.nz

Kepa, M., & Manuatu, L. (2007). *Fonua: Land, languages, teaching and learning*. Symposium conducted at the meeting of the BAAL Conference. Retrieved from http://www.baal.org.uk/proc07/17_mere_kepa.pdf

King, P., Maniapoto, M., Tamasese, T., Parsons, T. L., & Waldegrave. (2010). *Socio-cultural factors associated with food security and physical activity for Maori and Pacific people in Aotearoa New Zealand*. The Family Centre Social Research Unit. Retrieved February 8, 2012, from http://weightmanagement.hiirc.org.nz/page/21618/socio-cultural-factors-associated-with-food/?section=13878&contentType=166&tab=26

Kupa, K. (2009). Te Vaka Atafaga: A Tokelau assessment model for supporting holistic mental health practice with Tokelau people in Aotearoa, New Zealand. *Pacific Health Dialog, 15*(1), 156–163.

Mahina, O. (1992). *The Tongan traditional history tala-e-fonua: A vernacular ecology-centred historico-cultural concept*. Canberra: Australian National University.

Malo, V. (2000). *Pacific people in New Zealand talk about their experiences with mental health*. Wellington: Mental Health Commission.

Manuatu, L. (2005). Fonua, tu'ufonua mo e nofo fonua 'i Aotearoa, New Zealand. *Alternative, 1*(1), 137–149.

McFall-McCaffery, J. (2010). Getting started with Pacific research: Finding resources and information on Pacific research models and methodologies. *Mai Review, 1*. Retrieved from http://www.review.mai.ac.nz/index.php/MR/article/viewFile/332/367

Mental Health Commission. (2001). *Pacific mental health services and workforce: Moving on the blueprint*. Wellington: Mental Health Commission.

Ministry of Health. (2008). *Improving quality of care for Pacific peoples*. Wellington Ministry of Health.

Rush, E. (2009). *Food security for Pacific peoples in New Zealand. A report for the Obesity Action Coalition*. Wellington. Retrieved from http://www.ana.org.nz/sites/default/files/PacificfoodsecurityreportfinalMarch09_3.pdf

Statistics New Zealand. (2006). *QuickStats about Pacific people: 2006 Census*. Retrieved from http://www.stats.govt.nz.

Suaalii-Sauni, T., Wheeler, A., Saafi, E., Robinson, G., Agnew, F., Warren, H., et al. (2009). Exploration of Pacific perspectives of Pacific models of mental health service delivery in New Zealand. *Pacific Health Dialog, 15*(1), 18–24.

Taufe'ulungaki, A. (2004). *Fonua: Reclaiming Pacific communities in Aotearoa Symposium*. Pacific Health Symposium, Waipuna Hotel, Auckland, New Zealand.

Talemaitoga, A. (2011). Pacific peoples: Our health and wellbeing. *Vaikoloa: Journal of Primary Health Care, 3*(2), 167–168.

Tiatia, J. (2008). *Pacific cultural competencies: A literature review*. Wellington: Ministry of Health.

Wright, S., & Hornblow, A. (2008). Emerging needs, evolving services: The health of Pacific peoples in New Zealand. *Kōtuitui: New Zealand Journal of Social Sciences Online, 3*, 21–33.

REFERENCES

Ahio, L. L. (2011). *Vaevae Manava: Context and perception of food security for Tongan mothers and health workers*. Unpublished master's thesis, Auckland University of Technology, Auckland, New Zealand.

Anae, M., Coxon, E., Mara, D., Wendt-Samu, T., & Finau, C. (2001). *Pasifika education guidelines*. Wellington: Ministry of Education.

AUT University (2010). Pacific Island families: Aim of the PIF study. Retrieved May 10, 2013 from http://www.aut.ac.nz/study-at-aut/study-areas/health-sciences/research/pacific-islands-families/aim-of-the-pif-study

Fairbairn-Dunlop, P. (2011). Me and the Pacifc Islands Family Study—where it is now *Pacific Health Dialogue, 17*(2), 210–211.

Finau, S. (2006). Cultural democracy: The way forward for hard to reach New Zealanders. *New Zealand Family Physician Journal, 33*(5), 313–318.

Gray, A. (2001). *Definition and measurement of ethnicity: A Pacific perspective*. Wellington: Statistics New Zealand.

Health Research Council of New Zealand. (2005). *Guidelines on Pacific health research* (3rd ed.). Wellington: Author.

Helu-Thaman, K. (1999). *A matter of life and death: Schooling and culture in Oceania.* Keynote address paper delivered at Innovations for Effective Schooling Conference, Auckland, New Zealand.

Kupa, K. (2009). Te Vaka Atafaga: A Tokelau assessment model for supporting holistic mental health practice with Tokelau people in Aotearoa, New Zealand. *Pacific Health Dialog, 15*(1), 156–163.

Mahina, O. (July, 1992). Towards a general ta-va, 'time-space' theory of nature, mind and society. Paper presented at the Tongan History Association Conference, Nuku'alofa, Tonga.

Manu'atu, L (2000). Pedagogical possibilities for Tongan students in New Zealand Secondary Schooling: Tuli ke ma'u nono ngaahi malie. Unpublished doctoral dissertation, University of Auckland, Auckland, New Zealand.

Maua-Hodges, T. (2000). *Ako Pai ki Aitutaki: transporting or weaving cultures: Research report of field experiences to the Cook Islands.* Wellington New Zealand: Wellington College of Education.

McIntyre, L. (2003). *Food security: More than a determinant of dealth. Policy Options, 24*(3), 46–51.

Ministry of Health. (2008). *A portrait of health. Key results of the 2006/07 New Zealand Health Survey.* Wellington: Author.

Ministry of Health. (2011). *Tagata Pasifika in New Zealand.* Retrieved January 30, 2013, from http://www.health.govt.nz

Ministry of Health. (2012). *Tupu ola Moui: Pacific health chart book 2012.* Wellington: Author.

Ministry of Health and Ministry of Pacific Island Affairs. (2010). *'Ala Mo'ui: Pathways to Pacific health and wellbeing 2010–2014.* Wellington: Ministry of Health.

Pulotu-Endemann, F. K. (2001). *Fonofale model of health.* Retrieved from htpp://www.hpforum.org.nz/resources/Fonofalemodelexplanation.pdf

Rush, E. (2009). *Food security for Pacific peoples in New Zealand. A report for the Obesity Action Coalition.* Wellington. Retrieved from http//:www.obesityaction.org.nz

Smith, L. T. (2004). Building research capability in the Pacific, for the Pacific and by Pacific peoples. In T. L. Baba, O. Mahina, N. Williams, & U. Nabobo-Baba. (Eds.). *Researching the Pacific and indigenous peoples: Issues and perspectives* (pp. 4–16). Auckland: Centre for Pacific Studies, University of Auckland, Auckland, New Zealand.

Statistics New Zealand and Ministry of Pacific Island Affairs (2011). *Health and Pacific peoples in New Zealand*. Wellington: Statistics New Zealand and Ministry of Pacific Island Affairs.

Tamasese, K., Peteru, C., Waldegrave, C., & Bush, A. (2005). *O le taeao afua*, the new morning: A qualitative investigation into Samoan perspectives on mental health and culturally appropriate services. *Australian and New Zealand Journal of Psychiatry, 39*, 300–309.

Tamasese Ta'isi Efi, T. A. T. (November, 2007). *Bio-ethics and the Samoan indigenous reference.* Keynote paper presented at the UNESCO 2007 Regional Pacific ethics of knowledge production workshop. Tofamamao Conference Centre, Leauvaa, Samoa.

Taufe'ulungaki, A. (2000) *The role of research: A Pacific perspective.* Paper presented at the Research Unit in Pacific and International Education (RUPE) Conference, University of Auckland, Auckland, New Zealand.

Tu'itahi, S. (2005). *Langa Fonua: In search of success. How a Tongan kainga strived to be socially and economically successful in New Zealand.* Auckland: Massey University.

Vaioleti, T. M. (2006). Talanoa research methodology: A developing position on Pacific research. *Waikato Journal of Education, 12*, 21–34.

WEBSITES

Pacific Health Dialog:
http://www.pacifichealthdialog.org.fj

Ministry of Health:
http://www.health.govt.nz

Pacific Islands Family Study:
http://www.aut.ac.nz/study-at-aut/study-areas/health-sciences/research/
pacific-islands-families/about-us

CHAPTER 8

ABORIGINAL AND TORRES STRAIT ISLANDER PEOPLES OF AUSTRALIA AND RESEARCH

RAY GATES

CHAPTER OVERVIEW

This chapter covers the following topics:

- A long history
- Historical influences on Aboriginal and Torres Strait Islander health research
- Developing a research relationship with communities
- Building capacity through research
- Linking research to outcomes

KEY TERMS

Best practice
Capacity-building
Community
Critical
Empowerment
Partnership

It is important to recognise that Aboriginal and Torres Strait Islander cultures are distinct from each other; they are separate cultures and that even within each culture there are unique subgroups, each with its own distinct language and cultural practices and beliefs. Failure to appreciate this can reinforce the impact that colonisation, assimilation and institutionalisation has had upon Aboriginal and Torres Strait Islander peoples (Taylor & Guerin, 2010).

For this reason, the term 'peoples' is used to acknowledge and respect the cultural differences between and within these cultures. When both cultures are referred to collectively this is as 'Aboriginal and Torres Strait Islander peoples', rather than 'indigenous'. The term 'non-indigenous' is used when referring to those peoples who are not of Aboriginal nor Torres Strait Islander descent.

A LONG HISTORY

The Aboriginal and Torres Strait Islander peoples of Australia represent two of the oldest living cultures in our world. Researchers now believe that Aboriginal peoples have lived on the mainland for over 60,000 years and in the Torres Strait Islands for over 10,000 years (Pascoe, 2008). The invasion and consequent colonisation of Australia approximately 225 years ago could therefore be considered a relatively recent occurrence, yet nothing else in the history of these peoples has had such a profound, and in many ways detrimental, impact on their lives.

With the health and well-being of Aboriginal and Torres Strait Islander peoples recognised as one of the worst of any population within a First World nation, the need for research has been critical not only in determining the extent of the issues that need to be addressed, but also in discovering appropriate, culturally safe and relevant ways to address them (NATSIHC, 2004). However, the volume of research that has been undertaken, particularly within the last 40 to 50 years, is grossly disproportionate to the number of outcomes that have been achieved in improving the health and well-being of Aboriginal and Torres Strait Islander peoples. This chapter will explore issues related to developing effective research relationships, capacity-building and knowledge exchange, when working with Aboriginal and Torres Strait Islander peoples.

Critical
Of significance or a deliberate attempt to bring about social change.

HISTORICAL INFLUENCES ON ABORIGINAL AND TORRES STRAIT ISLANDER HEALTH RESEARCH

Until recently, the majority of research conducted within Aboriginal and Torres Strait Islander health, or any other field for that matter, has primarily been conducted by non-indigenous researchers. For much of the colonised history of Australia, research was conducted *on*, as opposed to *with*, Aboriginal and Torres Strait Islander peoples. This was in part due to the policies of the day, aimed as dispossessing Aboriginal and Torres Strait Islander peoples of their lands, culture and basic human rights (Gower, 2012; Laycock, Walker, Harrison, & Brands, 2011). No consideration was given towards cultural or societal differences, and in the non-indigenous viewpoint none needed to be. Their ethnocentric view of the world did not allow for variances based on cultural background or belief, and consequently much of the early research on Aboriginal and Torres Strait Islander peoples was misunderstood, and in many cases misrepresented (Gower, 2012; Laycock et al., 2011).

In addition, little to no consideration was given to informing participating communities of the results and outcomes of research being conducted. Neither was there any apparent benefit to communities for participating in research: despite providing researchers with the knowledge and information they wanted, nothing ever changed in terms of improving outcomes for communities or community members (NATSIHC, 2004). As late as the 1990s Aboriginal and Torres Strait Islander health research was still criticised as being research for the sake of research, and there was evidence of resistance to allowing research of any kind to be conducted within communities. Numerous reports and strategies on Aboriginal and Torres Strait Islander health have called for the need to link research with community-determined outcomes (AIATSIS, 2012; Gower, 2012), and while this has been recognised as critical for future research, translating this into practice has been a slow process (de la Barra, Redman, & Eades, 2009; NATSIHC, 2004). This has led to a reluctance, and in some communities active resistance, towards engaging with researchers on relevant and important issues (Burchill, et al., 2011).

Community
A group of people with defined commonality. This may include geographical location, belief systems or any other social construct.

RESEARCH ALIVE 8.1
REFLECTIONS ON MEANINGFUL INDIGENOUS RESEARCH PARTICIPATION

A recent study used participatory action research to explore Aboriginal and Torres Strait Islander communities' responses to pandemic influenza in rural and remote areas of Australia (Kelly et al., 2012).

When asked about research with and for indigenous peoples, Kylie, a community researcher from New South Wales, explained:

> I used to think that research was bad and it's still considered a dirty word to many Aboriginal people. Too much research in the past was done 'on' Aboriginal people that didn't benefit people at all. Usually the only benefits went to the non-Aboriginal researchers and academics (Kelly et. al., 2012, p. 46).

The establishment in 2010 of the Lowitja Institute (http://www.lowitja.org.au/about-knowledge-exchange), Australia's National Institute for Aboriginal and Torres Strait Islander Health Research, represents the culmination of work conducted over the last two decades to address the issues that have been present within Aboriginal and Torres Strait Islander health research, and thereby facilitate improvements in the health and well-being of Aboriginal and Torres Strait Islander peoples (Stewart, Sanson-Fisher, Eades, & Mealing, 2010). Some key ways it achieves this is by ensuring that research:

- follows rigorous quality assurance and ethical standards;
- promotes a collaborative approach between communities, researchers, service providers and policy-makers;
- is driven by Aboriginal and Torres Strait Islander communities, and maximises their input and control over research projects; and
- has a directly measurable impact.

In doing this, it is believed that research will not just provide information but lead to real outcomes in improving Aboriginal and Torres Strait Islander health and well-being (Lowitja Institute, 2013).

DEVELOPING A RESEARCH RELATIONSHIP WITH COMMUNITIES

Given the impact of historical influences on Aboriginal and Torres Strait Islander peoples' perceptions and involvement with researchers, undertaking research in communities can present quite a challenge. It is not simply a matter of going in and collecting data: researchers need to be willing to develop relationships based on trust, respect and partnership with the communities and all other participants or relevant stakeholders they plan to engage with (Jamieson, et al., 2012). In many instances this will involve establishing new relationships between the researchers and stakeholders. It may also involve repairing a relationship that has been damaged by poor past practices (Laycock et al., 2011).

Partnership
Genuine and respectful relationship between people.

A key factor in establishing an effective research relationship with communities is the investment of time. Time is not always on the researcher's side, with schedules to adhere to and deadlines to meet. However, investing time into developing and maintaining the research relationship is critical to ensure a successful outcome for all involved. This is especially true where the community has had negative past experiences with researchers (Jamieson, et al., 2012). While this may have nothing to do with your project, any residual mistrust and wariness from these experiences presents significant barriers that still need to be overcome. Doing this effectively will require an investment of time, and the amount of time required will be influenced by:

- any past or existing relationships with the community and other participants or stakeholders;

- the level of cultural knowledge and understanding of the researchers, and their ability to apply that in a culturally sensitive and safe manner;
- any barriers to effective communication, which may include what each party's first language is, but also includes being able to use terminology and concepts that can be understood by all involved;
- the learning curves of all parties involved in the project in relation to new information, ideas, concepts and ways of working; and
- access to those who can facilitate the building of effective relationships between all concerned—for example, community leaders or cultural mentors.

CASE STUDY 8.1

'ABORIGINALISING' THE RESEARCH PROCESS

A multidisciplinary research team investigating a culturally appropriate model of care for urban Aboriginal peoples with diabetes identified the need to embrace an Aboriginal approach to the project to ensure culturally appropriate outcomes (Burchill, et. al., 2011). In the establishment phase, the team established a project reference group with Aboriginal and non-indigenous key stakeholders, including health service providers, government and non-government representatives, and Aboriginal community members, to seek advice on culturally appropriate and feasible methods of engagement, data collection, communication and translation of findings into best practice. The reference group met at regular intervals throughout the project to assist in an advisory capacity.

Best practice
An approach to practice that has been investigated and has been acknowledged as enabling optimum outcomes.

The team engaged two Aboriginal researchers to lead the project in the exploratory phase to conduct and facilitate focus groups and interviews. These researchers used their knowledge of community, cultural protocols, and the time required to build mutual trust with participants in order to 'hunt' for suitable candidates for the focus groups, then 'gather' the data from the focus group discussions.

While the team discovered this approach challenged conventional academic methods and the ethical protocols that had been previously approved for the study, they concluded that the efforts made in developing relationships during the exploratory phase of their study not only benefitted their study, but also assisted in the development of an appropriate care model for Aboriginal peoples with diabetes.

Another key factor is the development of a true partnership between the community, participants and stakeholders, and the researchers. Consideration needs to be given to understanding the power relationships between all involved parties, and determining what these relationships should look like. The relationship between the researchers, the community and any other relevant participants or stakeholders should have solid grounding in cultural safety. Cultural safety has been defined as:

> An environment which is safe for people: where there is no assault, challenge or denial of their identity, of who they are and what they need. It is about shared respect, shared meaning, shared knowledge and experience, of learning together with dignity, and truly listening. (Eckermann et al., 2010, p. 174)

Just being aware of cultural differences is insufficient; the principles of cultural safety need to be applied to empower Aboriginal and Torres Strait Islander peoples to determine for themselves what sort of research is most important, valid and useful for their communities (Wilson, Gates, Samuela, & Weblemoe, 2012).

In Aboriginal and Torres Strait Islander communities, the greatest chance of having a successful research relationship exists where there is a sense of collaboration towards achieving a mutually desirable outcome. In the context of cultural safety, the community should determine what the priority issues and expected outcomes will be, as they are the ones with this level of knowledge and understanding (AIATSIS, 2012; Jamieson, 2012). Researchers need to be aware of how their own objectives and priorities can influence their collaboration with communities, and take measures to ensure this is not biasing the planning or implementation of the research project (AIATSIS, 2012; Jamieson, 2012).

BUILDING CAPACITY THROUGH RESEARCH

The need for and importance of self-determination for Aboriginal and Torres Strait Islander peoples has been widely publicised, particularly in relation to achieving improved outcomes in health (NHMRC, 2010). To achieve this, the capacity of Aboriginal and Torres Strait Islander communities—that is, the resources, skills, structures and empowerment—to achieve a state of self-determination must be developed and strengthened.

Empowerment
Giving or receiving the power in a particular situation.

Engaging a significant opportunity for capacity-building within Aboriginal and Torres Strait Islander communities at individual, organisational and community levels lies at the ethical core of good research practice. Some ways in which this can be achieved include:

Capacity-building
The process of developing knowledge and skills within a group.

- developing new skills, through on-the-job opportunities or undertaking formal training or education;
- identifying specific needs, and strategies to meet these needs;
- establishing systems and resources to improve service delivery;
- creating opportunities for leadership development and leadership groups; and
- encouraging self-determination and self-empowerment.

RESEARCH ALIVE 8.2
STRENGTHENING COMMUNITY CAPACITY

A fundamental feature of the Kelly, et al., (2012) participatory action research project was employing and training members from the local Aboriginal and Torres Strait Islander communities as a way of strengthening research capacities within the community itself.

Kylie, one of the community researchers, said:

> To see changes that are sustainable and have long term benefits to more people, you need to change not just the grass roots stuff, but also systems and infrastructure. (Kelly, et al., 2012, p. 45)

In addition, there exist opportunities for researchers to build their own capacity as well. Engaging in research projects with Aboriginal and Torres Strait Islander communities presents opportunities for researchers to develop their own broad knowledge and skills in planning and implementing effective research projects, as well as enhance specific skills such as cultural safety. In fact, cultural safety is regularly identified as a potential area of improvement for non-indigenous researchers (Burchill, et. al., 2011; Gower, 2012).

CASE STUDY 8.2

'YARNING' AS A METHOD FOR COMMUNITY-BASED HEALTH RESEARCH WITH INDIGENOUS WOMEN

Walker, Fredericks, Mills and Anderson (2013) discuss *yarning* as a culturally appropriate way to prompt discussion with Indigenous women about health and wellness. They used this technique in place of more traditional, Western-based data collection strategies such as one-on-one interviews, explaining that 'yarning is a conversational process that involves the sharing of stories and the development of knowledge. It prioritises Indigenous ways of communicating, in that it is culturally prescribed, cooperative and respectful' (p. 1). When reading about studies of Indigenous populations, take note of the researchers' levels of cultural sensitivity. Attention to this, or a lack of it, may indicate study quality.

LINKING RESEARCH TO OUTCOMES

Research for the sake of research, particularly within the context of Aboriginal and Torres Strait Islander health, is no longer acceptable, nor tolerated. Today, research must not only seek to provide an answer to a question, but it also must make use of that answer to effect change. To facilitate this, the Lowitja Institute advocates the use of knowledge exchange. Knowledge exchange is defined as 'a two-way process between researchers and the users of research, in which research is used to change what is done (policy and planning) or how things are done (practice and systems)' (Lowitja Institute, 2012, 'About Knowledge Exchange,' para. 1).

The key concept is that the transfer of information moves beyond dissemination of research findings in order to effect sustainable change for the users of the research (Laycock et al., 2011). It is an interactive process that extends beyond the time frame of the project: ideally it should commence prior to the start of the project while research priorities are being established, and continue well after the project's findings have been reported. To work effectively, it requires adequate time and resources, and appropriate skill sets within the research team, and this needs to be taken into consideration as early as possible. In Australia, the Lowitja Institute provides advice and assistance to help researchers plan for appropriate and effective knowledge exchange as part of their research project, and more information can be obtained from their website.

CLINICAL REFLECTION 8.1: CONSIDERING NORMS

The interaction of culture and health is known to affect health outcomes. Adding research processes into this interaction greatly increases complexity, and it can be challenging to conduct research that respects and accommodates the culture of participants. In Case Study 8.2, the research of Walker et al. (2013), who used yarning to collect data from Indigenous women, was discussed. With this in mind, reflect on your own ethnicity, cultural and social background and related beliefs and values. What would a researcher have to consider about your culture and beliefs if they were collecting data about your health?

SUMMARY

Numerous historical factors have influenced the way research has been conducted with Aboriginal and Torres Strait Islander peoples, and the response of those peoples to being researched. To successfully work with Aboriginal and Torres Strait Islander peoples, researchers need to invest time in developing strong, trustworthy relationships with communities and other key stakeholders, identify opportunities for capacity-building within the community, and ensure that the research being conducted can be utilised to produce real outcomes for those who have participated. A key concept is the idea of knowledge exchange, where research can be used to change either what is done or how it is done.

REFLECTION POINTS

- Why do you think historical factors such as colonisation, forced discriminatory policies and institutionalisation, not to mention cultural and social biases, have all had an impact upon Aboriginal and Torres Strait Islander peoples' perceptions of research?
- What are your thoughts on why establishing effective relationships with Aboriginal and Torres Strait Islander peoples is critical in ensuring a successful research project?
- What might you include in research designs so the projects are most likely to be successful when approached from within a framework of cultural safety and a spirit of collaboration?
- What comes to mind when considering how research provides an opportunity for capacity-building for all parties involved in the project?
- Why do you think it is vital that research be linked to producing outcomes for the communities being investigated?

STUDY QUESTIONS

1 How does your cultural identity shape your opinions, attitudes and beliefs towards peoples from other cultures? How might this influence your approach towards conducting research within Aboriginal or Torres Strait Islander peoples?
2 Who could you approach for assistance in developing an effective research project involving Aboriginal or Torres Strait Islander peoples?
3 What factors should you consider prior to obtaining funding and/or ethical approval for a project involving Aboriginal or Torres Strait Islander peoples?
4 What can you do once the project has been completed to ensure your findings are used to achieve outcomes for the community you've worked with?

ADDITIONAL READING

Laycock, A., Walker, D., Harrison, N., & Brands, J. (2011). *Researching Indigenous health: A practical guide for researchers.* Melbourne: Lowitja Institute.

NHMRC. (2010). *The NHMRC Road Map II: A strategic framework for improving the health of Aboriginal and Torres Strait Islander people through research.* Canberra: Author.

REFERENCES

AIATSIS. (2012). *Guidelines for ethical research in Australian Indigenous studies 2012.* Canberra: Author.

Burchill, M., Lau, P., Pyett, P., Kelly, S., Waples-Crowe, P., & Liaw, S. (2011). Reflections on 'Aboriginalising' the research process: 'hunting and gathering' as a focus group methodology. *International Journal of Critical Indigenous Studies, 4*(2), 29–39.

de la Barra, S. L., Redman, S., & Eades, S. (2009). Health research policy: a case study of policy change in Aboriginal and Torres Strait Islander health research. *Australia and New Zealand Health Policy, 6*(2), 1–11.

Eckermann, A., Dowd, T., Chong, E., Nixon, L., Gray, R., & Johnson, S. (2010). *Binaŋ Goonj: Bridging cultures in Aboriginal health* (3rd ed.). Sydney: Elsevier Australia.

Gower, G. (2012). *Ethical research in Indigenous Australian contexts and its practical implementation.* Paper presented at the Innovative Research in a Changing and Challenging World Conference, Phuket, Thailand, 16–18 May 2012 (pp. 1–12). Retrieved January 24, 2013 from http://www.auamii.com/proceedings_ Phuket_2012/Gower.pdf

Jamieson, L. M., Paradies, Y. C., Eades, S., Chong, A., Maple-Brown, L. Morris, P., et al. (2012). Ten principles relevant to health research among Indigenous Australian populations. *Medical Journal of Australia, 197*(1), 16–18.

Kelly, J., Saggers, S., Taylor, K., Pearce, G., Massey, P., Bull, J., et al. (2012). 'Makes you proud to be black eh?': Reflections on meaningful Indigenous research participation. *International Journal for Equity in Health, 11*(1), 40–47.

Laycock, A., Walker, D., Harrison, N., & Brands, J. (2011). *Researching Indigenous health: A practical guide for researchers.* Melbourne: Lowitja Institute.

Lowitja Institute. (2012). *About knowledge exchange.* Melbourne, Australia: Author. Retrieved January 8, 2013, from www.lowitja.org.au/about-knowledge-exchange

Lowitja Institute. (2013). *Our dreaming.* Melbourne, Australia: Author. Retrieved January 8, 2013, from www.lowitja.org.au/our-dreaming

NATSIHC. (2004). *National strategic framework for Aboriginal and Torres Strait Islander Health: Context.* Canberra: Office for Aboriginal and Torres Strait Islander Health.

NHMRC. (2010). *The NHMRC Road Map II: A strategic framework for improving the health of Aboriginal and Torres Strait Islander people through research.* Canberra: Author.

Pascoe, B., with AIATSIS. (2008). The little red yellow black book: An introduction to Indigenous Australia. Canberra: Aboriginal Studies Press.

Stewart, J. M., Sanson-Fisher, R. W., Eades, S. J., & Mealing, N. M. (2010). Strategies for increasing high-quality intervention research in Aboriginal and Torres Strait Islander health: views of leading researchers. *Medical Journal of Australia*, *192*(10), 612–615.

Taylor, K., & Guerin, P. (2010). *Health care and Indigenous Australians: Cultural safety in practice*. Sydney: Palgrave MacMillan.

Walker, M., Fredericks, B., Mills, K., & Anderson, D. (2013). 'Yarning' as a method for community-based health research with Indigenous women: The Indigenous women's wellness research program. *Health Care for Women International*, 1–11.

Wilson, D., Gates, R., Samuela, J. S., & Weblemoe, T. (2012). Culture. In S. Shaw, A. Haxell, & T. Weblemoe (Eds.), *Communication across the lifespan* (pp. 157–172). Melbourne: Oxford University Press.

WEBSITES

Australian National Health and Medical Research Council: http://www.nhmrc.gov.au/your-health/indigenous-health

Australia's National Institute for Aboriginal and Torres Strait Islander Health Research: http://www.lowitja.org.au

CHAPTER 9

IMMIGRANT AND REFUGEE COMMUNITIES: DIVERSITY IN RESEARCH

SHOBA NAYAR

CHAPTER OVERVIEW

This chapter covers the following topics:

- Aotearoa New Zealand: an immigrant nation
- Engaging diverse communities
- Research agenda—who benefits?
- Establishing researcher competence

KEY TERMS

Cross-cultural research

Ethics

Protection

Reflexivity

Relationships

Aotearoa New Zealand is a nation comprised of over 120 diverse ethnic communities, spanning indigenous, New Zealand-born, immigrant and refugee populations. Such diversity demands a range of services, including settlement support and health initiatives, which offer appropriate, accessible and effective assistance for all New Zealanders. Underpinning service and policy development is the need for research that uncovers and understands the needs of the multiple ethnic communities within society. Issues of engagement, the research agenda, questions about who benefits and researcher competence are central concerns when embarking on research with immigrant and refugee populations.

AOTEAROA NEW ZEALAND: AN IMMIGRANT NATION

Aotearoa New Zealand's history as an immigrant nation dates back to around ACE 800 with the arrival of the Polynesian settlers (Liu, Wilson, McClure, & Higgins, 1999). Next came the European immigrants in the early 1800s with a significant influx after 1840 and then again post World War II. From around 1840, a small population of Asian settlers (primarily from India and China) also began arriving; although it was not until the 1990s that their numbers grew with immigrants from Hong Kong, Korea and Japan. In 2006, one in five of New Zealand's population were born overseas, including people from Asia (28.6%), the Pacific (15.5%), and Europe (7.7%) (Statistics New Zealand, 2012).

The concept of 'immigrant' encompasses a complex blend of voluntary immigrants and refugees. Aotearoa New Zealand has been accepting refugees since the end of World War II. Approximately 1,000 refugees arrive annually in the country primarily through the quota category, which focuses on high protection cases, women at risk and people living with medical diagnoses and disabilities, and the Refugee Family Support immigrant category (Te Pou, 2008). It is acknowledged that the needs of refugees, particularly in relation to mental health, differ from those of voluntary immigrants. Yet although the reasons for coming to New Zealand may be different, across the immigrant communities the geographical changes in environment combined with cultural, psychological and social factors may affect all immigrants' health and well-being (Pernice, 1994).

Protection
The act of looking after or taking care of.

The diversity of immigrants has resulted in the creation of categories, for research purposes, in an attempt to capture multiple voices—for example, 'Asian', or more recently the MELAA (Middle Eastern, Latin American and African) category. While construction of such categories acknowledges the rapid growth of these communities in New Zealand society, mixing such diverse groups often means individual community voices are lost and research findings are potentially open to misrepresentation and misinterpretation. Thus what might seem a simple solution can be fraught with complexity. It is impossible to address the diversity of ethnic communities in Aotearoa New Zealand and their particular needs in a research context. However, concepts of engaging participant communities, who set the research agenda and researcher competence are pertinent across all immigrant and refugee communities.

ENGAGING DIVERSE COMMUNITIES

Successful research with immigrant and refugee communities involves establishing a relationship, which requires both time and trust. Some communities, such as refugee populations, may be more vulnerable than others; hence building trust is an important consideration. For example, with qualitative research, interviews are a common method for data collection; however, some refugees, who may have been persecuted for voicing political, religious or ethnic affiliations, may not feel safe or comfortable sharing their experiences (Pernice, 1994). Thus, the researcher needs to proceed slowly, utilising both professional and personal means to build a trusting relationship.

Ethically, the researcher may need to make multiple visits to explain the research both to the individual and the wider community, listening to and answering all questions, and subsequently adapting the research to meet the community's needs, while still ensuring the integrity of the research. For example, in 2008 Refugee Services Aotearoa New Zealand received funding from the Lotteries Community Sector Research Grant Fund for a project titled 'Research into the resettlement experience and special needs of women-at-risk'. Consultation with the refugee communities revealed their preference for the term 'women as sole heads of households'; thus this was the term used when talking with the women and subsequently in the research report (DeSouza, 2011).

In addition to professional practice, researchers may find they build better relationships through the use of self-disclosure. As a researcher, being prepared to discuss personal motivations for engaging in the research and spending time with communities sharing food, and engaging in cultural events and other activities not directly associated with the research, is critical for establishing trustworthiness as a researcher.

Relationships
The similarities and connections between people or variables in any given situation.

RESEARCH ALIVE 9.1
ENGAGEMENT IN PRACTICE

The ageing population in Aotearoa New Zealand is rapidly growing in size and ethnic diversity. However, a preliminary review of literature provides very little evidence of elder immigrants' participation in, and contribution to, families and/or community. There are some studies seeking to explore elder New Zealanders' community participation, including Māori; however, no studies specifically address elders from Asian immigrant communities.

A current study is exploring how senior Indian, Korean and Chinese immigrants participate in, and contribute to, New Zealand civic society.

[continued next page]

SHOBA NAYAR

As part of this current study, the researchers met with leaders of each community on multiple occasions to discuss the purpose of the study and processes for data collection. On the second visit, the community leader of the Central Auckland Chinese Association invited the researchers to provide feedback to the choir who were rehearsing for a celebration marking 40 years of New Zealand–Chinese diplomatic relations. This request was unexpected and the added time had not been factored in when making the appointment. However, the researchers, sensing the importance of the request, provided feedback which was met with applause from the choir and community members. On subsequent visits to the venue the researchers were greeted with smiles and welcomed into the community activities.

This research was carried out by Associate Professor Valerie Wright-St.Clair and Dr Shoba Nayar from Auckland University of Technology (AUT). The project was funded by an AUT Faculty of Health and Environmental Sciences Contestable Grant.

Building relationships is more difficult when researchers and community members do not share the same spoken language. Undertaking research with diverse communities may, therefore, require the use of interpreters during engagement and the subsequent processes of data collection and data analysis. Involving a third party (such as an interpreter) adds another layer of complexity when engaging communities; thus it is imperative that researchers factor in additional time to develop a working and trusting relationship between all parties.

RESEARCH ALIVE 9.2
LANGUAGE BARRIERS

When Esteban Nunez, a leader in the Auckland Latin American community, was asked about how people's first language influences their potential engagement in research, he said:

> Researchers or workers engaging in refugee and migrant communities experience frustrations derived from the language barrier. Lack of communication, along with the lack of understanding of the culture, habits, background and particular situations that refugees and migrants face when adapting to New Zealand society, affects the relation between the client and researchers. (personal communication, November 17, 2012)

Engagement with communities needs to commence well ahead of applying for research grants or submitting ethics applications, which will require evidence of community consultation. However, given the complexities of communication and relationship building, which include 'cultural awareness, patience and respect towards clients, consent of refugees/migrants to disclose information, and confidentiality at all times' (Esteban Nunez, personal communication, November 17, 2012), undertaking research with immigrant and refugee communities is not a quick process nor one that will necessarily progress as initially planned. Furthermore, engaging with communities extends beyond the initial steps of commencing research. Engagement needs to be maintained throughout the research process and beyond, including dissemination of findings.

Ethics
Moral values that are identified by any group of people, such as health professionals.

RESEARCH AGENDA—WHO BENEFITS?

As indicated in the introduction, research is necessary for informing the development of services and social policy that can support the health and well-being of all refugee and immigrant communities residing in Aotearoa New Zealand. However, it is not enough merely to engage with the communities and build a trusting relationship. Indeed:

> Once the leaders have been approached, the researcher needs to acknowledge that he or she is requesting favours from the community and therefore is in no position to set the agenda as to how the research should proceed. This preliminary interaction is critical in that it provides the community leaders with the opportunity to evaluate the trustworthiness of the research and to determine whether the project is likely to benefit the community. (Pernice, 1994, p. 211)

There is the risk of immigrants, as minority communities in Aotearoa New Zealand, being 'over-researched' and 'under-informed'. This issue has been raised by many refugee communities who have noted that they have been the subjects of many research projects yet have received little benefit as a consequence of the knowledge not going back to the community. A key element of engaging with communities, therefore, is learning about what immigrants and refugees perceive as community issues. Determining the research agenda, as identified by the communities themselves, is necessary for developing research that will result in tangible outcomes, such as changes to the ways services are delivered, in order to enhance their health and well-being. This is particularly important in qualitative research, where community consultation is pivotal for members checking and ensuring that findings accurately reflect community issues. In as much as time is required for developing relationships with communities and uncovering their needs, issues around 'timing' the approach to discuss research ideas with communities may also be pertinent.

RESEARCH ALIVE 9.3
PRESENTING THE RESEARCH AGENDA

For two researchers at AUT University, the interest in exploring how senior Indian, Korean and Chinese immigrants participate in, and contribute to, civic society emerged from a desire to combine the researchers' interests in ageing well in New Zealand (gerontology research) and immigrant and refugee resettlement. A brief review of the literature revealed a gap in current knowledge. Acknowledging that the research would not proceed without the communities' support, the researchers met with community leaders to present the proposal which coincided with media reports of Winston Peters, a New Zealand politician, describing senior immigrants from Asia as a 'burden to society'. Indeed one participant noted, 'Winston Peters in New Zealand First [political party] was the previous Foreign Minister. He has spoken some comments ignoring and despising Asian people' (Korean senior immigrant). Thus responses from the communities to participate in the study were overwhelmingly positive and highlight how pivotal the timing of the research proposal can be in facilitating community engagement.

Ensuring the research agenda is driven by community needs is critical for determining who benefits and, as with the process of engagement, it is important that the community benefits are ongoing. Benefits may range from increased knowledge gained by new insights raised through the research, and skill development with community members being named investigators or becoming researcher assistants within the research team. Thus underpinning engagement and who benefits from the research is the principle of 'inclusion', which requires the researcher to be proactive in the planning and implementing of the research process.

ESTABLISHING RESEARCHER COMPETENCE

Cross-cultural research
Research that takes place across more than one cultural context.

Defining the characteristics of a successful cross-cultural researcher is as impossible as developing a standardised approach to undertaking research with immigrant and refugee communities. As with any research, a blend of professional competence and personal characteristics is necessary; however, researchers interested in cross-cultural research need to demonstrate a capacity to be (1) reflexive, (2) open-minded, and (3) adaptable.

Research with immigrant and refugee communities demands that researchers have self-awareness and an 'honesty' with themselves regarding preconceived assumptions and biases. Shacklock and Smyth (1998) noted that:

> The process of reflexivity is an attempt to identify, do something about, and acknowledge the limitations of the research: its location, its subjects, its process, its theoretical context, its data, its analysis ... being reflexive in doing research is part of being honest and ethically mature in research practice. (pp. 6–7)

Thus reflexivity necessitates a constant questioning of the research process and the assumptions and beliefs of the researchers themselves.

Reflexivity
The process of using learning from a reflective process to inform development.

RESEARCH ALIVE 9.4
BREAKING STEREOTYPES

During a conversation about community-focused research with and for refugee and immigrant communities, Esteban Nunez, a leader in the Auckland Latin American community, reflected:

> Concerning refugee cases, the most general mistake of researchers/social workers is to be judgmental. Stereotypes are used to describe refugee and migrant behaviours and reactions to the process of adaptation to the country. In the case of public institutions in charge of supporting [refugees and migrants], the expectations are focused on them to be settled in a short time; thereby the support tends to be likewise. (personal communication, November 17, 2012)

CASE STUDY 9.1

RESEARCH INTO THE EXPERIENCES OF SINGLE REFUGEE WOMEN WITH CHILDREN

In an Australian study (Lenette, Brough & Cox, 2013), researchers used observations and interviews to explore the experiences of single refugee women with children in building new lives in Australia. The research results highlight the social complexity of stress and resilience, and the challenges these women experienced in being viewed as outsiders.

[continued next page]

These women interacted within a complex array of gendered roles, expectations and judgements, which speak to both the vulnerabilities associated with being single women with children from refugee backgrounds as well as the strengths they draw from … Furthermore, the women's stories on resilience in everydayness challenge the ongoing tendency of 'othering' refugees from mainstream Australian community (Lenette et al., p. 649).

Othering is achieved by distancing and stigmatising those who are different. It reinforces mainstream notions of 'normality' and promotes judgmental assumptions (Lenette et al., 2013). The study and its findings, which are too complex to be explained here, give an insight into the multifaceted nature of the refugee experience. It is also a good example of how research can inform a health worker's understanding of clients' experiences and how they can tailor the support they provide.

Being open-minded and adaptable are two further attributes essential for researchers engaging with immigrant and refugee communities. Researchers need to be aware that their 'research lens'—for example, critical, feminist, humanist—may not suit every community. This awareness requires, where necessary, an ability to step outside of your natural way of working and change paradigms to one that will best meet the needs of the community. Thus researchers need to be mindful that research plans with immigrants and refugees are often open to being changed as the needs of the community present themselves.

It can be easy for researchers to form stereotypes about communities and overlook the diversity that exists between and within cultural groups. For instance, the Indian community in New Zealand is diverse in terms of religion (Christians, Hindus, Muslims, Sikhs), geographical location of origin (for example, North or South India and, more specifically, state and region: Goa, Punjab, Gujarat) and length of time in Aotearoa New Zealand (first, second and third generations exist) (Nayar, Hocking, & Giddings, 2012). Thus to assume all Indian immigrants in New Zealand have the same experiences, without accounting for the wider context, would not respect the diversity within the community and the richness the diversity would bring to the research findings.

RESEARCH ALIVE 9.5
TRUSTING, LEARNING AND ENGAGING

For the AUT University researchers exploring how senior members of the three largest immigrant communities participate in, and contribute to, Aotearoa New Zealand civic society, the research process has presented learning opportunities for cross-cultural engagement and conducting research outside of a Western paradigm that have challenged pre-conceived ideas. Such opportunities have included:

- anticipating the arrival of additional participants who had 'heard about the study' and decided to join in the meeting—extra consent forms became a necessity;
- trusting that participants were comfortable with having their stories overheard by members of the community who were not part of the focus group but came in to use the hall when and where the groups were being conducted (Indian focus groups). These learnings centred around ethical challenges in a Western context including issues of 'informed consent' which requires participants to be fully informed before engaging in the research and concepts of 'confidentiality' and 'anonymity';
- learning food and service etiquette, such as only filling teacups halfway, beverage preference (men enjoy energy drinks and women like juice), men expect to be served food by women and women serve each other (Korean focus group); and
- engaging participants in gender-appropriate environments, for instance entering the 'table tennis' room (men) or the 'dance/exercise' room (women) (Chinese focus group). Opportunities for cross-cultural engagement required an openness and flexibility on behalf of the researchers to change actions in the moment, thus minimising any offence that might arise out of cultural misunderstanding.

CASE STUDY 9.2

RESEARCH INFORMING CULTURALLY APPROPRIATE SERVICES

Developing Culturally Responsive Services for Working with Refugee Youth with Mental Health Concerns (Sobrun-Maharaj, Nayar, & Choummanivong, 2011)

Objective: To examine issues faced by refugee youth presenting to mental health services in New Zealand and inform service development. *Method:* This qualitative descriptive study involved two phases. Phase one consisted of nine focus group interviews: four involving 20 mental health and community professionals, and five groups with 20 refugee youths and their caregivers or parents. Phase two comprised 16 individual interviews with additional youth participants. The study was conducted in the greater Auckland region. All interviews were audio-recorded and transcribed verbatim for analysis. *Findings:* Thematic analysis revealed four key challenges for refugee youth accessing mental health services: (1) personal and cultural—refugee youth encounter challenges related to premigration trauma, postmigration and settlement challenges, discrimination, adolescent development, lack of confidence and dignity, and homesickness; (2) family—family situations are often complex, with the family's mental health beliefs and knowledge influencing the help-seeking behaviour of refugee youth; (3) social and economic—access issues include service operating times, lack of transport and waiting lists; and (4) service capability—services face challenges with managing interpreters' and support people's responses, and liaising with other agencies, as well as gaps in mental health professionals' cultural knowledge and skills.

Recommendations for Practice

Personal and cultural: for some refugees, premigration trauma may include physical and mental torture; therefore it is important to be mindful of physical 'space' and touch, which may be more harmful than therapeutic.

Family: with many refugee and immigrant communities, family expectations are equally important as those of the individual; hence it is necessary to consider community beliefs in the choice and implementation of interventions.

Social and economic: be adaptable when it comes to planning interventions. This may mean delivering services outside of the 'hospital' environment.

Service capability: develop multiethnic teams, including cultural support workers. Where this is not possible, develop a resource kit which includes names and numbers of local organisations and community leaders who can be contacted for additional information and advice. Undertake training to work effectively with interpreters. Where possible, use the same interpreter for consistency, building trust and the therapeutic relationship.

SUMMARY

A researcher engaging in research with immigrant and refugee communities is on a journey of self-discovery, underpinned by opportunities for cross-cultural engagement and the formation of new understandings. Although there are complex and sensitive issues surrounding research with immigrants and refugees, these need not be obstacles provided the central concerns of engagement, research agenda, community benefits and researcher competence are given due consideration. Thus when critiquing the methodological trustworthiness in articles reporting immigrant and refugee studies, it is important to consider the elements for cross-cultural research as outlined in this chapter in determining the rigour and sensitivity of the research.

REFLECTION POINTS

- Research with immigrant and refugee communities requires ongoing engagement and time—before, during and after the research.
- Being a competent cross-cultural researcher requires setting aside your own needs— the research agenda—and forefronting the community needs.
- Cross-cultural research is as much about discovering yourself—reflexivity—as it is about understanding the complexities of multiethnic communities.

STUDY QUESTIONS

1   What is your cultural world view? How might this differ from communities that you engage with as a researcher and practitioner?
2   What professional and personal attributes do you consider essential for working with refugees and immigrants? Why?
3   You have a research proposal that involves an immigrant or refugee community of which you are not a member. What steps would you take to implement your study?

ADDITIONAL READING

Birman, D. (2006). Ethical issues in research with immigrants and refugees. In J. E. Trimble, & C. B. Fisher, *The handbook of ethical research with ethnocultural populations and communities* (pp. 155–177). Thousand Oaks, CA: Sage Publications.

Liamputtong, P. (2010). *Performing qualitative cross-cultural research*. Cambridge: Cambridge University Press.

Temple, B., & Moran, R. (2011). *Doing research with refugees: Issues and guidelines*. Bristol: Policy Press.

REFERENCES

DeSouza, R. (2011). *Doing it for ourselves and our children: Refugee women on their own in New Zealand. A report prepared for Refugee Services Aotearoa New Zealand*. Auckland. Retrieved from http://www.refugeeservices.org.nz/__data/assets/pdf_file/0003/7437/Doing_It_for_Ourselves_and_our_children-_Refugee_women_31_Jan_2012x.pdf

Lenette, C., Brough, M., & Cox, L. (2013). Everyday resilience: Narratives of single refugee women with children. *Qualitative Social Work, 12*(5), 637–653.

Liu, J. H., Wilson, M. S., McClure, J., & Higgins, T. R. (1999). Social identity and the perception of history: Cultural representations of Aotearoa/New Zealand. *European Journal of Social Psychology, 29*(8), 1021–1047.

Nayar, S., Hocking, C., & Giddings, L. (2012). Using occupation to navigate cultural spaces: Indian immigrant women settling in New Zealand. *Journal of Occupational Science, 19*(1), 62–75.

Pernice, R. (1994). Methodological issues in research with refugees and immigrants. *Professional Psychology: Research and Practice, 25*(3), 207–213.

Shacklock, G., & Smyth, J. (1998). *Being reflexive in critical educational and social research*. London: Falmer.

Sobrun-Maharaj, A., Nayar S., & Choummanivong, C. (2011). *Developing culturally responsive services for working with refugee youth with mental health concerns*. Auckland, New Zealand: Te Pou. Retrieved from http://www.tepou.co.nz/library/tepou/developing-culturally-responsive-services-for-working-with-refugee-youth-with-mental-health-concerns

Statistics New Zealand. (2012). *QuickStats about culture and identity 2006 census*. Wellington: Author. Retrieved December 7, 2012, from http://www.stats.govt.nz/Census/2006CensusHomePage/QuickStats/quickstats-about-a-subject/culture-and-identity/birthplace-and-people-born-overseas.aspx

Te Pou. (2008). *Refugee and Migrant Mental Health and Addiction Research Agenda for New Zealand 2008–2012*. Auckland: Te Pou.

WEBSITES

Asian Health Chart Book (New Zealand Ministry of Health):
http://www.health.govt.nz/publication/asian-health-chart-book-2006

Primary mental health for refugee and migrant communities:
http://www.primarymentalhealth.org.nz/section/18431/refugee-and-migrant

Health needs assessment of Middle Eastern, Latin American and African people living in the Auckland region:
http://www.refugeehealth.govt.nz/resources/articles/MELAA%20Health%20Needs%20Assessment%202010.pdf

PART 3

UNDERTAKING RESEARCH

CHAPTER 10

RESEARCH QUESTIONS

GRACE WONG

CHAPTER OVERVIEW

This chapter covers the following topics:

- Origin and nature of research questions
- Qualitative research questions
- Quantitative research questions
- Other research questions
- Evaluating research questions

KEY TERMS

Meta-analysis
Participants
Phenomenology
Systematic review
Theory
Variables

Every research project aims to answer a question. Without a question there is no study. The research question is a succinct statement about the aim, goal, purpose, intent or objective of the research. It quickly identifies what, and who, a study is about. It also provides clues about the type of study reported because different research designs start with different questions. The research question can be found in the abstract of a study and again, in more detail, in the paragraph immediately before the methods section.

ORIGIN AND NATURE OF RESEARCH QUESTIONS

The seeds of research questions lie in human curiosity. Just as students choose topics to focus projects on, so researchers choose topics to investigate. Some research questions come from practitioners who want to improve their practice. Others come from agencies which want information about specific topics. Some come from researchers interested in social change. Some topics are not researchable. For example, research studies cannot explore people's experiences of life after death—only people's thoughts about them—qualitative research may illuminate a range of human experience and understandings such as how they understand their experiences and cultures within the context of their daily lives. Some qualitative research questions seek to generate theory from the data in the study. A theory is an explanation of a phenomenon.

Theory
An explanation of a phenomenon.

Qualitative researchers believe that knowledge is subjective and constantly created in interaction with others and the environment. They ask open questions about general areas of interest and sometimes refine them as they learn more about the topic from the research participants. Therefore the question that appears in the research article may differ from the original question the researcher posed. This is not a problem for the reader because everything, including the research question, in the published article reflects the final research question.

Participants
People who choose to take part in research.

The process of looking for research which measures different factors about a topic of interest, calculates their relationship to one another, or tests whether something works or not, will locate studies with quantitative research questions. Many quantitative studies ask questions which test theories.

Quantitative researchers create questions which reflect their assumption that knowledge is a concrete, fixed entity which exists independently, can be measured and studied objectively, and can be incrementally added to. They create their questions by finding knowledge gaps in the research literature about their topics. They typically ask closed questions and use statistics to analyse numerical data to answer their questions. The research questions and processes stay exactly as originally planned throughout the study.

QUALITATIVE RESEARCH QUESTIONS

Just as there are different genres of music, art and movies, there are different genres of qualitative research questions. These overarching genres are 'interpretive', 'radical' and 'postmodern' (Grant & Giddings, 2002). Interpretive qualitative research questions aim to understand phenomena within their unique contexts. They include questions in the following research traditions: qualitative descriptive, phenomenology, grounded theory, ethnography and narrative inquiry.

Phenomenology
The study of human experience and consciousness.

Radical questions focus on interpreting phenomena in a way that facilitates emancipation from oppression for a group of people. They include questions in the critical and feminist research traditions. Postmodern questions aim to deconstruct social and cultural discourses. Other names for the postmodern genre of research questions are 'poststructuralist' and 'deconstructivist'.

Table 10.1 explains the aims of qualitative research questions that reflect different research approaches and provides some examples. There are more examples in Case Study 10.2 about using sticks to clean teeth and Research Alive 10.2 about achieving a smoke-free New Zealand by 2025.

TABLE 10.1 QUALITATIVE RESEARCH QUESTIONS

GENRE	METHODOLOGY	AIM	QUESTION EXAMPLE
Interpretive	Qualitative descriptive	To create a *straightforward textual account* of the participants' experiences or an event	What do parents think are the advantages and disadvantages of having pets for their children?
	Phenomenology	To reveal and explain human meaning by constructing an evocative description of the nature and essence of *lived experience*	What is the experience of living with a disabled spouse?
	Grounded theory	To *generate theory* out of data to explain human *processes*	How do elite sports people prepare to compete in the week before the event?
	Ethnography	To understand human behaviour and institutions by providing insights into the *culture*, perspectives and practices of groups	What are the customs, beliefs and behaviours of first year student nurses at AUT University?

[continued next page]

GRACE WONG

TABLE 10.1   QUALITATIVE RESEARCH QUESTIONS [*continued*]

GENRE	METHODOLOGY	AIM	QUESTION EXAMPLE
	Narrative inquiry	To describe how individuals make sense of life experiences	What are patients' stories of living with chronic back pain?
Radical	Critical social theory	To understand human experience in order to *change* the *inequitable* state of affairs existing in the social world	What are the experiences of refugees when they encounter health professionals in New Zealand?
	Feminist	To understand women's experiences in order to challenge the patriarchal nature of human institutions and *emancipate women*	What are midwives' experiences of being interviewed by the media?
Postmodern	Poststructuralist Deconstructivist	To *deconstruct* the naturalness of categories of meaning produced by discourses and to produce new narratives of the social world	What discourses underlie the choice of complementary therapies to treat depression?

QUANTITATIVE RESEARCH QUESTIONS

There are three basic categories of quantitative research questions. They are 'descriptive', 'relational' and 'experimental'. There are examples in Table 10.2, Case Study 10.2 and Research Alive 10.2.

DESCRIPTIVE

Variables
A factor that can be controlled or changed in an experiment.

Descriptive questions quantify and describe variables. Variables are factors that have different values. Descriptive questions aim to find out 'how many?', 'how often?', 'how long?', 'where?', 'what?', 'when?' and so on. The answers explain how many subjects are affected, how badly they are affected and how long they are affected for. They describe their characteristics, such as their age, sex, ethnicity, income levels and where they live. They may describe the composition of an intervention, such as a drug.

RELATIONAL

The second category of quantitative question is relational. The aim is to investigate the relationship between two or more variables. The researcher establishes whether change in the first variable (the predictor or explanatory variable) is *associated with change* in the second variable (the outcome variable). If there is no significant statistical relationship between the variables, the theory about the relationship is not supported.

CASE STUDY 10.1

THE RELATIONSHIP BETWEEN QUALITY OF LIFE, FATIGUE AND ACTIVITY IN AUSTRALIANS WITH CHRONIC KIDNEY DISEASE: A LONGITUDINAL STUDY

Chronic kidney disease (CKD) is a complex chronic illness which has a severe and negative impact on an individuals' quality of life and their ability to participate in everyday activities. A common symptom is extreme fatigue related to anaemia; this is treated with a medication (erythropoietin stimulating agent). Bonner, Caltabiano and Berlund (2013) used a longitudinal repeated measures design to investigate the relationship between commencement of the new medication and reported quality of life, activity and fatigue among 28 people with CKD. Participants completed surveys about their quality of life, activities and fatigue severity at a baseline point before they started taking the new medication, and then at 3, 6 and 12 months.

An example of a research question for this study is: 'Does the introduction of a new medication (erythropoietin stimulating agent) make a significant difference to participants' reported quality of life, fatigue and activity survey scores at baseline, 3, 6 and 12 months?' The researcher is looking for the impact of the new medication (the variable being tested) over 12 months on the experiences of the people with kidney disease (with several outcome variables—quality of life, activity and fatigue).

EXPERIMENTAL

The third category of quantitative research question is experimental. The aim of these research questions is to establish cause and effect by testing whether changing one variable (the independent variable) *causes a change* in the second variable (the dependent variable).

Experimental studies differ from non-experimental studies. In experimental studies the researcher actively manipulates (changes) the independent variable and measures the change in the dependent variable. In non-experimental studies the researchers cannot change the predictor or explanatory variable themselves for ethical or practical reasons. Any variation has happened already. It may be naturally occurring. For example, it is unethical to run a study which tests an experimental research question asking if people who smoke are more likely to get lung cancer than those who do not smoke. This is because subjects would be assigned either to a group which is directed to smoke or to a control group which would not smoke. It is unethical to put people at risk.

GRACE WONG

TABLE 10.2 QUANTITATIVE RESEARCH QUESTIONS

	QUESTION	SAMPLE	VARIABLES	HYPOTHESIS
Descriptive	What is the annual incidence of dog bite injuries among children in Auckland?	Children	Dog bite injuries	Not applicable
Relational	Is footwear associated with falling among residents in rest homes?	Residents in rest homes	Predictor variable—type of footwear Outcome variable—number of falls	There is a relationship between the type of footwear residents in rest homes wear and the number of times they fall.
Experimental	Does adding mobile phone reminders to an online exercise programme increase the amount that tertiary students exercise compared with an online exercise only programme?	Tertiary students	Independent variable—type of exercise programme Dependent variable—amount of exercise	Students on an online exercise programme who receive mobile phone reminders exercise longer than students on an online exercise programme who do not receive mobile phone reminders.

OTHER RESEARCH QUESTIONS

MIXED METHODS

Mixed methods research questions have qualitative and quantitative elements. Sometimes a single question encompasses both the quantitative and qualitative elements of the inquiry. Sometimes there are two separate questions: one that is qualitative and one that is quantitative. Sometimes the second question arises out of the answers to the first question.

RESEARCH ALIVE 10.1
WHY AREN'T YOU ON FACEBOOK?: PATTERNS AND EXPERIENCES OF USING THE INTERNET AMONG YOUNG PEOPLE WITH PHYSICAL DISABILITIES

Researchers (Raghavendra, Wood, Newman & Lawry, 2012) wanted to investigate if young people with disabilities were using internet-based social media in a similar way to young people without disability and to explore the young peoples' experience of this.

Quantitative descriptive question: 'What is the frequency, location, site type and length of internet access study participants do per week?' To answer this question the researchers collected data on how frequently participants used the internet per day, what device and location were used, the type of internet sites visited (social media, games, instant messaging) and for how long, as well as the total time in hours per week each person was online.

Qualitative question: 'What are young people with disabilities' perceptions, views and experiences of using the internet?' To answer this question the researchers interviewed 15 participants aged 11–18 years who had physical disabilities and asked about their experiences of using the internet and about their social media interactions.

KAUPAPA MĀORI RESEARCH QUESTIONS

The content of kaupapa Māori research questions reflects a Māori world view. Such questions can be qualitative and/or quantitative.

SYSTEMATIC REVIEW AND META-ANALYTIC RESEARCH QUESTIONS

Sometimes the question for which an answer is being sought is the same as the question in a systematic review or meta-analysis of many studies about the same topic. In this case the research question reflects the relevant questions in all of the studies. A systematic review question is usually quantitative. A meta-analytical question is always quantitative.

Systematic review
A specific process for analysing similar studies for the purpose of informing practice and practitioners.

Meta-analysis
The process of undertaking a quantitative analysis of similar research studies.

> ### CASE STUDY 10.2
>
> ### KEEPING YOUR TEETH CLEAN WHEN YOU FORGET YOUR TOOTHBRUSH
>
> In 2009 I went to India and saw little bundles of twigs for sale. The tour guide, Baddam, said that people use them to brush their teeth. He himself picked neem tree twigs to clean his teeth. He showed me a neem tree. I thought how handy it would be if I could pick a bit of shrub or tree to clean my teeth when I forgot my toothbrush. So I made 'cleaning teeth with sticks' a case study for this chapter about research questions.
>
> *[continued next page]*

I looked for relevant studies in the research database, Scopus. I used the search terms 'cleaning teeth' and 'sticks'. There were 53 results. After eliminating the 'commentaries', the non-English language studies and the off-topic studies, I categorised the studies by type of research question. This was not straightforward because some of the studies had more than one kind of question. I chose four studies. I analysed the questions so you can see what you can learn about the studies from their research questions. Finally I commented on the studies' results.

Study 1: A Qualitative Descriptive Research Question

Objective: 'The purpose of this study was to document the beliefs and perceptions and emerging oral health-care practices in parts of Nigeria' (Oke, Bankole, Denloye, Danfillo, & Enwonwu, 2011).

Comment: The abstract and methods show that this is a qualitative study. Both chewing sticks and toothbrushes are used in Nigeria.

Study 2: A Mixed Methods Research Question (Qualitative and Quantitative)

Aim: 'To describe traditional chewing-stick practices in a Ugandan rural community, and evaluate the antibacterial activity of the most commonly used plants' (Odongo, Musisi, Waako, & Obua, 2011).

Comment: The abstract and methods show that this is a mixed methods study. The qualitative component identifies plants people use to clean their teeth with. The quantitative part is experimental and shows that two plants have teeth-cleaning ingredients.

Study 3: A Relational Quantitative Research Question

Objectives: 'To measure the changing pattern of dental caries, periodontal health status and tooth cleaning behaviour among a cohort of Ethiopian immigrants to Israel between the years 1999–2005' (Vered, Zini, Livny, Mann, & Sgan-Cohen, 2008).

Comment: A group of people's dental health and practices are tracked over in time. The use of chewing sticks declines and dental health deteriorates when people migrate to a Westernised country. The non-experimental nature of the study means that the researchers cannot claim that changing from chewing sticks to toothbrushes causes poorer dental health.

Study 4: An Experimental Quantitative Research Question

Objectives: 'To compare the effects of the chewing stick miswak (from *S[alvadora] persica*) and toothbrush on subgingival plaque microflora among Saudi Arabian individuals. Further, to investigate whether components extracted from S. persica may interfere with the subgingival plaque micro-organisms' (Al-Otaibi et al., 2004).

Comment: The first research question was answered using a quantitative experimental design. The chewing sticks were as good as the toothbrushes (no toothpaste) in terms of reducing the levels of below-the-gum microflora.

Overall Comments

I found some interesting information in the studies above, but there are unanswered questions among the papers I located. One of them is whether or not there are New Zealand plants that I could use to clean my teeth effectively. Another is a rigorous systematic review to demonstrate conclusively how effective chewing sticks are. In conclusion, although commonly used chewing sticks may be effective, I cannot yet pick one to clean my teeth when I forget my toothbrush in Aotearoa New Zealand.

HYPOTHESES

An hypothesis is a special style of quantitative research question (see Table 10.2). It predicts a relationship between two or more variables. It is created out of the study question. Hypotheses are used to statistically test the relationship between variables in both non-experimental (relational) and experimental studies.

RESEARCH ALIVE 10.2

HOW CAN YOU HELP MAKE AOTEAROA NEW ZEALAND SMOKE-FREE BY 2025?

This section shows how research questions lead to studies which contribute to the evidence base for delivering brief smoking cessation interventions in your daily practice as a health professional.

[continued next page]

BACKGROUND

The New Zealand government is committed to a goal of a smoke-free Aotearoa/ New Zealand by 2025 (New Zealand Government, 2011). The aim is a tobacco smoking prevalence rate of 5 per cent. As the current smoking rate is 17 per cent currently, at least 400,000 smokers need to quit (Ministry of Health, 2012). No one should start smoking. One important strategy for increasing the quit rate is for all health professionals to trigger supported quitting attempts among their clients/patients who smoke (Ministry of Health, 2011).

TABLE 10.3   APPROPRIATE RESEARCH QUESTIONS

TOPIC AREA	EXAMPLE OF RESEARCH QUESTION	TYPE OF QUESTION (IN EXAMPLE)
Significance of the issue		
Establishing harm	What is the mortality of doctors in relation to their smoking habits? (Doll, Peto, Boreham, & Sutherland, 2004)	Quantitative—relational
The size of the problem	How many people are current smokers in New Zealand? (Ministry of Health, 2010)	Quantitative—descriptive
Contribution to health inequalities	Is smoking associated with gender, age, ethnicity and neighbourhood deprivation? (Ministry of Health, 2010)	Quantitative—relational
Why people smoke		
The addictive nature of tobacco	Does nicotine renal excretion rate influence nicotine intake during cigarette smoking? (Benowitz & Jacob, 1985)	Quantitative—experimental
Why individuals smoke	What is the meaning of nicotine addiction among teenage girls? (Moffat & Johnson, 2001)	Qualitative—Narrative inquiry
Addressing the issue		
Benefits of quitting	What is the relationship between continuing-to-smoke versus quitting smoking with the subsequent risk of lung cancer? (Peto et al., 2000)	Quantitative—relational
Desire to quit	How many smokers have tried to quit in the past five years? (Ministry of Health 2010)	Quantitative—descriptive

TOPIC AREA	EXAMPLE OF RESEARCH QUESTION	TYPE OF QUESTION (IN EXAMPLE)
Support to quit Meaning/process of quitting smoking for individuals	Does a combination of smoking cessation medication and behavioural support help smokers to stop? (Stead & Lancaster, 2012)	Quantitative—experimental (systematic review)
	What are Māori women's views on smoking cessation initiatives? (Fernandez & Wilson, 2008)	Qualitative—Kaupapa Maori
*Health professionals' practice**		
Effectiveness of interventions by health professionals	What is the effectiveness of interventions for tobacco cessation delivered by oral health professionals? (Carr & Ebbert, 2012)	Quantitative—experimental (systematic review)
Smokers' perceptions of help from health professionals	What are midwives' perceptions of providing stop-smoking advice and pregnant smokers' perceptions of stop-smoking services? (Herberts & Sykes, 2012)	Qualitative
Health professionals who smoke	How do nurses who smoke manage the contradictions they encounter when caring for tobacco-dependent patients? (Radsma & Bottorff, 2009)	Qualitative—grounded theory

The New Zealand Smoking Cessation Guidelines for health professionals are based on a comprehensive literature review (Ministry of Health, 2007, 2008).

EVALUATING RESEARCH QUESTIONS

Research questions can be evaluated by asking the following questions:

- Is the topic researchable?
- Is there a sound reason for asking the research question?
- Does the question logically arise from the literature review (quantitative studies)?
- Is the research question clearly written? Can you understand it?

Other points of interest are:

- Are the study approach and methods congruent with the study question?
- Do the study findings and discussion address the research question as it is expressed in the abstract and before the methods?

SUMMARY

The research question expresses the intent of the inquiry and dictates the study design. Research questions can be qualitative or quantitative. Qualitative research questions aim to analyse aspects of being human in the context of everyday living. Quantitative research questions aim to quantify phenomena and, where relevant, to attribute cause and effect.

REFLECTION POINTS

- Why is understanding research questions a good start to comprehending research articles?
- Explain in your own words how research questions can be sequenced to track the development of evidence which underpins practice.

STUDY QUESTIONS

1   Where can you find the research questions written in a journal article?
2   What are the differences between qualitative and quantitative research questions?
3   What kind of research questions do you look for when you want to find out if a treatment or practice is effective or not?

ADDITIONAL READING

Bryman, A. (2012). *Social Research Methods*. Oxford: Oxford University Press.

REFERENCES

Al-Otaibi, M., Al-Harthy, M., Gustafsson, A., Johansson, A., Claesson, R., & Angmar-Mansson, B. (2004). Subgingival plaque microbiota in Saudi Arabians after use of miswak chewing stick and toothbrush. *Journal of Clinical Periodontology, 31*(12), 1048–1053.

Benowitz, N. L., & Jacob, P., 3rd. (1985). Nicotine renal excretion rate influences nicotine intake during cigarette smoking. *Journal of Pharmacology and Experimental Therapeutics, 234*(1), 153–155.

Bonner, A., Caltabiano, M., & Berlund, L. (2013). Quality of life, fatigue and activity in Australians with chronic kidney disease: A longitudinal study. *Nursing and Health Sciences, 15*(3), 360–367.

Carr, A. B., & Ebbert, J. (2012). Interventions for tobacco cessation in the dental setting. *Cochrane Database Syst Rev, 6*, CD005084.

Doll, R., Peto, R., Boreham, J., & Sutherland, I. (2004). Mortality in relation to smoking: 50 years' observations on male British doctors. *British Medical Journal, 328*(7455), 1519.

Fernandez, C., & Wilson, D. (2008). Maori women's views on smoking cessation initiatives. *Nursing Praxis in New Zealand, 24*(2), 27–40.

Grant, B. M., & Giddings, L. S. (2002). Making sense of methodologies: a paradigm framework for the novice researcher. *Contemporary Nurse, 13*(1), 10–28.

Herberts, C., & Sykes, C. (2012). Midwives' perceptions of providing stop-smoking advice and pregnant smokers' perceptions of stop-smoking services within the same deprived area of London. *Journal of Midwifery Womens Health, 57*(1), 67–73.

Ministry of Health. (2007). *New Zealand smoking cessation guidelines.* Wellington: Author. Retrieved from http://www.nzgg.org.nz/guidelines/0148/nz_smoking_cessation_guidelines.pdf

Ministry of Health. (2008). *Literature review for the revision of the New Zealand smoking cessation guidelines.* Retrieved June 2008, from http://www.moh.govt.nz/moh.nsf/indexmh/literature-review-for-the-revision-of-the-nz-smoking-cessation-guidelines

Ministry of Health. (2010). *Tobacco use in New Zealand: Key findings from the 2009 New Zealand Tobacco Use Survey.* Wellington: Author.

Ministry of Health. (2011). *Health targets 2012/13: Better help for smokers to quit.* Retrieved from http://www.health.govt.nz/new-zealand-health-system/health-targets/2012-13-health-targets/health-targets-2012-13-better-help-smokers-quit

Ministry of Health. (2012). *Annual report for the year ended 30 June 2012 including the Director-General of Health's annual report on the state of public health.* Wellington: Author.

Moffat, B. M., & Johnson, J. L. (2001). Through the haze of cigarettes: teenage girls' stories about cigarette addiction. *Qualitative Health Research, 11*(5), 668–681.

New Zealand Government. (2011). *Government response to the report of the Māori Affairs Committee on its inquiry into the tobacco industry in Aotearoa and the consequences of tobacco use for Māori (final response).* Retrieved from http://www.parliament.nz/NR/rdonlyres/3AAA09C2-AD68-4253-85AE-BCE90128C1A0/188520/DBHOH_PAP_21175_GovernmentFinalResponsetoReportoft.pdf.

Odongo, C. O., Musisi, N. L., Waako, P., & Obua, C. (2011). Chewing-stick practices using plants with anti-streptococcal activity in a Ugandan rural community. *Frontiers in Pharmacology, 2,* 13.

Oke, G. A., Bankole, O. O., Denloye, O. O., Danfillo, I. S., & Enwonwu, C. O. (2011). Traditional and emerging oral health practices in parts of Nigeria. *Odonto-stomatologie tropicale (Tropical Dental Journal)*, *34*(136), 35–46.

Peto, R., Darby, S., Deo, H., Silcocks, P., Whitley, E., & Doll, R. (2000). Smoking, smoking cessation, and lung cancer in the UK since 1950: combination of national statistics with two case-control studies. *British Medical Journal*, *321*(7257), 323–329.

Radsma, J., & Bottorff, J. L. (2009). Counteracting ambivalence: nurses who smoke and their health promotion role with patients who smoke. *Research in Nursing & Health*, *32*(4), 443–452.

Raghavendra, P., Wood, D., Newman, L., & Lawry, J. (2012). Why aren't you on Facebook?: Patterns and experiences of using the internet among young people with physical disabilities. *Technology and Disability*, *24*, 149–162.

Stead, L. F., & Lancaster, T. (2012). Combined pharmacotherapy and behavioural interventions for smoking cessation. *Cochrane Database Syst Rev*, *10*, CD008286.

Vered, Y., Zini, A., Livny, A., Mann, J., & Sgan-Cohen, H. D. (2008). Changing dental caries and periodontal disease patterns among a cohort of Ethiopian immigrants to Israel: 1999–2005. *BMC Public Health*, *8*, 345.

WEBSITES

Hints on how to develop a research question:
http://www8.esc.edu/htmlpages/writerold/menus.htm

Resources for behavioural science researchers:
http://theresearchassistant.com/tutorial/2-1.asp

CHAPTER 11

DEVELOPING A PROPOSAL

NICOLA KAYES AND ALICE THEADOM

CHAPTER OVERVIEW

This chapter covers the following topics:

- Getting started
- Writing the proposal
- Next steps

KEY TERMS

Data	Purpose
Design	Research proposal
Guidelines	Sampling
Interviews	Treatment
Limitations	Writing
Methods	

A considerable amount of time can be spent learning about the why, when and how of different methodological approaches, the many and varied analytical strategies, and associated issues of scientific reliability, validity, rigour and credibility. While these are clearly fundamental issues, applying that knowledge to the acquisition of new knowledge in any given field requires another set of skills. It requires being able to ask a clearly focused question that can be answered in a scientifically robust way, within the financial and logistical constraints of the real world. Central to this process is the development of a research proposal.

So, what is a research proposal? For many students, a research proposal will simply be that dreaded assignment required for a compulsory research paper or to gain approval for proposed postgraduate research. In many cases, it is the one opportunity to sell an idea to a funder—the very people who hold the future of a research project in their hands. In this sense, a research proposal may be equated with a sales pitch. Put simply, though, a research proposal 'follows a set of sequential steps that provide structure to the prospective study. It is a written submission which spells out the design of the intended project' (Hollins Martin & Fleming, 2010, p. 791). A well-constructed, detailed research proposal is the ultimate application of research skills and knowledge. Bradley (2001) aptly suggests that 'developing good research ideas is both a science and an art' (p. 569).

GETTING STARTED

Before starting to write a research proposal, there are a number of things to consider. As a starting point there are four key questions to ask:

1   Does this identify a clear research gap?
2   Is there a clearly focused research question?
3   What is the purpose of this proposal?
4   Who are the intended audience of this proposal?

If the first two questions cannot be answered affirmatively there is work to do because these questions form the foundation on which any proposal should be built. One of the key roles of a research proposal is to clearly articulate the state of knowledge with regard to the topic area, identify the limitations of this (in terms of scope, purpose and methodological approach), and highlight the research gap that the proposed research aims to address (Bordage & Dawson, 2003; Hollins Martin & Fleming, 2010; Inouye & Fiellin, 2005; Jonker & Marshall, 2010; Verhoef & Hilsden, 2004). This provides the scientific rationale for the work and helps the reader to get a sense of why this work is worth pursuing and why now. Familiarity with the relevant literature is imperative to the development of a proposal.

Perhaps even more crucial is the development of a clearly focused research question (Bordage & Dawson, 2003). This has already been addressed in detail in Chapter 10 but warrants mention here given its fundamental importance in the context of developing a research proposal. The downfall of many research proposals is a lack of clarity and

Research proposal
A document that outlines the intention and design of a study.

Design
The process of planning and creating a solution to a problem.

Purpose
The intended outcome, reason or goal.

Limitations
Restrictions on applicability or consequences.

detail (see Case Study 11.1) with such proposals described as 'nebulous' and 'diffuse' (Inouye & Fiellin, 2005; Landsberger, 2011; Verhoef & Hilsden, 2004). More often than not, this issue stems from the lack of a clearly focused research question on which to hang the proposal. The research question provides a central point to keep coming back to while developing the proposal, to keep it focused. Internal consistency, or 'fit' between the research question and proposed design and methods, is an important component of a well-developed research proposal (Klopper, 2008). On the surface, developing a clear research question seems like a very simple thing to do. In reality, it is frequently identified as one of the most difficult parts of the research process.

The remaining two questions related to getting started ('what is the purpose of this proposal?' and 'who is the audience?') are to do with targeting the proposal and ensuring it is fit for the purpose. Depending on the purpose of the proposal (for example, for an assignment or to seek approval for funding) the target audience will differ. The proposal may be being reviewed by a lecturer or university board, non-government organisation, ethics committee or government funding body. There is always a need to tailor the approach in terms of both the emphasis and the language adopted. Clayton (1982) referred to this as 'pitching to the catcher' (p. 629). Table 11.1 gives an example of how the emphasis and language might change in each of these cases. If there are guidelines available (for example, many universities and research funders set out clear standards for what they expect to be covered in a research proposal) it is important to become familiar with the guidelines and ensure they are followed. In many instances, failing to adhere to guidelines (such as those for presentation, format, word count and page limits) may mean the proposal simply gets discarded before it has even been read or, worse, a fail grade is awarded for the assessment.

Methods
Systematic procedures for undertaking an inquiry.

Guidelines
Information providing advice on how to interpret policy or procedure.

TABLE 11.1 COMPARISON OF WRITING STYLES FOR DIFFERENT AUDIENCES

PURPOSE	EMPHASIS	LANGUAGE
Assignment	Meeting learning outcomes of the paper	Formal academic writing
Thesis proposal	Demonstrating potential of research to meet graduate profile of the qualification	Formal academic writing
	Feasibility of completion within enrolment timeframes	
Funding	Targeting investment priorities	Formal academic style using lay language
	Demonstrating capacity of the research team to deliver on the project	
Pitch an idea	Fit with organisation strategic plan and ethos	Lay language
Ethics	Key ethical considerations pertinent to the proposed research	Responding to specific queries via closed and open ended questions

NICOLA KAYES AND ALICE THEADOM

In summary, a good research proposal requires careful preparation and planning. While it can be tempting to hurry and get the proposal written, knowing the topic, being able to articulate a clearly focused research question, and becoming familiar with the target audience and their expectations are important first steps. Spending time on these key things at the outset will enhance the finished product.

RESEARCH ALIVE 11.1
CREATING A MIND MAP

There are a number of tools and strategies you can draw on to firm up your ideas in the early phases, such as preparing a one-page overview of your initial thoughts, having a brainstorming session with peers, or using a 'mind map'. The following mind map is an example prepared through the development of a qualitative project seeking to explore the perspectives of people living with multiple sclerosis (MS) to identify things that help or hinder their engagement in physical activity. Some key aspects of this mind map worth orienting to are:

a   The research question sits at the centre of the map—it is crucial that all components of the project have 'fit' with the research question;

b   The content of the map is concerned with advancing thinking beyond the 'what' to the 'how' and the 'why'—this is central to demonstrating *how* you might put your research idea into action; and

c   Viewing the research project in this way allows for a closer examination of the core components of the proposed research to identify gaps, possible issues and any limitations that may be inherent in the design—this allows for consideration of how one might overcome identified issues OR to acknowledge that as a limitation of the proposed work. Mind mapping is also a good time-saving device—there is nothing worse than writing a whole proposal and then realising that a different approach is needed to overcome an issue later on.

WRITING THE PROPOSAL

Research proposals are commonly structured using sections as outlined below. Depending on the area of interest and discipline, different subheadings can be used; however, the same information is inherently required. To help address this diversity the most commonly used section headings are included below, along with a description and key things to think about for each section.

FIGURE 11.1 MIND MAP OF PART OF THE THINKING PROCESS FOR
DEVELOPING A PROPOSAL

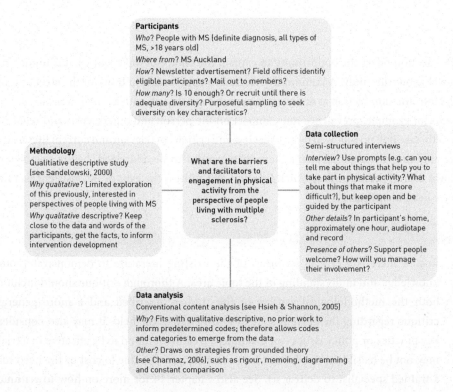

Participants

Who? People with MS (definite diagnosis, all types of MS, >18 years old)

Where from? MS Auckland

How? Newsletter advertisement? Field officers identify eligible participants? Mail out to members?

How many? Is 10 enough? Or recruit until there is adequate diversity? Purposeful sampling to seek diversity on key characteristics?

Methodology

Qualitiative descriptive study (see Sandelowski, 2000)

Why qualitative? Limited exploration of this previously, interested in perspectives of people living with MS

Why qualitative descriptive? Keep close to the data and words of the participants, get the facts, to inform intervention development

What are the barriers and facilitators to engagement in physical activity from the perspective of people living with multiple sclerosis?

Data collection

Semi-structured interviews

Interview? Use prompts (e.g. can you tell me about things that help you to take part in physical activity? What about things that make it more difficult?), but keep open and be guided by the participant

Other details? In participant's home, approximately one hour, audiotape and record

Presence of others? Support people welcome? How will you manage their involvement?

Data analysis

Conventional content analysis (see Hsieh & Shannon, 2005)

Why? Fits with qualitative descriptive, no prior work to inform predetermined codes; therefore allows codes and categories to emerge from the data

Other? Draws on strategies from grounded theory (see Charmaz, 2006), such as rigour, memoing, diagramming and constant comparison

ABSTRACT

In the structure of a research proposal this section almost always comes first, despite the fact that it is usually best if this is the last section to be written. The purpose of the abstract, often fewer than 300 words, is to provide a summary of the proposal. During the process of writing a proposal the details and logistics of carrying out the project become clearer therefore it can be helpful to write or revisit this section at the end of the writing process. This section will determine if people decide to read the whole proposal so it is important to be clear, concise and persuasive so that people want to read more.

Writing
The process of developing a written piece of work.

Some agencies or disciplines prefer structured abstracts where there are set subheadings (background, methods, results and conclusions) while others prefer one single paragraph without subheadings. Either way, the content required is the same. The key elements to get across are:

• What are the aims/objectives of the research?

• Why is this research question important?

- How will the question be answered (both methods and analysis)?
- What is the possible impact of any findings?

INTRODUCTION OR BACKGROUND

This section offers the opportunity to explain the choice of topic and what is unique or novel about the study. A commonly referred to approach is to think of the structure of the introduction section as an inverted pyramid starting off with a broad overview of the area (for example, prevalence rates, impact on the person and others, costs and relevant health-care policy) followed by an overview and critique of relevant and current literature, highlighting any gaps or inconsistencies that need to be addressed, before narrowing down to the specific project which (ideally) will address the gaps or inconsistencies that have been identified.

KEY POINTS OF THE INTRODUCTION OR BACKGROUND

- Ensure there is a critical synthesis of the existing literature to demonstrate your knowledge and understanding of the topic area. A thorough critique should include both the methodological aspects of the studies described and a more general critique regarding the current state of knowledge in the field. It may also consider key practice or policy issues (for example, a treatment found to be effective in a trial may not be feasible to implement into everyday practice due to cost or the need for a trained specialist to deliver it). See also Chapter 14 for more on how to critique research.
- Highlight any gaps or unanswered questions in the literature to show what is different or unique about the planned study and what it will add to the existing body of knowledge.
- Include the details or rationale for any theoretical perspectives that will underpin the study.
- Keep the research question in mind while writing and make sure each paragraph directly relates to that question to keep the proposal on track and relevant.
- Focus on the key points, rather than trying to illustrate a range of knowledge about the subject.
- The key argument to get across in the introduction is answering the 'so what?' question. There are many attractive research ideas that could yield some interesting results—but is it really worth the time and effort and money if nothing is really going to change as a result of the research? Think about how the research could make a difference such as improving health-care delivery and patient outcomes and/or informing policy or health-care planning, or whether this is an important

first step in the development of other studies that will lead to a novel approach or breakthrough.

AIMS AND OBJECTIVES

The main focus of the planned research project can be explained in terms of research aims and objectives. Aims and objectives are often confused, but are quite distinct. Aims are a broad statement to describe what the researcher hopes to achieve at the end of the project, whereas an objective is the plan of how to achieve it.

It is important to be as specific as possible. Drafting the aims and rechecking them for meaning is a useful process. For example, if the aim is to identify how sleep and daytime fatigue interrelate following a stroke, is the project really looking at interrelationships or would it be more accurate to state that it is looking at associations? The aims and objectives should clearly link back to the research question.

DESIGN AND METHODS

The 'design and methods' section is one of the largest sections of the proposal and accordingly it can be useful to use subheadings to orient the reader to particular sections. Sufficient information needs to be provided to enable the reader to determine that the research will be methodologically sound (of good quality), and to show that all possible factors that may affect the research have been considered (and addressed). Someone else should be able to replicate the study from the details given in this section (not unlike a recipe) so details of the 'how' and 'why' are important.

RESEARCH DESIGN AND METHODOLOGY

- Specify and justify the type of research planned, such as 'a retrospective, cross-sectional questionnaire' or 'focus groups guided by a semi-structured interview schedule drawing on a grounded theory approach'.
- Identify the research paradigm or methodological approach that underpins the research.
- Provide a justification of the particular approach drawing on evidence (and citing references). If a method other than what may be considered 'ideal' will be used to answer the research question, then it is important to state why an alternate approach is being used. For example, the most rigorous and robust method is often not the most cost-effective, practical or ethical approach.

RESEARCH PARTICIPANTS

- Be specific about who (for example, a specific diagnostic group or a particular age group) and how many participants to recruit into the study, and why.

- Specify any people to be excluded to prevent certain factors (confounders) affecting the results (for example, setting an upper age limit to prevent age-related decline affecting the results).
- Think about whether there needs to be a comparison group (and, if so, who that might be)?

Sampling
The process of identifying participants for a study.

- Specify how (for example, random selection, convenience sampling or purposive sampling) and where participants will be recruited, and whether the target sample size can be expected to be met from these sources.

APPARATUS, EQUIPMENT, QUESTIONNAIRES AND OUTCOME MEASURES

Data
Information that is gathered for the purpose of analysis and research.

Interviews
Conversations held for the purpose of gathering information.

The information to be included in the section on data collection depends on the type of study, but in summary an outline of the tools that will be used to collect the data (such as interviews, focus groups or a self-report questionnaire) is required:

- For questionnaire-based studies, provide details of each questionnaire to be included and outline why each has been selected. It can help to provide details of previous research that has found the measure to be reliable and valid in the population of interest.
- For some qualitative approaches, provision of details on the questions to be asked and how these were derived will be required.
- Be clear at what time points (specify all if more than one), in what setting (context), and by whom the data will be collected.
- Detail any equipment to be used (such as the type, make and model of a heart-rate monitor).

PROCEDURE

The 'procedure' section is best written as if the study was underway. Writing this section as if the study is being carried out step by step enables the reader to follow the procedure in a logical way. This can also help to highlight areas where there is a need to add more information about the logistics; for example, who will search the database to identify people from a clinical service?

- Be specific about the setting (where the research will be done and where participants will be recruited from).
- Acknowledge any limitations or any anticipated problems honestly and consider including backup plans if things do not work out (for example, additional recruitment sites which could be drawn on).
- Ask whether all the services and people who will be important to the delivery of the project have been contacted. Identifying this early can prevent delays and adjustments later on.

INTERVENTION OR TREATMENT

If testing a new treatment or intervention, it needs to be described in detail, for example dosage, frequency of administration, content, who will deliver it and, if it is a treatment programme, an outline of what will be covered in each session.

Treatment
The act of carrying out an intervention for the purpose of alleviating or curing a problem.

DATA ANALYSIS

The data analysis section involves explaining the plans to analyse the data in order to show that the research question can indeed be answered. Predefining the analyses also helps to prevent what is known as 'data fishing trips' where many different analyses are conducted in the search for a significant result.

FOR QUANTITATIVE STUDIES

- Include details of specific analyses that will be done (for example, the specific statistical tests that will be used), and what each statistical test is and why that analysis has been chosen.
- Consider types of data that will be collected (think back to those research methods lectures) and whether they are likely to meet parametric assumptions (for example, have a normal distribution and be ratio or interval level data) to enable related statistical tests to be used. If the data will not meet these assumptions (as is often the case with health questionnaire data), what tests could be used to analyse the data? It can be helpful when unsure to specify what will be done in each case; for example, if data meet parametric assumptions, a t-test will be used to explore differences between the two groups. If data do not meet parametric assumptions, a Mann–Whitney U test will be conducted.

FOR QUALITATIVE STUDIES

- Specify 'how' the specified analytic approach will be implemented. This will be largely dependent on the approach chosen but could include the following: how many people will code transcripts and will this be done independently if more than one? How will themes be derived from codes?

FOR ALL TYPES OF STUDIES

- Justify the sample size. Although not all studies need a formal sample size calculation, there is a need to justify the rationale behind the number of participants recruited (whether this be related to the methodological approach, logistical or resource issues, or indeed all of these).

- Specify any expectations that participants may drop out of the study and how this attrition will be managed, for example over-recruit by expected attrition rate. Drop-out rates specified from previous studies can be used as a guide.

ETHICAL, CULTURAL AND SAFETY ISSUES

Any research studies that involve humans or animals will need ethical approval before the project commences, with consideration of the potential ethical, cultural and safety issues. Thinking about these issues in advance enables the inclusion of strategies to manage these issues in the proposal.

- Confirm the requirements for the local area (either by talking to the supervisor or contacting a relevant ethics committee) as procedures can be different based on the location of the research. In some locations researchers may need to go to more than one committee (such as a university committee and a health and disability committee). Specify how the data will be securely stored and kept confidential.
- Consider if there could be any potential safety issues; for example, could participants become distressed from answering the questions. If they do, what is the appropriate response? If testing a new intervention and adverse effects are observed (this is always a possibility with new treatments), how will this be addressed?

TIME SPAN

This section is often short, but is important to show the study will indeed be possible to conduct in the time frame available. Things often take longer than expected (particularly the recruitment of participants) so it is better to over- rather than underestimate the time needed. If the time span does not look feasible this may suggest a need to narrow down the proposal to ensure a particular deadline can be met. Flow charts or Gannt charts can be a good way of presenting this information (see Table 11.2).

RESOURCES AND BUDGET

Even paper and pens cost money and costs can quickly add up when looking at the numbers of participants in research studies, so it is important to think about how to fund the research. Working out how much each resource will cost per participant and then multiplying this for the total number of participants (and also by time point if relevant) is a useful strategy for outlining costs.

For example:

Consent forms (2 per participant) and a patient information sheet = 10 pages.

10 pages @ 10 cents per page × 462 participants = $462

TABLE 11.2 EXAMPLE OF A GANNT CHART FOR A CROSS-SECTIONAL QUESTIONNAIRE STUDY

Activity	MONTH									
	Mar	Apr	May	Jun	Jul	Aug	Sep	Oct	Nov	Dec
Ethics submission	■									
Participant recruitment		■	■	■	■	■	■			
Data collection			■	■	■	■	■	■		
Data analysis							■	■	■	■
Report writing		■	■	■	■	■	■	■	■	■

- Check what resources and funds are available. Some institutions and charitable organisations offer funds to support student projects so it helps to ask around. If seeking funding, check if there are any restrictions on funding—some may not cover equipment or salary costs or have annual limits that must be adhered to.
- Fully cost all resources needed to run the project, such as postage, cost of telephone calls, transport/mileage and transcription. If these cannot be funded by a grant, think about how to cover the cost in ways such as borrowing equipment or using a free online questionnaire package rather than printing the questionnaire.

DISSEMINATION

Many interesting and useful research studies have been written up and left to sit in a library or online archive for people to seek out if they wish to. However, considerable evidence now suggests that active dissemination (sharing of information) is needed to create change (Graham et al., 2006). As such, a dissemination plan is becoming an expected element of a good research proposal. Dissemination options are varied and could include publishing in an academic journal, a presentation to a clinical service, a talk with a patient support group, and/or sending a short summary of the findings to study participants. Including theses or dissertations in academic commons is another option worth considering (universities often have online repositories for research so it can be accessed by the public). Another consideration is whether or not to tailor the dissemination approach to different audiences (such as different cultures or population groups).

CASE STUDY 11.1

REASONS FOR REJECTION

While applying for grant funding is not the only context in which a research proposal is written, examining reasons why grant proposals may fail to get funded gives an idea of the common pitfalls. A Google search was carried out using a combination of search terms ('grant proposal', 'common problems', 'pitfalls' and 'reasons for rejection') and the first 20 hits examined. Of these 20 hits, 10 expressly identified a list of common pitfalls in grant writing. Sources ranged from resources available on institutional websites, reports from funding bodies, or tips from non-profit organisation websites. Table 11.3 lists the key reasons for rejection and/or pitfalls identified by these sources ranked according to the frequency of citation.

TABLE 11.3   KEY REASONS FOR REJECTION OF PROPOSALS AND/OR PITFALLS RANKED ACCORDING TO THE FREQUENCY OF CITATION

RANK	REASON FOR REJECTION/PITFALL	NUMBER OF CITATIONS
1	Poorly written, unstructured proposal (in particular a lack of flow, clarity, conciseness and excessive repetition)	8
2	Lack of 'fit' with funder goals and/or priorities	7
3	Lack of rationale for proposed methods or methods poorly explained or inappropriate	6
4	Unrealistic (too high, or too low) or confusing budget or the budget does not match activities described in the proposal	6
5	Deviation from guidelines (e.g. page limits, submission deadlines, format)	5
6	Literature reviewed out of date or key references overlooked (considered indicative that the writer does not know their topic)	5
7	Lack of a clear research question and/or objectives	4
8	Mechanical errors (e.g. grammatical errors, typos, formatting errors)	4

RANK	REASON FOR REJECTION/PITFALL	NUMBER OF CITATIONS
9	Proposed timeline lacks detail or appears overly ambitious	4
10	Lack of originality or innovation	4
11	Capacity of the research team or host organisation to undertake the proposed research in question	4
12	Overuse of jargon	3
13	Overemphasis on the 'why' and not enough on the 'how'	2
14	Cost-benefit of the proposed research not apparent	2
15	Hypotheses not testable or unsound	2
16	Possible constraints to carrying out the research not identified or addressed	1
17	Lack of engagement with key stakeholders	1
18	Title misleading or poorly written	1
19	Insufficient time allowed for peer review and rewrites	1

NEXT STEPS

Writing the first draft of a proposal is not the end. There are a number of steps to go through beyond the first draft to help refine the proposal (and avoid some of those pitfalls identified in Case Study 11.1). Often this refinement phase takes longer than people expect so it is important to: (1) plan adequate time for this phase at the outset; (2) expect that the proposal will go through several iterations before it is a finished product; and (3) be flexible and allow room for change to the proposal through this process. Table 11.4 outlines four key steps and associated questions to consider during this refinement process.

TABLE 11.4 STEPS TO REFINE A PROPOSAL

Step 1: Read through your proposal with a critical eye
- Is the proposal clear and well-reasoned? Does it flow well?
- Is there 'fit' between the key components of the proposal (e.g. between the research question, methods, budget, timeline, proposed outcomes of the research)?
- Have you given adequate weighting to the different components of the proposal (e.g. the 'why', and the 'how')?
- Is the proposed research logistically viable?
- Have you made any assumptions about the reader (i.e. their knowledge, understanding of key terms)?

[continued next page]

NICOLA KAYES AND ALICE THEADOM

TABLE 11.4 STEPS TO REFINE A PROPOSAL *(continued)*

Step 2: Ask a colleague to read through the proposal
- Have they understood the proposal?
- What questions does the proposal raise for them?
- Can they identify any issues you may not have considered?

Step 3: Check formatting
- Does the formatting of the proposal meet the guidelines for submission (e.g. page numbers and limits, word count, heading formats)?
- Does the formatting help or hinder the reader to access the key points (e.g. appropriate use of bullet points, bold font, tables, white space)?
- Have you used the correct referencing style?

Step 4: Proofread
- Have you corrected any typos, spelling and/or grammatical errors?
- Have you checked your references for accuracy?

SUMMARY

Writing a research proposal is a test in the application of research skills—it is about moving beyond a description of 'what' the intention is to a detailed rationale ('why' this question, 'why' now and 'why' this approach) and plan of 'how' to do it. It requires careful planning, a structured approach and adequate time for refinement. While the content of the proposal (that is, a research plan) is clearly important, how it is presented in terms of clarity, flow and 'fit' is critical. A good research proposal is the first step in making research ideas a reality, as the door to research funding, the basis of subsequent ethics submissions or the protocol that drives decision-making and task allocation when researchers are ready to put it into action. As such, the time spent at this phase of the research is time well spent.

REFLECTION POINTS

- Have I found a gap in the literature to ensure my study is needed?
- Have I got a clear, focused research question?
- Do all sections of my research proposal relate directly to my research question?
- Will my proposal be feasible to carry out in everyday life?

STUDY QUESTIONS

1   What are the key sections that need to be included in a research proposal and why?
2   What can be done to avoid some of the common pitfalls of proposal writing?

ADDITIONAL READING

Bordage, G., & Dawson, B. (2003). Experimental study design and grant writing in eight steps and 28 questions. *Medical Education, 37*(4), 376–385.

Hollins Martin, C. J., & Fleming, V. (2010). A 15-step model for writing a research proposal. *British Journal of Midwifery, 18*(12), 791–798.

Inouye, S. K., & Fiellin, D. A. (2005). An evidence-based guide to writing grant proposals for clinical research. *Annals of Internal Medicine, 142*(4), 274.

Punch, K. F. (2006). *Developing effective research proposals*. London: Sage Publications.

REFERENCES

Bordage, G., & Dawson, B. (2003). Experimental study design and grant writing in eight steps and 28 questions. *Medical Education, 37*(4), 376–385.

Bradley, D. B. (2001). Developing research questions through grant proposal development. *Educational Gerontology, 27*(7), 569–581.

Charmaz, K. (2006). *Constructing grounded theory: A practical guide through qualititative analysis*. London: Sage Publications.

Clayton, B. (1982). The other side of proposal writing: People. *Personnel and Guidance Journal, 60*(10), 629.

Graham, I. D., Logen, J., Harrison, M. B., Straus, S. E., Tetroe, J., Caswell, W., & Robinson, N. (2006). Lost in knowledge translation: Time for a map? *Journal of Continuing Education in the Health Professions, 26*, 13–24.

Hollins Martin, C. J., & Fleming, V. (2010). A 15-step model for writing a research proposal. *British Journal of Midwifery, 18*(12), 791–798.

Hsieh, H. F., & Shannon, S. E. (2005). Three approaches to qualitative content analysis. *Qualitative Health Research, 15*(9), 1277–1288.

Inouye, S. K., & Fiellin, D. A. (2005). An evidence-based guide to writing grant proposals for clinical research. *Annals of Internal Medicine, 142*(4), 274.

Jonker, L., & Marshall, G. (2010). Writing a research proposal. *Synergy, 9*, 22–25.

Klopper, H. (2008). The qualitative research proposal. *Curationis, 31*(4), 62–72.

Landsberger, J. (2011). *How to write a reseach proposal*. Retrieved March, 6, 2013, from http://www.studygs.net/proposal.htm

Sandelowski, M. (2000). Whatever happened to qualitative description? *Research in Nursing and Health, 23*(4), 334–340.

Verhoef, M. J., & Hilsden, R. J. (2004). *Writing an effective research proposal.* Calgary: University of Calgary.

WEBSITES

Youtube clip on writing a research proposal:
http://www.youtube.com/watch?v=uyoU4BwTHmo

Study guides and strategies—how to write a research proposal:
http://www.studygs.net/proposal.htm

CHAPTER 12

ETHICS

TINEKE WATER AND ROSEMARY GODBOLD

CHAPTER OVERVIEW

This chapter covers the following topics:

- Why is ethics important to research?
- Research principles: protection, participation and partnership
- Future directions in ethics and research

KEY TERMS

Behaviour

Biomedical

Ethics

Informed consent

Partnership

Philosophy

Protection

Science

Treaty of Waitangi

WHY IS ETHICS IMPORTANT TO RESEARCH?

Philosophy
The study of thought, meaning and existence.

Ethics
Moral values that are identified by any group of people, such as health professionals.

Behaviour
The response of a living thing (including people) to stimulation.

Informed consent
The process where research participants, having been fully informed, agree to engage in the study; also used in clinical settings to ensure patients are informed and agree to procedures or treatments.

Biomedical
Relating to a way of thinking about health and illness with a focus on diseases as physical entities that affect physical bodies. This is the dominant Western model of health care.

Ethics is a branch of philosophy that is intrinsically embedded in everything people do—including research. In our everyday lives people constantly use ethics or moral principles to guide their behaviour or the choices they make. Ethics is defined as a body of theoretical knowledge pertaining to which principles, duties or obligations should be taken into account when a person is making a choice around what to do or how to act (Johnstone, 1994; Lutzen, Dahlquvist, Erikson, & Norberg, 2006; Thompson, Melia, & Boyd, 1994).

The point of research is to improve the situation of human beings. Human participants must never be treated as a means to an end but seen as an 'end in themselves'. In other words, they should not be used as objects for others' gains. Therefore ethical research is very important to make sure that no harm comes to any participant in research; it is the concern and responsibility, and within the capability, of every researcher.

To understand ethics in research it is useful to look at the past and what the catalysts were for what is understood as research ethics today. A good starting point is World War II and the 'research' experiments that were carried out on prisoners in the concentration camps. The human experiments were carried out on mainly Jewish prisoners (including children) in concentration camps during the Nazi Germany regime. In some cases these experiments resulted in disfigurement, permanent disability and death. The prisoners were not willingly participants and there was no informed consent.

In 1946 physicians and administrators were indicted before the War Crimes Tribunal at Nuremberg for their willing participation in the systematic torture, mutilation and killing of prisoners in experiments and for 'crimes against humanity'. In 1947 the Nuremberg Code was established, laying down strict guidelines of 'permissible medical experiments' which included a very strong emphasis on 'voluntary informed consent'. This was followed with the Declaration of Helsinki 1964, which was adopted by the World Medical Association as a guiding set of principles for the medical profession in relation to clinical research again with an emphasis on informed consent. The Declaration of Helsinki makes consent a central requirement of ethical research and contains statements of ethical principles for human participation in biomedical research.

Although it is easy to look back and think this would never happen in modern times, Aotearoa New Zealand has its own dark history of 'unfortunate' experiments. In 1987 it was revealed that a research project at National Women's hospital was studying the natural trajectory of cervical cancer in a group of women who had abnormal cells found on a smear test. One group was treated while the other was not, even though international evidence suggested treatment. The women themselves did not know that they were taking part in the study, and 22 per cent of the untreated women developed invasive cancer, compared to the 1.5 per cent among women who were treated (Coney, 1988).

A national outcry saw the establishment of the Cartwright Inquiry in June 1987. The inquiry also uncovered practices of vaginal examinations by medical students on anesthetised women without their knowledge, and the mass taking of vaginal smears on newborn girls without their parents' knowledge or consent. Williams (2004) says what was shocking was this was not the Middle Ages—there were in fact international guidelines set out in the Nuremburg Code in 1948 and Declaration of Helsinki 1964 following the atrocities of the Nazi experiments during World War II. The Cartwright report led to establishing of the Code of Health and Disability Services Consumers' Rights under the *Health and Disability Commissioners Act 1994*, in effect implementing a doctrine of informed consent for health care consumers. By 2004, there were 15 health and disability ethics committees established in Aoteraroa New Zealand, chaired by a layperson and with significant non-health-professional representation on the committee (Pinnock & Crosthwaite, 2004). The main obligations which all ethics committees in Aotearoa New Zealand operate under are to protect all participants of research and innovative practice; protect consumers of health and disability services; and ensure that Māori ethical practices and standards are included in any ethical review.

RESEARCH ALIVE 12.1
HEALTH RESEARCH ETHICS IN AUSTRALIA

In Australia the National Health and Medical Research Council (NHMRC) is a federal government organisation that funds research and promotes the development and maintenance of public and individual health standards for research practice. Australian health researchers are guided by nationally recognised standards, similar to the New Zealand legislation discusssed in this chapter, which detail acceptable research practices that protect participants. Key documents and guidance are available from the NHMRC website (www. nhmrc.gov.au) and include the *Human research ethics handbook* and *Values and ethics: Guidelines for ethical conduct in Aboriginal and Torres Strait Islander health research.*

CASE STUDY 12.1

STUDIES INVOLVING HUMAN PARTICIPANTS

Jim is an oral health therapist who wants to formally evaluate the antenatal oral health promotion programme he's been running with a group of 30 new migrants at the city's new migrant centre and write it up as a journal article. To gather his data, he would like to survey the women and then follow up

[continued next page]

TINEKE WATER AND ROSEMARY GODBOLD

with interviews. Jim decides to speak to his ethics advisor about the ethical dimensions of the methods and design of his study.

Ethics Advisor (EA): So, Jim, tell me a bit about your research.

Jim: I've been working with an antenatal class to provide an oral health promotion programme which gives guidance on optimal oral health care for pregnant women and their babies. I have a strong sense that the programme has been well received and the informal feedback has certainly been great. Now I would like to do a formal evaluation of the project and publish the results in our national oral health journal. I believe I need ethics approval?

EA: Yes, that's right. This is a research project and all studies involving human participants need to come through an ethics committee. As you are working with a staff member from this university you should come through our ethics committee. Have you thought about what methods you will use?

RESEARCH PRINCIPLES: PROTECTION, PARTICIPATION AND PARTNERSHIP

Treaty of Waitangi
The founding document of Aotearoa New Zealand signed between indigenous Māori and the British Crown in 1840.

Partnership
Genuine and respectful relationship between people.

Protection
The act of looking after or taking care of.

Three principles closely linked to the Treaty of Waitangi—partnership, participation and protection—are integral in the implementation of the treaty in any research with Māori. There are specific issues identified that should be considered under each of the principles in relation to research with Māori (Hudson & Russell, 2010). However, thinking about and applying the three principles even more broadly provides a robust framework for the consideration of the ethical dimensions of all research projects involving human participants (not just research with Māori). The following case study and dialogue between a novice researcher and an ethics advisor demonstrates how this can be achieved.

RESEARCH ALIVE 12.2
THE TREATY OF WAITANGI CONSIDERED IN RELATION TO ETHICS AND RESEARCH

PROTECTION
Jim: I'm a bit worried. I really want to do this research. But while I've done a research methods paper in my degree and a health promotion evaluation paper, I'm not very confident.

EA: You are right to be cautious. The ethics committee will be concerned about whether you are adequately trained to carry out the research project and if there is any guidance or support there for you. Many people believe that poor research is unethical research; it wastes people's time and results in no tangible benefits for the participants, the researcher, the production of knowledge, or benefits for the people.

Jim: Right, I see that. I'm working on this project with one of my old university lecturers who is experienced in this area and has offered to provide guidance and support.

EA: That's great. Who are your research participants going to be?

Jim: They are new migrants, mostly women, but some men, partners and husbands of the women.

EA: That is a vulnerable group, but you must already have their trust because you've been working with them for some time. How will you invite the group members to participate in your research? Because of your position leading this programme they may feel they have to participate or have to somehow pay you back. How will you ensure that they are participating because they want to, not because they feel they have to?

Jim: I did think that I might get good numbers in my study because of the positive relationships I've built with the antenatal group, but I hadn't thought of that. How can I tackle that?

EA: There are a number of ways you can address this. Ultimately, you need to remove yourself from the recruitment process, emphasise that participation in your research is entirely voluntary and that participants can withdraw from the project at any time without giving reasons. You could ask someone not associated with the programme or the new migrant centre—perhaps your colleague from the university—to introduce the project and get the consent from participants. And do you think you're the best person to do the interviews? I think you need to think carefully about the ethical issues that may arise from working with this group of vulnerable participants.

Jim: Yes, I wondered about that. The people in the group come from a wide range of cultures and not all of them speak English. That's been fine in the group because family members have come to interpret. I think they can do the same for the questionnaires, consent forms and information sheets. But I was thinking of excluding people who can't speak English from the interviews. I just don't have a budget for translation.

EA: That is your decision, but that does raise issues of equity and accessibility to your research. It doesn't seem fair to exclude people on those grounds, but if you

[continued next page]

haven't got funding, it's hard to see a way round it. There may also be cultural issues relating to a male interviewing female participants which you need to think about. And how will people get to your interviews? Money may well be an issue for this group of participants; will you be compensating them for any costs?

PARTICIPATION

Jim: I would like to perhaps give them a petrol voucher which would cover their travel costs but also show my appreciation for their participation. But, again, funding is an issue.

EA: I think that's a really great idea; offering koha (a small gift) and ensuring your participants do not incur costs as a result of participating in your research are important. Can you source funds from somewhere? Perhaps your sponsoring organisation? You will need to tell your participants who is providing funding and whether there are any potential benefits to them from the research. Usually you don't tell participants about koha prior to their participation in the research as it may constitute an inducement, but it seems reasonable to let them know you'll cover any travel expenses. Have you started on your information sheet?

Jim: Not yet. How much information should I give to participants and how should I give it to them?

EA: These are important questions. Voluntary, informed consent is the linchpin of ethical research involving human participants, and ensuring they have enough information and the freedom to choose whether or not they wish to participate is crucial to upholding the principle of autonomy—the right to self-determination. The Code of Health and Disability Services Consumers' Rights [http://www.hdc. org.nz/the-act--code/the-code-of-rights] provides valuable guidance about how much information should be given. Remember that Right 9 extends all of the rights in the code to all health consumers participating in research. Right 5 is the right to effective communication which must be in a form, language and manner which is understandable (including the use of an interpreter when necessary and practicable). Right 6 is the right to be fully informed and gives explicit guidance on how much information is required to achieve this; before making a choice or giving consent, every consumer has the right to the information that a reasonable consumer in their circumstances needs to make a decision. Right 7 is the right to make an informed choice and give informed consent and provides significant guidance for health researchers who are working with groups, such as children or others, who may have diminished capacity to give consent to participate. Some key advice is that these participants still retain the right to take part in the decision-making process 'to the extent appropriate to his or her level of competence'.

So, in summary, you have to give your participants as much information as they need to be able to make a fully informed decision about whether they wish to participate. You've talked about providing an introduction session delivered by your colleague. You will also need to give them a written information sheet that they can take away with them and plenty of time for them to consider your invitation. They should know that if they do decide to participate, they can withdraw at any time without giving a reason. You should be very clear about why you are doing the research and what benefits or risks there are likely to be. For example, if you were doing the research for an academic qualification or if there may be potential commercial gain. The focus of your research does not seem controversial, but what will you do if one of your participants becomes distressed? Or reveals something untoward about themselves?

PARTNERSHIP

Jim: I think the potential for participant distress is unlikely given my research focus. What do you think?

EA: I agree. But this is a vulnerable group who are new to the country. It wouldn't hurt to offer free counselling services to participants as a safety net just in case anything comes up for them, particularly during the interviews. And what about you—have you thought about where you will conduct the interviews and how you will maintain your own safety? Researcher safety is becoming more of a concern, particularly if you're doing the interviews in people's homes, for example. A simple safety protocol in which you consider issues like carrying a mobile phone, letting people know when you arrive and when you have finished is sensible. Guidance on this is available [see for example the UK Social Researchers Association's safety code for researchers: the-sra.org.uk/wp-content/uploads /safety_code_of_practice.pdf; and Cardiff University's research fieldwork policy: cardiff.ac.uk/socsi/research/researchethics/resources/fieldwork-has.pdf]. We haven't talked about privacy and confidentiality yet.

Jim: No, and I know that's important in maintaining trust and respecting the autonomy of my participants. I was thinking about making the questionnaire anonymous. I could give it out at one of my last sessions and ask participants to return it either in a prepaid envelope or to a drop box at the migrant centre.

EA: Yes, I think that's a good idea. You would not need to get participants' written consent for that either, as long as your participants knew upfront that their agreement to participate was indicated by their completing the questionnaire. How about using an online instrument like Survey Monkey?

Jim: Access to technology may be an issue for my participants. Actually, there a number of issues coming up here. I'm starting to wonder if I should involve them in the planning of this project.

[continued next page]

EA: Yes, I think that is an excellent idea. Consultation with communities has a number of benefits for your research [Dickert & Sugarman, 2005]. I think because of the culturally diverse make-up of your target group, talking to them about how you're planning to carry out your research would ensure that it is culturally appropriate for all of your participants. There are a number of other ways you can act in partnership so that your research is with, rather than on, your participants. For example, asking your interviewees to check the transcripts of their interviews not only ensures that the data are true to what they have expressed, but also involves participants in the research process. And it ensures that participants have a meaningful say over any information that may identify them, or someone else. And have you thought how you will disseminate your findings? While getting your findings out there (whether they are what you wanted to find or not) is an important principle of research it is also a way of honouring your participants. Reciprocity is an important principle in research with Māori and refers to ensuring there are mutual benefits between researchers and participants (Hudson & Russell, 2010). If you kept your participants informed about your findings and any changes that may have resulted they may gain satisfaction from their part in that, particularly if there were benefits for future migrants.

EA: You could also talk to them about issues like translation and whether they would like to have a support person with them for the interview. Both of these issues take us back to privacy and confidentiality. If others are present at the interviews, confidentiality needs to be considered. Perhaps with your research focus it is not so important, but if you were discussing high-risk topics, such as domestic violence or elder abuse, you'd have to think more carefully about this. Other issues that need consideration are how you will store your data, whether you will use them in the future, whether they will be shared and how they will be destroyed. New Zealand's Health Information Privacy Principles provide help here [http://www.privacy.org.nz/the-privacy-act-and-codes/privacy-principles]. For example, Principle 10 states that 'personal information obtained in connection with one purpose must not be used for another'. So if research data are collected for your study, you cannot share those data with anyone else without getting the consent of the participants. Sharing data with other researchers and keeping them for future projects is advocated more and more for a number of reasons, including better value for money spent on research (Olds, 2011). This is fine, and may even be seen as best practice in the future, as long as you get full, informed consent from your participants to do this.

Jim: Wow, there's a lot to think about here. And what about storing the data? My colleague said he had facilities at the university.

EA: That's good, as long as your data are securely stored separately from the consent forms to maintain confidentiality. Also, the university will have a policy about how long research data should be kept in case anyone wants to check the validity of your findings. You should check that, while bearing in mind that Principle 9 of the Health Information Privacy Principles reminds us not to maintain personal information longer than necessary.

Jim: Can you offer me any other tips?

EA: It's really great that you're thinking about the ethics of your research at the beginning of the development of your design and I would advise all researchers to do it this way. Careful consideration of the ethical dimensions of your research from the outset will influence the way you do things, as will consultation with your target population, stakeholders or experts in the area. You should also check other guidelines, in particular the National Ethics Advisory Committee guidelines for observation and intervention studies [http://neac.health.govt. nz/publications-and-resources/neac-publications/streamlined-ethical-guidelines-health-and-disability] and Te Ara Tika guidelines for Māori research ethics (http://www.hrc.govt.nz/news-and-publications/publications/maori#te-ara-tika—guidelines-for-m%C4%81ori-research-ethics:-a-framework-for-researchers-and-ethics-committee-members).

CLINICAL REFLECTION 12.1: CONDUCTING RESEARCH WITH PEOPLE

Consider the core ethical concept from this chapter of conducting research *with* people rather than treating research participants as objects. Compare this with concepts of partnership with people and community who are participating in research, which is a strong theme in two of the previous chapters (Chapter 8: Aboriginal and Torres Strait Islander Peoples of Australia and Research; Chapter 9: Immigrant and Refugee Communities: Diversity in Research) and in Research Alive 12.2. What are your conclusions about the potential vulnerabilities of research participants? How might the vulnerability of a research participant be magnified when the person is already experiencing disadvantage or is part of a minority or marginalised group?

CASE STUDY 12.2

THE EXPERIENCE OF COUPLES FOLLOWING DIAGNOSIS OF A FOETAL ANOMALY

Imagine the emotional turmoil a couple would experience after being told by medical specialists that their foetus has a major abnormality. Then imagine being asked to participate in research and to be interviewed about this experience. What would your reaction be? Might being asked to be involved in such research about this awful time be harmful or distressing?

Australian researchers (deVitry-Smith, Dietsch & Bonner, 2013) explored the experiences of 31 couples who were in this situation and, using interviews, sought to understand the couples' experiences and how they coped. The core ethical principles of informed consent and protecting participants from further harm were major challenges in gaining ethics clearance for this study and the researchers had to be mindful of these principles while conducting it.

FUTURE DIRECTIONS IN ETHICS AND RESEARCH

Science
The body of processes used to develop and extend knowledge (often with an emphasis on empiricism and positivism).

Ethics is embedded in all aspects of human lives and as science and technology evolve, there are likely to be more ethical issues arising in relation to what it means to a human being. Society now has to consider questions such as: just because technology is available, should it be used (for example, saving extremely premature neonates)? What are the implications of genetic testing and the human genome project? What are the ethical issues around ownership of genetic material, the implications for health insurance and the disclosure of information to family members who may not realise they carry a particular gene (Water, 2008)? How might routine antenatal or genetic screening have the potential to deconstruct and reconstruct physical and social identities (Water, 2008)? There are also ethical questions around the implementation of the findings of research because these are always within the financial context of a community or country. Because of financial constraints, researchers also may have to consider whether their research will benefit a few (justice) or the many (utilitarianism). Essex (2004) argues that science and knowledge have not always kept up with ethical and legal guidance. This makes it even more important that all researchers are able to consider the ethical implications of not only planning and carrying out research, but also the possible future consequences.

SUMMARY

'Researchers are guests in the private spaces of the world' (Stake, 2003, p. 154). As such, they are privileged to be given entry into the lives and experiences of participants which they entrust to the researcher. The intention of participation in research may be to make a difference, add to knowledge and improve the health and lives of people, perhaps not even for themselves but for others. Therefore the onus of responsibility for the respectful and fair treatment of research participants and the integrity of the research process lies with every researcher.

REFLECTION POINTS

- What are the particular ethical issues you would need to consider related to your research project?
- Are there particular ethical issues that would come up because of your study design, participant group or topic?

STUDY QUESTIONS

1 Why is ethics in research so important?
2 Who is responsible for ethics in research?

ADDITIONAL READING

Davidson, C., & Tolich, M., (2003). *Social science research in New Zealand: many paths to understanding*. Auckland: Pearson Education NZ Ltd.

Wiles, R. (2012). *What are qualitative research ethics?* London: Bloomsbury Publishing.

REFERENCES

Coney, S. (1988). *The unfortunate experiment*. Auckland: Penguin Books.

deVitry-Smith, S., Dietsch, E., & Bonner, A. (2013). Pregnancy as public property: The experience of couples following diagnosis of a foetal anomaly. *Women and Birth, 26*(1), 76–81.

Dickert, N., & Sugarman, J. (2005) Ethical goals of community consultation in research. *American Journal of Public Health, 95*(7), 1123–1127.

Essex, C. (2004). Home ventilation creates huge issues. *New Zealand Doctor*, 8 September, 26.

Hudson, M., & Russell, K. (2010). The Treaty of Waitangi and research ethics in Aotearoa. *Journal of Bioethical Inquiry, 6*, 61–68.

Johnstone, M. J. (1994). *Bioethics: A nursing perspective.* Sydney: WB Saunders/Balliere Tindall.

Lutzen, K., Dahlqvist, V., Erikson, S., & Norberg, A. (2006). Developing the concept of moral sensitivity in health care practice. *Nursing Ethics, 13*(2), 187–196.

Olds, R. (2011). Sharing research data to improve public health: A joint statement by funders of health research. Auckland: Health Research Council. hrc.govt.nz/sites/default/files/Ethics-May2011.pdf

Pinnock, J., & Crosthwaite, J. (2004). The Auckland hospital ethics committee: The first seven years. *New Zealand Medical Journal, 117*(1205).

Stake, R. (2003). Case studies. In N. K. Denzin, & Y. S. Lincoln (Eds.), *Strategies of qualitative inquiry* (2nd ed.) (pp. 134–164). Thousand Oaks, CA: Sage Publications.

Thompson, I. E., Melia, K. M., & Boyd, K. M. (1994). *Nursing ethics.* Melbourne: Churchill Livingstone.

Water, T. (2008). *The meaning of being in dilemma in paediatric practice: A phenomenological study.* Unpublished doctoral dissertation, AUT University, Auckland, New Zealand.

Williams, L. (2004). Looking back at the 1987 Cervical Cancer Inquiry. *The New Zealand Medical Journal, 117*(1202).

WEBSITES

Code of Practice for the Safety of Social Researchers: http://the-sra.org.uk/wp-content/uploads/safety_code_of_practice.pdf

Cardiff University's research fieldwork policy: http://www.cardiff.ac.uk/socsi/research/researchethics/resources/fieldwork-has.pdf

Health Information Privacy Principles: http://www.privacy.org.nz/the-privacy-act-and-codes/privacy-principles HRC (Health Research Council of New Zealand)—Maori Research—*Te Ara Tika— Guidelines for Māori research ethics: A framework for researchers and ethics committee members*: http://www.hrc.govt.nz/news-and-publications/publications/maori#te-ara-tika—guidelines-for-m%C4%81ori-research-ethics:-a-framework-for-researchers-and-ethics-committee-members

National Health and Medical Research Council:
  www.nhmrc.gov.au

NEAC (National Ethics Advisory Committee) *Streamlined ethical guidelines for health and disability research*—guidelines for observation and intervention studies:
  http://neac.health.govt.nz/publications-and-resources/neac-publications/
  streamlined-ethical-guidelines-health-and-disability

Code of Health and Disability Services Consumers' Rights:
  http://www.hdc.org.nz/the-act–code/the-code-of-rights

CHAPTER 13

BEGINNING THE RESEARCH PROCESS

BARBARA McKENZIE-GREEN, DEBORAH PAYNE
AND SHOBA NAYAR

CHAPTER OVERVIEW

This chapter covers the following topics:

- Entering the field
- Determining data
- Gathering the data

KEY TERMS

Experimentation

Interviews

Mind

Relationships

Researcher attributes

World view

The research process is not as linear as people often think. Depending on methodology, there may be constant movement between particular stages of the research process. Ways of working with data, including data collection and data analysis, will be examined in the chapters related to the specific research methodologies. This chapter focuses on three umbrella notions related to beginning the research: 'entering the field', 'determining data', and 'gathering the data'. Within these three notions, the focus is on conducting research in a respectful manner. This includes an awareness of researcher attributes and researcher-participant relationships. Over time, the authors have come to learn that research cannot be rushed—it requires thinking time.

Researcher attributes
The characteristics of a researcher.

Relationships
The similarities and connections between people or variables in any given situation.

ENTERING THE FIELD

Entering the field is about engagement and interaction between researcher and participants. Conducting a research study, therefore, is always a dynamic, complex process; thus, the process of 'entering the field' commences from the moment the researcher begins conceptualising the research proposal. Designing the research requires thinking about, and reflecting on, the *who*, *why*, *when*, and *how* of the study. Each of these questions leads to the other; for example, studying populations living with or in vulnerable situations (*who*), demands considering *how* and *when* in relation to interaction with participants in order to gain the information to answer the research question (*why*). The two key factors to be considered alongside each other, from the outset, are the 'who' and the 'why'.

Who: this is about the self and participants. As many experienced researchers will testify, the researcher is always part of the research. Knowing this, regardless of methodology, each researcher requires a degree of reflexivity in their work. Understanding the personal world view leads to recognition that world views influence approaches to data gathering and to participants. The 'who' also invites a consideration of the research participants. What particular features of the participant population need to be taken into account when designing a research study? Questions that the researcher might ask may pertain to issues of gender, age, sexuality, ability and disability, culture, socio-economic status and location. Each of these issues, generally grounded in personal world views, has the potential to facilitate or inhibit the development of relationships, close or detached, and interactions between researcher and participants.

World view
A set of beliefs or concepts held by an individual informing how they interpret their environment and experience.

Why: It is imperative that the rationale for the study extends beyond the researcher's need to solve a problem in the field of study. Thus, entering the field demands that the researcher consult. The consultation process involves discussions and negotiations with participant representatives to ensure safe passage for the participants in the ensuing process, and establishes that the study is congruent with the population need. In Aotearoa New Zealand, there are established processes for consulting with Tangata Whenua. Accepted bicultural processes established in New Zealand ensure that consultation also

CASE STUDY 13.1

HAVING DISABILITY ADVISORS

'Right from the beginning, in our national study of mothers with physical or sensory impairments experiences of the New Zealand maternity system, it was imperative that we consulted with the disability community. Our study aimed to improve the interventions and support for disabled mothers in Aotearoa New Zealand.

'Firstly, the disability community affirmed the importance of the study: that there was a real need for disabled mothers' experiences to be collated. Secondly, they asserted the need for us to have disability advisors as part of our team. These advisors' input was critical in planning and preparing the study. For example, they suggested which disability organisations we needed to contact to assist in recruiting our participants; what formats our 'information sheets' had to be for women with visual impairments; how the 'information sheets' were to be worded for women with hearing impairments; where we could hold our focus group meetings so that they would be accessible to women with physical impairments.

'Through this process we grew as researchers in understanding the issues that confront disabled people. Everyday activities that we had previously taken for granted, such as going to a café, going to the doctors, reading advertorial flyers or the newspaper assumed a different significance. But more importantly, it allowed our research to become more accessible and also more credible to the community.'

Source: D. Payne, personal communication, November 12, 2012.

occurs when the research involves ethnic groups. Such consultation should extend to particular populations and communities—for example, disabled, Lesbian Gay Bisexual Transgender (LGBT) or aged care groups.

When: 'When' mainly refers to those doing prospective studies and not necessarily to those gathering data from de-identified data banks. Entering the field is a process that commences with the conceptualisation of the study. However, due consideration needs to be given to the actual timing. Many novice researchers tend to insufficiently plan to achieve the necessary practicalities associated with time and location for engaging participants, and also the length of time required to build the relationship. Building relationships may not happen in one meeting.

How: Knowing who participants are going to be and having a sound rigorous rationale for conducting the study, the **mind** turns to 'how'. The dimensions of how include the method and nature of data collection.

Mind
That which thinks, reasons and perceives.

RESEARCH ALIVE 13.1
ENTERING THE FIELD

Here is an example of entering the field for an interview-based study with health professionals (McGilton, Bowers, McKenzie-Green, Boscart, & Brown, 2009). Figure 13.1 depicts the circular nature of the process.

FIGURE 13.1   THE CIRCULAR NATURE OF ENTERING THE FIELD

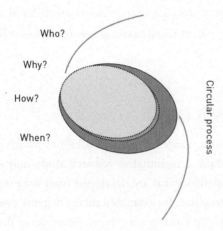

Who: I was a team member for a study that was focused on registered nurses (RN) working in residential aged care in Canada. Our aim was to study in depth the work that these RNs do during a shift. However, RNs are responsible to a range of administrators who in turn are responsible for managing the facility as a whole and their actions can influence RN work. Our 'who' for this study ended up including RNs and managers.

Why: Residential aged care in many countries has difficulties in attracting and keeping RNs. RNs themselves, in other studies, have indicated that there is a tension between meeting the needs of residents and families, the facility management and government-required documentation. We figured that this study may show us a way that RN work could be restructured so that high-quality resident care could be delivered and structural requirements could be met.

[continued next page]

BARBARA McKENZIE-GREEN, DEBORAH PAYNE AND SHOBA NAYAR

How: We chose a methodology that would provide us with in-depth qualitative data which would reveal the processes the participants used to solve their concerns—grounded theory. We also decided that participant interviews would be the most effective way to gather data taking into consideration the funding that was available to us. The 'how' included discussions of the team roles as the research team comprised colleagues from Canada, Australia and the US. Canadian team members gathered data while the Australian and the US team members were involved in planning, data analysis and publication.

When: We were mindful of the busy lives of RNs and took care to schedule interview times that would not disrupt the delivery of resident care. Because of our team make-up, there were many 'whens'. Our decision-making through this process occurred by conference phone with team members in their various countries at various times of the day due to time differences. This study shows that careful thinking through these processes can facilitate an in-depth, worthwhile study.

B. McKenzie-Green, personal communication, November 12, 2012.

DETERMINING DATA

Research involves a wide range of data possibilities which are closely linked to methodology. For example, a quantitative research study may include collecting data measurements and/or statistics that are developed from data that have not necessarily involved participant interaction, for example a survey of gyms' open hours on advertising material. On the other hand, a quantitative research study may also involve measurement testing and **experimentation** which does involve close physical connection with participants. It is worthwhile exploring *what constitutes data* and how the forms of data collection shape *researcher–participant relationships*.

Experimentation
A process of testing hypotheses.

WHAT CONSTITUTES DATA?

Depending on the methodology, numbers, words or other modes such as photographic images may constitute data. When researchers aim to examine people's experiences or the meaning they give to particular events, or the strategies used, or the power relations within a field of study, they are more likely to choose in-depth **interviews** as their data collection method in order to gather such rich contextual data. Observations of seemingly mundane everyday activities, social engagement and interactions with environments may all provide valuable insights in relation to health and health-care practice. Measurements

Interviews
Conversations held for the purpose of gathering information.

of anatomical structures or physiological functions may produce knowledge regarding disease processes and possible interventions. Regardless of the method of data collection, each approach requires rigorous examination of its fit with the research question—can the data actually answer the research question? For example, questionnaires can produce more effective data when they adhere to a reliable, valid scientific process of questionnaire development.

CASE STUDY 13.2

CHOOSING TYPES OF DATA

In 2008, the Council of Occupational Therapists Registration Boards (Australia and Aotearoa New Zealand) examined new graduate and recent migrant occupational therapists' perspectives on work preparedness, professional development and work environment issues. Findings revealed that only 9.3% of Aotearoa New Zealand graduates felt very well prepared for practice. An equal percentage reported feeling not prepared at all to fulfil their current work requirements (Nayar, Blijlevens, Gray, & Moroney, 2011). The research reported here sought to determine new graduate occupational therapists' preparedness for practice based on the Occupational Therapy Board of New Zealand (OTBNZ) competencies for registration in Aotearoa New Zealand.

It was determined that two types of data collected in two phases would best answer the research question:

1 An *online survey* was designed and sent to all New Zealand registered occupational therapists via the OTBNZ website. Advantages of an electronic survey included: (a) reduced costs associated with paper mail outs; (b) increased ease of follow-up reminders; and (c) ease of collating response for analysis. Challenges included the time required to designing the questionnaire to meet software requirements.

2 Following the survey a total of five *focus groups*, two in Auckland and one each in Palmerston North, Nelson and Dunedin, were held with participants representing new graduate occupational therapists, senior practising occupational therapists, educators and managers. Advantages of focus groups included: (a) the gathering of multiple, in-depth perspectives; and (b) the opportunity to explore concepts arising from the survey. Challenges included: (a) the time and expense associated with travel; (b) participant recruitment in regions where the research team were not based; and

[continued next page]

BARBARA McKENZIE-GREEN, DEBORAH PAYNE AND SHOBA NAYAR

(c) limited responses due to mixed participant groups—for example, new graduates may not have fully participated in the presence of senior practitioners.

Ultimately both forms of data gathering were necessary to ensure opportunities for participants to have a voice on the issue.

RESEARCHER–PARTICIPANT RELATIONSHIPS

Research may involve close or detached connection with participants depending on context. Getting up close and personal may involve interviews and/or observations, whereas a more detached connection could be developed through analysis of texts. However, it is not a black and white choice. Even for quantitate researchers who may not interact directly with participants and deal primarily with de-identified data, personal world views can influence the construction of questions that may unwittingly cause distress or raise unanticipated issues for participants. Thus, all researchers need to be mindful of the responsibilities and power relations that sit with the researcher throughout the research process.

RESEARCH ALIVE 13.2
A CONTINUUM OF FORMS OF DATA

Figure 13.2 illustrates how the type of data gathered, the form of the data, and the proximity of the researcher to participants all occur on a continuum.

FIGURE 13.2   THE CONTINUUM OF FORMS OF DATA

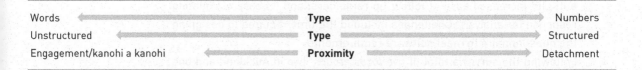

Words	←	Type	→	Numbers
Unstructured	←	Type	→	Structured
Engagement/kanohi a kanohi	←	Proximity	→	Detachment

GATHERING THE DATA

Once a decision has been made on the type of data to be collected in the study, the next question becomes how to actually proceed with data gathering. The researcher needs to consider factors such as time and place, the equipment required, human resources, issues of confidentiality or anonymity, and participant-related features.

Time and place are also important to consider, especially in relation to face-to-face interviews or telephoning participants for questionnaires. Examples are deciding what time of day is best when interviewing busy RNs at work or mothers with disabilities, and what the best location is for data gathering. Be mindful about who might be in the vicinity of data collection—who might overhear the interview, such as co-workers or family members, or see what questions are being answered.

RESEARCH ALIVE 13.3
ISSUES TO CONSIDER WHEN GATHERING DATA

The following are examples of issues researchers have considered in recent studies:

- Would it be best to interview the parents of children when the children are awake and playing or when the parent can give due attention to the interview?
- What facilities are required at locations for focus groups with disabled people, such as disability parking, wheelchair-friendly toilets and toileting facilities for guide dogs?
- What is likely to be the best time of day for interviewing older people, considering issues of impaired senses (for example, sight and hearing), as well as fluctuating energy levels, particularly for those in advanced older age?

None of the potential data-gathering issues should lead researchers to avoid including such populations because it is very important that these groups have access through a voice to research. Often particular groups are marginalised and because of their particular situations are placed in the 'too hard basket' when it comes to being included.

A wide range of equipment is used to manage information and data in research studies. Equipment can range from very expensive measuring devices—for example, body scanning equipment—to the simpler tools of pen and paper. However, in today's world, where technology permeates everyday human interactions, conducting qualitative interviews has moved from large, intrusive, interview-recording machines to unobtrusive electronic data-gathering mechanisms, from which the recorded interview can be uploaded and secured electronically. Quantitative data may now also be collected using iPads or other devices rather than paper. Be mindful, though, that data gathering cannot rely solely on technology and even the best devices will inevitably fail when least expected. Be prepared with extra batteries and make sure you actually turn the device on! Equipment supports data gathering; however, it does not replace it and the most important piece of equipment for gathering data is the researcher.

BARBARA McKENZIE-GREEN, DEBORAH PAYNE AND SHOBA NAYAR

The human resources involved in any research project need to be identified and managed carefully. Sometimes data collection involves other people in addition to the researcher and participants. These people may include research assistants to help facilitate focus groups, or support people to be with participants as they engage in the study. Additionally, organisations support researchers in developing skills, assisting with generating funds and disseminating news about the study. There are occasions when the researcher him- or herself may encounter distressing situations owing to the nature of the data collected; on these occasions, the parent organisation will most likely have mechanisms in place for researcher support. It is important that the researcher learn about the supports available even though they may not be required.

Confidentiality and/or anonymity are of prime importance when dealing with people and information about them, and this takes on special significance when participants are potentially identifiable. It is important to acknowledge that researchers are the holders of participants' private information. In Aotearoa New Zealand, the *Privacy Act* and the related code for the health sector (Privacy Commissioner, 1994; *Health and Disability Commissioner's Act 2009*) and health research and health professionals' codes of ethics require careful attention to the collection, storage and dissemination of research data. Prior to consenting to take part in the research study, participants themselves are provided with information about the mechanisms by which researchers will store their data and the use to which that data will be put. No human research study is undertaken without rigorous ethics applications and approval. For further details see Chapter 12 on research ethics.

CASE STUDY 13.3

WARMING UP TO DATA GATHERING

'Much of my research has focused on those who live and work in residential aged care. Those in residential aged care live with a wide range of disability and ability. Many are very busy, which belies the popular notion that older people rest all day. As I conducted research studies in this setting, I came to realise that the data I collected were more in-depth and rich if I paid attention to the relationships first; when I spent time getting to know the person rather than moving straight into my 'questions'. Conversational interviewing works well with this group of people. What I have found in my research is that people in residential aged care are very generous with their limited time, are willing to talk about situations of difficulty and wish to have a voice. To my delight, they are also in charge. They have set the time and the place for meeting with me.

In some cases, they have set the number of times they wish to talk to me. One person opted to see me three times.

'However, before even beginning the conversation I needed to consider how I would work with people who may have sensory impairment (sight, hearing), functional impairment (difficulty sitting for any length of time) or who were living with multiple comorbidities. Medications can cause dry mouths which make it difficult to talk for lengthy periods. In all instances I have learned to negotiate with the participant before I begin. I ask them to stop the conversation at any time they require fluid or a change of position or have any reason to cease the interview. Never be afraid to stop the tape yourself if you sense that the participant is unwell or distressed. On occasions, I have stopped the tape and rechecked that they are willing to continue to talk on particular subjects that might be distressing. Many times, they have indicated a willingness to continue and many times they have said that it helped to 'get things off their chest'.

'I would encourage you to conduct research with older people. They will teach you more than you could ever dream. They have certainly taught me and I have been privileged to have them as research participants on many occasions'.

Source: B. McKenzie-Green, personal communication, November 12, 2012

Matching the researcher characteristics with those of the participants can facilitate equitable and rich data gathering; however, this does not mean that the researcher has to always be of the same gender, age or ethnicity as the participants. What it does mean is that the researcher needs to adopt the perspective of the 'naïve inquirer' (Morrow, 2005, p. 254).

RESEARCH ALIVE 13.4
PARTICIPANT-RELATED FEATURES

Considerations for how acceptable the researcher may be to participants are important, but are there reasonable limits? What are your thoughts on these?

1   The researcher who grew her hair in order that she might be more acceptable to a particular ethnic group ... is it right or wrong?
2   Interviewing cultural groups with the support of an interpreter can facilitate understandings of the nuances of verbal and body language?
3   The appropriateness for the interviewer to be the same or different gender for some cultures (Liamputtong, 2010)?

Underpinning all these considerations and plans is the nature of the relationship between the researcher and participants which emphasises the need to think about power relations when entering the field and throughout the research process.

RESEARCH ALIVE 13.5
RESEARCH–PARTICIPANT RELATIONSHIPS

The closer the research relationship, the more the researcher needs to be aware of the power that they hold within that relationship. Figure 13.3 aligns appropriate data-gathering methods with the relational closeness of the researcher and participants.

FIGURE 13.3   THE RELATIONSHIP BETWEEN DATA-GATHERING
             METHODS AND THE CLOSENESS OF THE RESEARCHER
             AND PARTICIPANTS

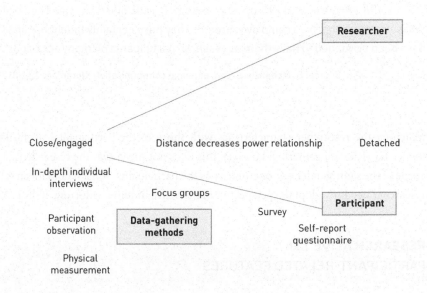

SUMMARY

When embarking on the research process, issues of *entering the field*, *determining data* and *gathering data* are key elements for consideration. Shaping the research project takes considerable thinking time. Most compelling, however, is the notion that who researchers are as people, and how they conduct themselves as researchers, will have immense impact on the process and outcome. While researchers may feel pressured to rush through beginning the research process, the time spent planning at the outset brings immeasurable rewards. It is a privilege to conduct research. It can be very enlightening and humbling to learn from participants when researchers genuinely engage in the research process.

REFLECTION POINTS

Reflect on the attributes that you bring to a research study as a researcher. How are these going to be helpful in the beginning of the research process?

STUDY QUESTIONS

1   Think about a research study you would like to conduct.
2   What population would you access to conduct the study?
3   Would you use a qualitative or quantitative approach? Why?
4   What would you need to consider when preparing to begin this study?
5   How would you prepare yourself?
6   What power dynamics would you need to think about?

ADDITIONAL READING

Health and Disability Commissioner. (2009). *Code of Health and Disability Services Consumers' Rights.* Wellington: Author. http://www.hdc.org.nz/media/24833/leaflet%20code%20of%20rights.pdf

Hudson, M., Milne, M., Reynolds, P., Russell, K., & Smith, B. (2010). *Te ara tika: Guidelines for Māori research ethics: A framework for researchers and ethics committee members.* Wellington: Health Research Council of New Zealand.

Lowe, M. (2007). *Beginning research: A guide for foundation degree students.* London: Routledge.

REFERENCES

Liamputtong, P. (2010). *Performing qualitative cross-cultural research.* Cambridge: Cambridge University Press.

McGilton, K. S., Bowers, B., McKenzie-Green, B., Boscart, V., & Brown, M. (2009). How do charge nurses view their roles in long-term care? *Journal of Applied Gerontology, 28*(6), 723–742.

Morrow, S. L. (2005). Quality and trustworthiness in qualitative research in counseling psychology. *Journal of Counseling Psychology, 52*(2), 250–260.

Nayar, S., Blijlevens, H., Gray, M., & Moroney, K. (2011). *An examination of the preparedness for practice of New Zealand new graduate occupational therapists.* Prepared for the Occupational Therapy Board of New Zealand. Auckland: AUT University.

Privacy Commissioner. (1994). Health Information Privacy Code. Wellington: Author. Retrieved from http://privacy.org.nz/the-privacy-act-and-codes/the-privacy-act

WEBSITES

The encyclopaedia of informal education:
http://www.infed.org/research/participant_observation.htm

Ethnographic and field study techniques (University of Cambridge):
https://camtools.cam.ac.uk/wiki/site/e30faf26-bc0c-4533-acbc-cff4f9234e1b/ethnographic and field study.html

Journal of Intellectual Disability Research:
http://bbi.syr.edu/_assets/staff_bio_publications/McDonald_Research_Participants_View_2012.pdf

CHAPTER 14

IDENTIFYING AND EVALUATING MULTIPLE SOURCES OF INFORMATION

RHODA SCHERMAN

CHAPTER OVERVIEW

This chapter covers the following topics:

- Information literacy
- Identifying sources of knowledge
- Primary and secondary sources
- Scoping and filtering the information
- Evaluating the content
- Growth of the internet
- The role of social media as a source of knowledge
- What to do when the research has limitations

KEY TERMS

Filter

Information literacy

Library databases

Peer-review

Primary sources

Scholarly

Secondary sources

Social media

Systematic reviews

Even before developing a research question and (if required) applying for ethical approval, there is a need to see what has already been written on a topic. In fact, whether researching attitudes toward paraplegic athletes, looking at the evidence for promoting breastfeeding, comparing therapeutic practices, or just wanting to be better informed about global warming, getting started requires knowing what research has already been undertaken, what information is already available on the topic, and knowing where to go to get the information.

INFORMATION LITERACY

Information literacy
Competence to access and understand information from appropriate sources.

The ability to identify the best sources, consider how to use the information, and evaluate the material for its quality, rigour, validity and reliability has been referred to as information literacy (Behrens, 1994). According to the American Library Association (1989), 'Ultimately, information literate people are those who have learned how to learn' (p. 1).

Adapting the information literacy definitions, as approved by the Society of College, National and University Libraries and the Chartered Institute of Library and Information Professionals, McMillan and Weyers (2013, p. 120) summarised the seven key thinking skills as the ability to:

1   identify a personal need for information (*identify* information);
2   assess current knowledge and identify gaps (*scope* information);
3   construct strategies for locating information and data (*plan* information);
4   locate and access the information and data needed (*gather* information);
5   review the research processes and compare and evaluate information and data (*evaluate* information);
6   organise information professionally and ethically (*manage* information); and
7   apply the knowledge gained: present the results of personal research, synthesise new and old information and data to create new knowledge, and disseminate in a variety of ways (*present* information).

With so much information available, and from so many different sources, this task might seem insurmountable. Yet, for university students especially, it is an essential skill. It requires considering how to identify sources of knowledge, scope and filter that information, and evaluate the content of the information obtained. It also requires having a critical perspective on the role of the internet and other social media sources.

Filter
Sort elements into categories.

IDENTIFYING SOURCES OF KNOWLEDGE

Information comes to people all the time, in myriad ways, but, quite simply, ideas and facts come from research or scholarship that has been published or otherwise communicated. It is the medium of that publication that varies, usually depending on the discipline from which it originates (McMillan & Weyers, 2013). While not restricted to written sources, in the current academic context most of the sources of information are in written form (see Table 14.1). This is related to what is valued as acceptable *ways of knowing*. Historically, ways of knowing included such mediums as hearsay (accepting the comments of others as truth), authority (as in proclamation of the King or Queen), belief (or faith), and intuition—to name just a few (DePoy & Gitlin, 2011). Nowadays a much higher value is placed on knowledge that is logical, understandable, confirmable and useful—all aspects of the scientific method of research-based knowledge (DePoy & Gitlin, 2011).

TABLE 14.1 SOME EXAMPLES OF MOSTLY WRITTEN SOURCES OF KNOWLEDGE

SOURCE	TYPE
Books	Edited books; textbooks; non-fiction books; experiential stories
Reference books	Encyclopaedias; dictionaries; directories; atlases
Academic journals	Subject-specific publications (print or electronic)
Newspapers	Daily; weekly; national; local
Magazines or periodicals	National; international; discipline-specific
Reports	Research; private; public
Dissertations and theses	Doctoral; Masters; Honours
Internet*	Blogs; wikis; columns; commentaries; social media
Non-written	Lectures; podcasts; presentations; recorded talks

*Internet sources can be all of the above (for example, a portal to those works) or can be works beyond this list. See below for more on the internet.

PRIMARY AND SECONDARY SOURCES

Another common distinction when considering sources of knowledge is that of primary and secondary sources (Cottrell, 2005; McMillan & Weyers, 2013). While these distinctions will vary, depending on the discipline from which the information comes, generally speaking, primary sources are first-hand sources, from the time and place of the events being considered. They present original thought that has not been filtered or otherwise interpreted. (see Table 14.2).

Secondary sources References to publications or research that are found within another publication or source.

Primary sources Acknowledged research findings traceable to their original sources.

TABLE 14.2 EXAMPLES OF PRIMARY AND SECONDARY SOURCES OF
KNOWLEDGE

PRIMARY	SECONDARY
Peer-reviewed journal articles	Books (or other writings) from an after-the-fact perspective
Conference or meeting proceedings	Textbooks
Newspaper articles	Biographies
Surveys and other raw research data	Meta-analyses of other studies
Interviews	Magazine articles
Letters and diaries	Secondary interviews (e.g. what was heard from the witnesses)
Audio and video recordings	Dictionaries and encyclopedias
Works of art and photographs	Commentaries
Books and autobiographies	Histories

Peer-review
The process of appropriately qualified individuals evaluating work for the purpose of maintaining quality.

Systematic reviews
A specific process for analysing similar studies for the purpose of informing practice and practitioners.

Secondary sources, on the other hand, are usually materials with an after-the-fact, filtered perspective. These are interpretations, analyses or evaluations of the primary sources. However, this is not an absolute distinction; for example, a biography of a world leader would generally be considered a secondary source, but might include original interview materials, which would be primary sources. Even peer-review journal articles can be secondary sources if there is a reliance on the interpretation of another person's research. On the other hand, meta-analyses and systematic reviews would be examples of secondary data that, due to the robustness associated with these methods, are considered more like primary sources, as they provide comprehensive evidence.

Primary sources are always preferred over secondary sources. For example, it is better to access the original journal article than to cite the textbook in which the information was found. Nonetheless, sometimes a secondary source is all that can be obtained.

SCOPING AND FILTERING THE INFORMATION

Once the appropriate sources have been identified and locating the information has begun there is a need to filter the information, since there will probably be much more information available on any given topic than will be needed or that there will be time to review. This does not involve evaluating the *quality* of the materials, but rather sorting through the information for its scope, relevance and usefulness—in other words, determining what sources might be useful, how they might be useful and where the information might sit. For example, a newspaper clipping might not be the best source of empirical evidence for a literature review, but it might offer some local context (Cottrell, 2005). Likewise, a journal article is the logical place to find research evidence but may lack the scope of the overarching topic. It is important to understand that while there should be a goal to work from reliable and valid sources, not all information will originate from within academic, peer-reviewed experimental reports. Each source, regardless of where it is published, requires evaluation.

CASE STUDY 14.1

THE EXAMPLE OF CYBER BULLYING

Imagine that you are writing a paper on cyber bullying. You suspect that the library must have something about it, so you jump on your computer and, after getting into the electronic AUT Library, you find an eBook and a journal article on the subject. You then put the word 'cyberbullying' into your favourite search engine, and from that you get a link to Wikipedia and find an article in the *New Zealand Herald*.

Below are excerpts from all four of these different sources (Wikipedia, newspaper, book and journal article, respectively), each of which offers some information on the topic of cyber bullying. Read over each excerpt and then consider: (1) what kind of information it can offer your report; and (2) where it might be used in your report, if at all.

Cyberbullying

From Wikipedia, the free encyclopedia

Cyberbullying is the use of the Internet and related technologies to harm other people, in a deliberate, repeated, and hostile manner. As it has become more common in society, particularly among young people, legislation and awareness campaigns have arisen to combat it ...

Cyberbullying vs. cyberstalking

The practice of cyberbullying is not limited to children and, while the behavior is identified by the same definition when practiced by adults, the distinction in age groups sometimes refers to the abuse as cyberstalking or cyberharassment when perpetrated by adults toward adults. Common

(continued next page)

RHODA SCHERMAN

tactics used by cyberstalkers are performed in public forums, social media or online information sites and are intended to threaten a victim's earnings, employment, reputation, or safety...

Anon. Retrieved from http://en.wikipedia.org/wiki/Cyber-bullying

Govt speeds cyber bullying laws

By Simon Collins

6:49 AM Thursday Apr 4, 2013

Inciting someone to commit suicide will be punishable with up to three years in jail under tough new cyber-bullying laws to be unveiled today. The new laws, fast-tracked by Justice Minister Judith Collins after a Herald campaign to 'stop the bullying' last year, will also create a new offence of using a communications device to cause harm, punishable with up to three months in jail or a $2000 fine ... The proposed new offence of incitement to suicide will apply to all forms of incitement, not just through texting or the internet. It is already a crime to incite someone to suicide if the victim does actually attempt.

Collins, S. (2013) Govt speeds cyber bullying laws. *New Zealand Herald.* Retrieved from http://www.nzherald.co.nz/nz/news/ article.cfm?c_id=1&objectid=10875273

Confronting cyber-bullying: what schools need to know to control misconduct and avoid legal consequence

As technologies evolve and advance at rapid rates and children are immersed in them at increasingly younger ages—and as adolescents become proficient and comfortable with social networking sites, blogs, chat rooms, and mobile phones—many adults, whose use of computers is limited to e-mail and word processing, find themselves incapacitated and left behind ... This book also discusses the extent and potential of cyber-bullying to spread in countries with large populations such as India and China. The international research also discloses a tendency in Asia, like the West, to adopt a punitive rather than educational approach, although a number of interesting cultural nuances are disclosed.

Shariff, S. (2008). *Confronting Cyber-bullying: What Schools Need to Know to Control Misconduct and Avoid Legal Consequences.* New York: Cambridge Books Online. Retrieved from http://ebooks.cambridge.org/ ebook.jsf?bid=CBO9780511551260

Students' perspectives on cyber bullying

Abstract

The aim of this study was to gain a better understanding of the impact of cyber bullying on students and the possible need for prevention messages targeting students, educators, and parents. A total of 148 middle and high school students were interviewed during focus groups held at two middle and two high schools in a public school district ... We found that students' comments during the focus groups suggest that students—particularly females—view cyber bullying as a problem, but one rarely discussed at school, and that students do not see the school district personnel as helpful resources when dealing with cyber bullying...

Agatston, P. W., Kowalski, R., & Limber, S. (2007). Students' perspectives on cyber bullying. *Journal of Adolescent Health, 41* (6 Suppl.), S59–S60.

EVALUATING THE CONTENT

After locating the literature and beginning to filter and sort through the materials, it is time to begin evaluating the content. This stage in the process requires critical thinking skills to carefully examine and analyse the evidence to assess its validity and worth (O'Shea, 2000); this involves being systematic and persistent, and other attributes, including:

- objectivity;
- scepticism;
- intellectual curiosity;
- open-mindedness;
- flexibility of thought;
- tolerance of uncertainty;
- intellectual honesty; and
- reflection.

Reduced to its essence, there are five basic steps to evaluating research (Burton, 2010; Law, Stewart, Letts, Pollock, Bosch, & Westmorland, 1998; Law, Stewart, Pollock, Letts, Bosch, & Westmorland, 1998a; O'Shea, 2002). (See Table 14.3 for the five steps along with a breakdown of each step.)

TABLE 14.3 FIVE BASIC STEPS TO EVALUATING RESEARCH EVIDENCE*

1 Identify the source.	Where	• The most important of the three questions about the source. • Peer-reviewed or refereed sources are best, as they undergo a rigorous examination process before acceptance for publication. • Sources such as newspapers, magazines and some internet sources often lack scrutiny.
	When	• This is the date of publication. • In general, you want to review more recent literature (currency), as it will be more up-to-date and relevant. • However, past (seminal) research can also be important as it will have shaped current research.
	Who	• Not as important as *Where* and *When* from a 'critical thinking' perspective. • It is still useful information, as it may provide insight into a study, especially if the author is well-published. • It may also be important from an ethical standpoint, to ensure no conflicts of interest.
2 Analyse the arguments.		Critical questions to ask: • Does the evidence support the argument? • Does it support what I already know? • Does it contradict other evidence? • Have both/all sides of the argument been addressed? • Have alternative explanations been offered?
3 Examine the research methodology.	Sample	• Who were the participants and how were they recruited? • Was there justification for the quantity (size) of participants? • Were they 'representative'—broadly or narrowly? • (*If not*) Why were they sought or selected? • Are there any stated or observed limitations?
	Measures	• Were the constructs clearly defined? • What tests were used? Were they valid and reliable? • If involving surveys, was the construction explained? Tested? • If qualitative, did the researcher explain how data were collected?

	Procedure	• What steps were involved in gathering the data? • How rigorously were the tests/tools administered? • Was there consistency with research methodology or protocols?
4 Evaluate the results.		• Do you understand the analyses? • Are the results presented clearly? • Have the appropriate analyses been used? • Do the results appear to support the hypothesis? • (*If not*) Has the researcher acknowledged this? • Are the results interpreted with insight? • (*If quantitative*) Are the *p*-values or statistical significance stated? • (*If qualitative*) Is the method of interpretation explained?
5 Analyse the conclusions.	Interpretations	• In the final discussion section, researchers share their interpretation of the findings. • Here the researchers can be creative, but their conclusions must still be anchored in logic and evidence. • You need to assess their conclusions, as well as the importance of the study's findings, weighed against any limitations (stated by the author or noted by you).
	Limitations	Does the author acknowledge the study's limitations? Possible areas of discussion include: • Generalisability of findings; • Sample size and representativeness; • Extraneous variables; • Validity/reliability (*quantitative*); • Trustworthiness (*qualitative*).

*See Law, Stewart, Pollock, Letts, Bosch, and Westmorland (1998b) for useful critical review forms for interpreting and evaluating quantitative research.

In the spirit of teaching *critical thought*, I note here that the research literature on 'how to critique research literature' has a major limitation of its own, in that it favours quantitative research over qualitative research. This is evident in the stage summaries above, which emphasise the review processes for the features of quantitative analyses, such as the use of measures, confirming or refuting hypotheses, and concepts like validity and reliability. Far less has been written on the process of critically reviewing qualitative research, which requires the same level of critical thought, but which may involve a different set of analytic tools. See Chapter 3 for more on qualitative research, and Chapter 18 for a look at other critiquing tools.

GROWTH OF THE INTERNET

For people who have studied more than a decade or so ago, the primary source of information was that found in physical libraries. However, locating information now is as close as a computer keyboard, where the internet may be the first—if not only—source of knowledge people are familiar with. There are a lot of benefits to living in the current *information age*, with the internet offering quick, easy and convenient access to literally thousands of knowledge sources. There is a downside, however, as that ease can lead to the temptation for academic dishonesty and plagiarism (Ross, 2005), such as 'cutting and pasting' through countless websites and electronic pages. In light of the many limitations associated with using online sources—an uncertainty of the truth of what is posted, who has written it, and how current or reliable the information is—the question arises of whether or not lecturers should exclude the internet from the allowable sources for academic assignments. At a minimum, a higher level of critique is required when using these tools. In response to that question, Anderson (2012) had this to say:

> The reality is we use Google for our own information needs, so why should we expect the students to only use what we want them to use? The consensus on this is that we should teach students how to search both Google and databases effectively. (p. 20)

With a similar aim in mind, Jerz (2012) outlines a couple of important questions to ask of the online articles:

- Does the article conclude with a bibliography or a reference list?
  - A *bibliography* is a list of any information sources that an author may consult in preparation for the article, but it does not guarantee that any of that information made it into the paper.
  - A *reference list* is the list of information sources that should link up to the 'in-text' citations. The reference list allows the reader to locate those sources directly, and verify what the author has said.
- Does the source specify the author, publisher, and date?
  - If *no*: it is not the kind of information source for an academic paper.
  - If *yes*: the next question you should ask is: 'Is the author someone trustworthy?' To answer that, revisit the steps to reviewing literature in Table 14.3.

People looking online for academic, peer-reviewed literature are much less likely to find it via a standard search, as it is often locked behind the 'pay walls' (Jerz, 2012, p. 1) of subscription-based publications, and only accessible through libraries, which often pay for access to the most popular journals. On the other hand, it might be challenging to locate scholarly articles on current or local events. In such cases, the internet might be the perfect place to locate non-academic literature, such as newspaper articles, magazine stories, and opinion pieces, that can provide insight into local or current events, while the scholarly articles provide the research evidence (Jerz, 2012). Another option is to consider the choice of search engine, as not all search engines are alike. *GoogleScholar* is an example of a search engine that gives preference to the 'scholarly' articles, and while it is not as comprehensive or robust as the library databases, most of the items it finds will be academic and probably peer-reviewed sources.

Scholarly
Relating to rigorously exploring, sharing and developing knowledge.

Library databases
Tools for cataloguing information that enable many sources to be searched.

THE ROLE OF SOCIAL MEDIA AS A SOURCE OF KNOWLEDGE

The internet is more than just Google or Wikipedia. It is the home of a host of social media sites that sometimes serve as information sources. (See Table 14.4 for a list of the major social media websites).

Social media
Technological tools that enable communication to be interactive.

TABLE 14.4 SOME SOCIAL MEDIA SITES

CATEGORIES	EXAMPLE SITES
Collaborative projects	Wikipedi; Basecamp; GoogleDocs; Yammer; Huddle
Blogs and microblogs	Twitter; Tumblr; Weibo; Ping.fm
Content communities	YouTube; Flickr; Travbuddy; SlideShare; Vimeo; iTunes (podcasts)
Social networking sites	Facebook; MySpace; Tagged; Bebo; MyYearbook; LiveJournal; Blauk
Professional networking	LinkedIn; ResearchGate; XING; Viadeo
Social bookmarking	Pinterest; Digg; Delicious; Diigo; StumbleUpon
Social news	Digg; Reddit; Newsvine; Mixx
Virtual worlds	World of Warcraft; Second Life; Vitrue; Gaia Online

The above list is neither comprehensive nor definitive. The categories and examples are loosely based on the work of Kaplan and Haenlein (2010) and Hodges, Jones, and Morgan (2010).

Facebook, for instance, is one of the most popular and most accessed social media sites on the internet (Fowler, 2012); and while it may fuel our need to belong, give us a self-esteem boost when people 'like' our posts, or even offer some social capital (the accumulation of social support, including career leads, that come from having a Facebook profile; Winerman, 2013), is it a place to get information? Apparently it is, as an increasing number of university academics are creating class-based Facebook pages. According to Chamberlin (2013), 'while some begrudge the ubiquitous distraction of social media, others are using Facebook to build community in their classes' (p. 60). Using Facebook to connect with students, the lecturers can offer study tips, post amusing and interesting facts and clips, and answer assignment questions—all of which seems to boost learning, promote solidarity and create a deeper appreciation for the subject matter (Chamberlin, 2013). Innovative academic environments are also tapping into other social media sites like iTunes U, where lectures are uploaded, allowing people from all over the world to 'sit in' on a class (Miller, 2013). YouTube is another social media site where students can find information of a visual nature. The internet is growing daily (Finley, 2011) and as a consequence it is changing the way we access, view and use information—and possibly even the way we think (Carr, 2012). Despite the easy access, now more than ever there is a need to approach online information with a very critical lens.

RESEARCH ALIVE 14.1
WIKIPEDIA: IS IT A RELIABLE SOURCE?

Raise your hand if you've ever used Wikipedia as an information source while doing research. Now look around. Well, of course you can't see the others, but trust me when I tell you that there are a lot of raised hands—mine included!! This clever, collaborative, social networking site is one of the most contentious subjects in the realm of information literacy.

> While some would argue that it is not a scholarly tool, Wikipedia is a good example of how openness and social productivity can be used to create a knowledge resource ... Since its creation in 2001 Wikipedia has ... allowed more than 77,000 contributors to create 22 million articles in 285 languages ... [and] has become the encyclopedia of choice for much of the world attracting 470 million unique visitors a month as of February 2012. (Lewis, 2013, p. 166)

Believing it to be an interesting social experiment in the compilation and coding of knowledge, Denning, Horning, Parnas and Weinstein (2005) argue that 'without more formal content-inclusion and expert review procedures' (p. 152)

Wikipedia will never attain the status of a true encyclopaedia. They've outlined the six major risks associated with Wikipedia as an information source:

Accuracy: not knowing the accuracy of the content, which can be exacerbated by lack of references;

Motives: not knowing the motivations or biases of editors;

Expertise: not knowing the expertise of editors;

Stability: not knowing the stability of an article and how much it may change between viewings;

Coverage: irregular coverage of topics;

Sources: citation information is unreliable and may come from hidden or non-independent sources.

Yet, despite knowing that the quality of the information will vary enormously, a large percentage of university students continue to rely on Wikipedia as an information source for academic purposes (Denning et al., 2005; Head & Eisenberg, 2010; Kim, Sin & Yoo-Lee, 2013; Kittur, Suh, & Chi, 2008).

Encouragingly, research has also found that when students do access Wikipedia, it is not as a singular source of knowledge. Instead, it is used to quickly assess background information and to check against other sources (Kim et al., 2013), as well as to find the meaning of related terms (Head & Eisenberg, 2010). As for why this unauthenticated, seemingly unreliable site is so popular, Fast and Campbell (2004) suggest that when compared with other web-based online public access catalogues (those that our libraries use), students prefer the simpler and more useable interface offered by Wikipedia, Google and other internet search engines.

So what do students do to check the trustworthiness and rigour of information gleaned from Wikipedia? Some students will compare the content against other sources; others check the references provided for indicators of quality (Kim et al., 2013), and many use the information in combination with other sources (Head & Eisenberg, 2010).

These studies are not without their own limitations, related primarily to both being based on North American university student populations only. And while they make an important contribution to a fairly new field of study, much more research is needed to better understand the information literacy needs, trends, and perceptions of university students.

Nonetheless, based on the current body of research, it's been suggested that:

1   students know the limitations associated with using Wikipedia as a source of knowledge;

2   students are in no hurry to stop using it and other social network sites as sources of evidence; and

[continued next page]

RHODA SCHERMAN

3   teachers of research and information literacy need to acknowledge the appeal of such sites and, instead of trying to pry students away from them, should aim to arm students with the skills to be more critical consumers of the information gleaned from these internet sites.

One possibility is that distrust of wiki content is not due to the inherently mutable nature of the system but instead to the lack of available information for judging trustworthiness...Given the right information, readers can make more informed judgments of the trustworthiness of content, which may increase overall trust in the system. (Kittur et al., 2008, p. 4)

It might surprise you to know that the Gerald R. Ford Presidential Library and the British Museum both have a 'Wikipedian in Residence' whose jobs it is to link between their institutions and the Wikipedia community (New, 2013). This is one example of how Wikipedia might eventually gain some of the credibility that it currently lacks.

WHAT TO DO WHEN THE RESEARCH HAS LIMITATIONS

Having considered how to identify, filter and evaluate literature, it is also important to know what to do when it seems impossible to find the answers to questions or the information available is obviously flawed, weak or incomplete.

Finding weak or poorly written work *is a good thing*! Identifying weaknesses in available work provides an opportunity for critical thinking and the development of an argument or debate.

SUMMARY

The concept of information literacy has key components of identifying, filtering and evaluating literature. The process of *identifying* literature requires an appreciation of different sources of knowledge—both traditional, written sources and the more recent online sources. It also encompasses a sound understanding of the differences between *primary* and *secondary* sources of knowledge. *Filtering* information involves determining how best to utilise a resource, and where it might fit in a research report or essay.

The last step, once literature has been identified, located and filtered, is to critically *evaluate* it. This includes identifying and critiquing the source (or author), the arguments, the methodology, the results and the conclusions. The growth of the *internet* and its many *social media* sites, means more sources of knowledge are available to us than ever before. The ease of access and the uncertainty of the quality of the information available from the internet require that we be even more cautious with online resources. Therefore, students are encouraged to learn how to judge the quality of information coming from the internet and other social media sites like Facebook and Wikipedia.

REFLECTION POINTS

- How information-literate are you?
- What skills do you need to locate, filter and evaluate literature?
- How confident are you at critically evaluating internet sources?
- Should students be allowed to cite from the internet's non-academic sources?
- How confident would you be to use video-based online sources?
- What do you do when you don't find the quality research you seek?

STUDY QUESTIONS

1   What are the skills associated with information literacy?
2   Why is it better to use primary (as opposed to secondary) sources of data?
3   What's the value in scoping or filtering research literature after it has been located, but before it is evaluated?
4   When writing an essay or research report, what kinds of information would be easily obtained from the internet and which elements would be better retrieved from the library databases?
5   How do university students use Wikipedia and other internet sources when completing academic assignments?
6   What are the major concerns with using Wikipedia as a source of knowledge for an academic assignment?
7   Can internet sources ever be reliable enough to use in academic assignments?
8   What are the main steps to critically reviewing and evaluating research literature?

ADDITIONAL READING

Baker, R., Matulich, E., & Papp, R. (2007). Teach me in the way I Learn: Education and the internet generation. *Journal of College Teaching and Learning*, 4(4), 27–32. Retrieved from http://journals.cluteonline.com/index.php/TLC/article/view/1613

Beal, V. (2010). The difference between the Internet and World Wide Web. *Webopedia*. Retrieved from http://www.webopedia.com/DidYouKnow/Internet/2002/Web_vs_Internet.asp

Block, J. J. (2008). Issues for DSM-V: Internet addiction. *American Journal of Psychiatry, 156*(3), 306–307. Retrieved from http://ajp.psychiatryonline.org/article.aspx?articleID=99602.

Facione, P., & Gittens, C. A. (2013). *Think critically.* Pearson: New York.

Griffiths, J. R., & Brophy, P. (2005). Student searching behavior and the Web: Use of academic resources and Google. *Library Trends, 53*(4), 539–554. Retrieved from https://www.ideals.illinois.edu/handle/2142/1749

Sparrow, B., Liu, J., & Wegner, D. M. (2011). Google effects on memory: Cognitive consequences of having information at our fingertips. Science, *333*(6043), 776–778.

REFERENCES

Agatston, P. W., Kowalski, R., & Limber, S. (2007). Students' perspectives on cyber bullying. *Journal of Adolescent Health, 41*(6 SUPPL.), S59–S60.

Anon (n.d.). Cyberbullying. *Wikipedia.* Retrieved from http://en.wikipedia.org/wiki/Cyberbullying#cite_ref-definitions.uslegal.com_1-1

American Library Association (1989). *Presidential Committee on Information Literacy. Final report.* Retrieved from http://www.ala.org/acrl/publications/whitepapers/presidential

Anderson, M. A. (2012). Google literacy lesson plans: Way beyond 'just Google it'. *Internet@Schools, 19*(4), 20–22,4. Retrieved from http://ezproxy.aut.ac.nz/login?url=http://search.proquest.com/docview/1039289315?accountid=8440

Behrens, S. J. (1994). A conceptual analysis and historical overview of information literacy. *College and Research Libraries, 55*(4), 309–22.

Burton, L. (2010). *An interactive approach to writing essays & research reports in psychology.* Milton: John Wiley & Sons.

Carr, N. (2012). Is Google making us stupid? What the Internet is doing to our brains. *The Atlantic.* Retrieved from http://www.theatlantic.com/magazine/archive/2008/07/is-google-making-us-stupid/306868

Chamberlin, J. (2013). 'Like' it, or not. *APA Monitor, 44*(3), 60.

Collins, S. (2013, 4 April). Govt speeds cyber bullying laws. *New Zealand Herald.* Retrieved from http://www.nzherald.co.nz/nz/news/article.cfm?c_id=1&objectid=10875273

Cottrell, S. (2005). *Critical thinking skills: Developing effective analysis and argument.* New York: Palgrave MacMillan.

Denning, P., Horning, J., Parnas, D., & Weinstein, L. (2005). Wikipedia risks. *Communications of the ACM, 48*(12), 152.

DePoy, E. & Gitlin, L. N. (2011). *Introduction to research: Understanding and applying multiple strategies* (4th ed.). St. Louis, MO: Mosby.

Fast, K. V. & Campbell, D. G. (2004). 'I still like Google': University student perceptions of searching OPACs and the Web. *Proceedings of the American Society for Information Science and Technology, 41*(1), 138–146.

Finley, K. (2011). Was Eric Schmidt wrong about the historical scale of the Internet? *ReadWrite*, 7 February. Retrieved from http://readwrite.com/2011/02/07/are-we-really-creating-as-much

Fowler, G. (2012, 4 October). Facebook: One billion and counting. *The Wall Street Journal*. Retrieved from http://online.wsj.com/article/SB10000872396390443635404578036164027386112.html.

Head, A. J. & Eisenberg, M. B. (2010). How today's college students use Wikipedia for course-related research. *First Monday, 15*(3). Retrieved from http://www.firstmonday.org/htbin/cgiwrap/bin/ojs/index.php/fm/article/viewArticle/2830/2476

Hodges, A., Jones, G., & Morgan, N. (2010). *The complete guide to social media: From the social media guys*. Retrieved from http://www.thesocialmediaguys.co.uk/resources

Jerz, D. G. (2012). *Research essays: Evaluating online sources of academic papers. Jerz's Literacy Weblog, Seton Hill University*. Retrieved from http://jerz.setonhill.edu/writing/academic1/research-essays-evaluating-online-sources

Kaplan, A. M. & Haenlein, M. (2010). Users of the world, unite! The challenges and opportunities of social media. *Business Horizons, 53*, 58–68.

Kim, K. S., Sin, S. C. J., & Yoo-Lee, E. Y. (2013). Undergraduates' use of social media as information sources. *College and Research Libraries*. Retrieved from http://crl.acrl.org/content/early/2013/02/06/crl13-455.short.

Kittur, A., Suh, B., & Chi, E. H. (2008). Can you ever trust a wiki? Impacting perceived trustworthiness in Wikipedia. *Proceedings of the Computer Supported Cooperative Work (CSCW) Conference*, 8–12 November, San Diego, California, USA. Retrieved from http://dl.acm.org/citation.cfm?id=1460563&picked=prox&CFID=278590549&CFTOKEN=57845011.

Law, M., Stewart, D., Letts, L., Pollock, N., Bosch, J., & Westmorland, M. (1998). Guidelines for the critical review of qualitative studies. McMaster University Occupational Therapy Evidence-Based Practice Research Group. Retrieved from http://www.musallamusf.com/resources/Qualitative-Lit-Analysis-pdf.pdf.

Law, M., Stewart, D., Pollock, N., Letts, L., Bosch, J., & Westmorland, M. (1998a). *Guidelines for critical review of the literature: Quantitative studies.* McMaster University Occupational Therapy Evidence-Based Practice Research Group. Retrieved from http://fhs.mcmaster.ca/rehab/ebp/pdf/quanguidelines.pdf.

Law, M., Stewart, D., Pollock, N., Letts, L., Bosch, J., & Westmorland, M. (1998b). *Critical review form—Quantitative studies. McMaster University.* Retrieved from http://www.srs-mcmaster.ca/Portals/20/pdf/ebp/quanreview.pdf

Lewis, D. W. (2013). From stacks to the Web: The transformation of academic library collecting. *College and Research Libraries, March,* 159–176. Retrieved from https://scholarworks.iupui.edu/bitstream/handle/1805/3252/DLewis%20Stacks%20to%20Web.pdf?sequence=1.

McMillan, K. & Weyers, J. (2013). *How to improve your critical thinking & reflective skills.* Essex: Pearson.

Miller, A. (2013). Tuning to psychology. *APA Monitor, 44*(1), 28.

New, J. (2013, 28 January). Ford Presidential Library hires a 'Wikipedian in Residence'. *Chronicle of Higher Education.* Retrieved from http://chronicle.com/article/U-of-Michigan-Masters/136847

O'Shea, R. P. (2000). *Writing for psychology: An introductory guide for students* (3rd ed.). Sydney: Harcourt.

Ross, K. A. (2005). Academic dishonesty and the Internet. *Communications of the ACM, 48*(10), 29–31.

Shariff, S. (2008). *Confronting cyber-bullying: What schools need to know to control misconduct and avoid legal consequences.* New York: Cambridge Books Online. Retrieved from http://ebooks.cambridge.org.ezproxy.aut.ac.nz/ebook.jsf?bid=CBO9780511551260

Winerman, L. (2013). What draws us to Facebook? *APA Monitor, 44*(3), 56.

WEBSITES

Basic and advanced search tips:
    http://www4.uwm.edu/secu/policies/upload/Search-Tips.pdf

Boolean search tips:
    http://talent.linkedin.com/assets/Product-Pages/Training/TipSheet-BooleanSearching.pdf

Editing Wikipedia:
    http://en.wikipedia.org/wiki/Help:Editing

Google in education:
http://www.google.com/edu

Google lesson overview:
http://www.google.com/insidesearch/searcheducation/lesson-overview.html

Google lesson plan map:
http://www.google.com/insidesearch/searcheducation/lesson-map.html

iTunes U:
https://edu-vpp.apple.com/qforms/start/itu?dst=enroll_
marcom&pdname=itunesu#main:enroll_marcom:NEW_RECORD@itunesu@null@
null@true

Presidential Library gets a 'Wikipedian in Residence':
https://chronicle.com/blogs/wiredcampus/michigan-student-is-first-wikipedian-in-
residence-at-a-presidential-librarySearch tips and tricks:
http://www.google.com/insidesearch/tipstricks/index.html

YouTube TED talk on the new media:
http://www.youtube.com/watch?v=LeaAHv4UTI8

CHAPTER 15

PRESENTING AND PUBLISHING RESEARCH

KEITH TUDOR

CHAPTER OVERVIEW

This chapter covers the following topics:

- Reading
- Writing
- Editing
- Presenting
- Publishing
- Future directions

KEY TERMS

Editing
Presenting
Publishing
Reading
Writing

It is tempting to think that undertaking research is the ultimate goal, and its completion is the final stage or process and achievement. From a perspective that focuses only on research, study and findings, that may be true. On the other hand, when research is not published in the public domain, it is inaccessible and, therefore, in a sense does not exist. For the purposes of this chapter, the concept of research encompasses clinical, conceptual, empirical and experimental, and interdisciplinary research (Leuzinger-Bohleber, 2006), and the chapter discusses and offers practical guidance as to what happens *after* the student completes their assignment or paper, or the researcher completes their research. It is based on distinguishing between, on the one hand, research itself, and, on the other hand, writing, editing, presenting and publishing as four distinct phases of a process from research to publication—and, by means of practical exercises and tips about these processes, to encourage those who may get stuck at any of the phases prior to publication.

There are a lot of myths about writing. One is that everyone and anyone can write; another is that writing is easy; and another is that writing is difficult! This chapter is based on three assumptions: first, that writing for publication requires a set of skills that people need to understand and develop; second, that most students and researchers, in addition to having something to say and being inspired to say it, need to learn both the craft and the discipline of writing; and, third, that writing can be fun and a great expression of creativity which can be done anywhere, anytime.

Writing
The process of developing a written piece of work.

Editing
Selecting and preparing information in a variety of media for publication or presentation through a process of review and crafting. It involves correction, condensation and other modifications of the original text or medium.

Presenting
The process of sharing information.

Publishing
The process of having research scrutinised and promulgated to an audience in a particular medium.

READING

CASE STUDY 15.1

INSIGHTS INTO READING

Stephen King, one of the most successful fiction writers of all time explains that reading assists with the writing process: 'If you want to be a writer, you must do two things above all others: read a lot and write a lot. There's no way around these two things that I'm aware of, no shortcut' (King, 2000, p. 164). With regard to reading, the student and researcher need to read and in some way analyse or process the literature which forms the background to their research, source material and data, but, beyond that, it is also useful to read newspapers, novels, poetry, blogs and so on, in order to appreciate and learn about what makes for good—and bad—writing. Apart from the particular content, reading helps writers appreciate language, the use of metaphor, sentence structure and, even in relatively short pieces, how to structure a piece of writing, whether a newspaper column, an article, a chapter or a poem.

Reading
The process of engaging with published information.

KEITH TUDOR

Reading gives the reader an *experience* of what they like and *what* works, at least for them. A reader does not have to know that the first line of Shakespeare's Sonnet XII— 'When I do count the clock that tells the time'—is an iambic pentameter, but knowing and studying form and structure can help understand *how* things work (of which more in the section below on editing).

RESEARCH ALIVE 15.1
EXERCISES TO ASSIST WITH READING

Exercise 1: Find in something you read every day (such as a newspaper, magazine or website) a sentence that you like. Think about why you like it. What is good about the sentence? How and why does it work?

Exercise 2: Find in the same sources a sentence that you do not like. Think about why you don't like it. What is not so good about it? How and why does it not work?

Tip 1: Collect favourite writings: sayings and quotations.

This tradition, of having a 'commonplace book' dates back to the fifteenth century CE and can, over time, become a great source of inspiration and a practical resource of quotations for the student, researcher and author.

WRITING

Writers write. A good working definition of a writer is someone who always has some means of writing to hand, whether this is a laptop, electronic tablet, smart phone, or paper and pen or pencil. One of the many ways in which people can put off or procrastinate about writing is not to write or not to have the means for writing to hand.

Part of the discipline of and commitment to becoming and being a writer is that you find a way of writing anywhere, anytime. At the same time, it is true that every writer has their own preferences about writing: typing on a computer keyboard or writing with a pen or pencil in a book; writing on a desk or curled up on a sofa; being inside or outside; writing in the morning, afternoon, evening or at night; writing in silence or with radio or music in the background; writing alone or with others; writing in a 'room of one's own', as Virginia Woolf (1929) proposed, or in public, as did J. K. Rowling when she wrote the first Harry Potter novel in Nicholson's café in Edinburgh, Scotland. A number of writers have written about writing, and all of them in one way or another describe the discipline of writing.

CASE STUDY 15.2

WRITING IS DOING

On one writing workshop, after spending some time in which we had gathered, checked-in with each other and had lunch, my co-facilitator and I began to set up a writing exercise when one of the participants interrupted and said: 'You mean we're going to write? I thought we were going to *talk* about writing'! After a pause, the participant laughed as she realised what she had said, and this was followed by more shared laughter; importantly, my co-facilitator and I set up the first writing exercise and got the participants writing. While it was tempting to talk further *about* writing, it was more important to facilitate people actually *writing*.

While it is important that the student, researcher and writer find their own room or space, one of the myths about writing is that people always need long, uninterrupted time and, although this is often both welcome and useful, for most people it is unaffordable. Interestingly, Woolf's other proposition for women writers—she was writing in the context of giving lectures to women students about literal and figural space for women writers—was an income. For some people who are trying to write, having extended periods of time simply means that they spend more time procrastinating. A useful discipline is to write in short time frames, right down to 10 minutes and, indeed, some people do better having only a short period of time such as half an hour and then stopping or pausing.

RESEARCH ALIVE 15.2
EXERCISES TO ASSIST WITH WRITING

Exercise 3: If you tend to edit yourself and/or be a bit of a perfectionist, experiment with just writing on a particular subject—without editing! If you tend to let the writing flow (and perhaps too much so), then experiment with writing a particular word length, say 500 words, or for a specific time, say 20 minutes, on a specific subject.

Exercise 4: Experiment with writing with different means, in different places and at different times. Find what works for you.

Writing involves both creativity and discipline (that is, inspiration and perspiration) and different people, and people at different times, need these in different proportions: some people need encouragement to flow and others need structure to write to task and within word limits. There are many techniques, tips and exercises to help with this and writers, both budding and experienced, can benefit from participating in writing workshops—there is great learning to be had from writing, and learning about writing, in groups, and in sharing the fears and joys of writing. Another great writer who also wrote about writing was George Orwell, the English essayist. In his essay on 'Politics and the English Language' (Orwell, 1946), he identified a number of 'rules' for writing (see Case Study 15.3).

CASE STUDY 15.3

RULES FOR EFFECTIVE WRITING

George Orwell expounded his own rules for effective writing (Orwell, 1946):

- Never use a metaphor, simile, or other figure of speech which you are used to seeing in print.
- Never use a long word where a short one will do.
- If it is possible to cut a word out, always cut it out.
- Never use the passive where you can use the active.
- Never use a foreign phrase, a scientific word, or a jargon word if you can think of an everyday English equivalent.

And Orwell added that these rules should be broken rather than saying—or writing—anything 'outright barbarous'.

In terms of the micro-skill of writing and crafting sentences and paragraphs, the days of learning grammar and of parsing a sentence—that is, analysing a sentence by its component categories and functions—have, by and large, gone, with the result that perhaps the majority of people writing simply do not know or are unfamiliar with parts of speech (the noun, pronoun, verb, adjective, adverb, preposition, conjunction, and interjection), or the correct use of punctuation marks (the comma, semicolon, colon, apostrophe) (see Case Study 15.4 below). Again, while these specifics, skills and structures are rarely taught, information about them is now widely retrievable through the internet (see the Additional Reading and Website sections at the end of this chapter).

CASE STUDY 15.4

PUNCTUATION

It is common for writers to misunderstand or misuse basic English punctuation. Understanding the definition and usage of punctuation marks can assist with the writing process and add to the quality of the writing. Table 15.1 gives examples.

TABLE 15.1 PUNCTUATION MARKS AND THEIR USES

PUNCTUATION MARK	NAME	DEFINITION/USE
,	Comma	Used to separate elements within the grammatical structure of a sentence; when there is or needs to be a pause; to separate a series of words.
;	Semicolon	Used to connect independent clauses of a sentence; for long lists (following a colon).
:	Colon	Used to introduce or direct attention to matter: a list, an explanation, a quotation, or such.
.	Full stop or period	Used to mark the end of a sentence.
?	Question or interrogation mark	Used at the end of a sentence to indicate a direct question.
!	Exclamation mark	Used after an exclamation or interjection to indicate a forceful utterance, by thunder!
'	Apostrophe	Used to indicate the omission of a letter or letters from a word ('don't', 'fish "n" chips'), or the possessive case, singular and plural (the author's table, Wayne's conditions, the editors' book).
-	Hyphen (en dash)	Used to connect continuing numbers, such as 1955–2013, or a compound adjective, such as peer-review.
—	Dash (em dash)	Used to denote a sudden change—a wind of change, perhaps, blowing through the common usage of punctuation marks—in construction and sentiment; for oratorical effects, and emphasis; sometimes used instead of parentheses.

[continued next page]

KEITH TUDOR

PUNCTUATION MARK	NAME	DEFINITION/USE
...	Ellipsis	Used to indicate an omission of letters or words (four dots or periods are used to indicate the end of a sentence followed by an omission).
" ... "	Quotation marks	Used as a pair to mark the beginning and end of a quotation from another author or source.
(...)	Parentheses (sometimes referred to as brackets)	Used to amplify or explain a word or phrase in a sentence; to make an aside or a note.
[...]	Brackets	Used for technical notation or explanation, thus: '[sic]'; for a bracketed word or phrases within parentheses (American Psychological Association [APA]).
{ ... }	Braces	Used, principally in mathematics and computer programming, to show that two or more lines or listed items are considered as a unit.
/	Slash or oblique (sometime referred to as a forward slash to distinguish from the backslash ['\'] in general typography)	Used as a substitute for the word 'or' to indicate a choice, often mutually exclusive such as he/she; also to bring things together, as in s/he; to indicate a line break when quoting multiple lines of poetry in prose.

EDITING

All writing—or, at least, all writing for publication—involves editing, and editing again. It requires discipline and attention to detail. Writing for publication also involves other people such as reviewers, editors, publishers and, ultimately and most importantly, readers. This means that, if the writer wants to communicate, then they need to have or to develop empathy for the reader, features of which include making the piece readable (clear, grammatical, and well-structured); and accessible (with the accurate citing and referencing of source material, so that the reader may find and consult it). Submitting a well-written and well-edited manuscript or draft is not only considerate or courteous to the editor or copy-editor, but it is also the mark of a researcher and writer who takes themselves and others seriously.

CASE STUDY 15.5

INSIGHTS INTO EDITING

The process of developing a piece of work for publication takes time and careful consideration. Here are some examples of how well-respected authors experienced the editing process.

Oscar Wilde, the Irish poet, is reported to have said: 'I was working on the proof of one of my poems all the morning, and took out a comma. In the afternoon I put it back again'.

Eric Berne (1966), the founder of transactional analysis, said:

> [Authors] should regard the reputable publication of an article as an honor.... [Their] obligations are the same as those of all writers. The first is integrity, whether it be scientific or artistic, and the second is craftsmanship. Craftsmanship here is almost synonymous with literacy ... By maintaining ruthlessly high literary standards ... [authors] are forced to express themselves gracefully. (p. 194)

Learning to edit helps craft what to say and refines the writing. Some people—and this appears to be a trend among university students—tend to give away or subcontract the editing of their work to someone else. There are two problems with this:

1   If the editor has to do extensive work on the original draft, not only is this time-consuming and irritating, but also there comes a point when the piece becomes so edited that it is, in effect, co-authored. This may then present a problem in terms of authorship, attribution and, particularly, the submission of individual work for assessment or publication.
2   By giving away the task of editing, the author does not learn a crucial part of the craft or skill of writing.

RESEARCH ALIVE 15.3
FURTHER EXERCISES TO ASSIST WITH WRITING

Exercise 5: Take any sentence you have written and cut a word from it.

If you were to do that with the sentence above, you might end up with: 'Take any sentence you have written and edit out a word'.

Exercise 6: Write a poem.

Writing poetry helps to synthesise expression (of thoughts and emotions) and therefore helps to develop editing skills.

Exercise 7: Once you have your final edited draft, print it; find somewhere where you can read it out aloud, and edit it by hand as you read it through.

In doing this, you will pick up mistakes and omissions, particularly in punctuation, and improve the quality of the final version. The longer the piece, the more important this process is. In this process, you may find yourself moving and/or deleting whole sections, and/or realising that you need something else such as another section. Sometimes, extensive deletions may form the basis of another article or publication.

It is tempting not to do this, especially when you are trying to finish something, and especially late at night—but, in any case, just do it! (In following this discipline with regard to this chapter, the author found seven mistakes and two omissions, and made 36 edits and 32 additions!)

Tip 2: Build your experience, competence and capacity as an editor: offer to edit a colleague's work; or offer your services as a peer reviewer to a journal in your area of research, expertise, and/or interest.

All publishers have a 'house style' and word limits so it is important for students, researchers and writers to know what these are and to observe them.

PRESENTING

When writing for publication, the final presentation is usually the responsibility of the publisher—with regard both to the house style and the overall 'look' of the finished product. Within that, the author or contributor to an edition still retains responsibility for the initial finishing and presentation of their piece, for instance, with text interspersed in some way—with pictures, diagrams or, in this present case, text boxes. This is also the case with regard to oral presentations of research with some visual input such as PowerPoint. This perspective is informed by ideas about multiple intelligences (Gardner, 1983), which include spatial intelligence, and about learning styles, which, alongside auditory and kinaesthetic learners, includes visual learners who learn best through linguistic and spatial channels. Eric Berne was clearly a visual learner—and presenter—as he insisted that every piece of transactional analysis theory should be presented with a diagram. His most famous diagram was that of the representation of human personality, based on the three ego states of personality: Parent, Adult and Child (Berne, 1975).

In the book in which this first appeared, Berne (1975) commented on the features of the ego state model as presented in the two-dimensional medium of a diagram on paper, reflecting that 'the Parent was put at the top and the Child at the bottom intuitively' (p. 60). This speaks to the significance of presentation and, in this instance, the importance of both the design and presentation of theory.

RESEARCH ALIVE 15.4
EXERCISES TO ASSIST WITH CHECKING THE FINAL PRESENTATION

Tip 3: Following on from the points about editing (in Research Alive 15.3), check that all figures, tables and boxes in the text have a title, that all authors and works cited in the text appear in the list of references, and that all items in the reference list are referred to in the text.

Tip 4: If, when submitting an article to a journal, you are required to supply key words (for indexing purposes), ensure that you chose words that are key or central to your article—and that they appear in the text!

Tip 5: After you have made all the changes as a result of your final edit, make sure that these changes are integrated into the whole piece.

PUBLISHING

When writing for publication, in whatever form, whether a refereed journal article, a complete journal, a book (edited or authored), a chapter, a thesis, a dissertation, a magazine article, a report, or a review, you are writing in context. Indeed, the order in which these different forms of publication are noted here represent a particular context: in this case, a hierarchy of what is generally considered, at least from an academic perspective, influenced by funding bodies, as the most to the least important type of publication. In any case, the writer is, in effect, writing to task: to have their work published in a particular publication with, usually, a specific audience in mind—and, always, a word limit.

RESEARCH ALIVE 15.5
EXERCISES TO ASSIST WITH SUBMITTING WORK
FOR PUBLICATION

Before submitting an article to a publication and peer review, the researcher and author are advised to:

- research the field thoroughly, a process which is made much easier these days as almost all journals and publishers now have websites;
- compare journals, what the editors say about them, and the type and length of articles they consider;
- check the requirements and 'house style' of respective journals, and read other articles that have been recently published in them.

Different publications have different requirements of the different forms; a 'scientific' journal would rarely accept a poem as part of an article and, if it did, it would pay it little attention; a poetry journal would subject even the shortest submission to rigorous review and generally give detailed feedback. Research of the kind referred to in this book is usually published in peer-reviewed journals—that is, journals in which submitted articles are subjected to review by at least two peers (colleagues in the relevant field). Usually, the process is 'double-blind', a term which refers to the fact that neither the submitting authors or the reviewers are known to each other. This mutual anonymity is designed to ensure fair and unbiased consideration of the submission, to make the process of review, evaluation and feedback rigorous and, thereby, to ensure the quality and integrity of the product—both the article and the publication. This process, however, is under scrutiny in the age of increasing internet publication (Ware, 2008), and in the context of other, cultural considerations, including indigeneity (Street, Baum, & Anderson, 2009).

Following peer review, the editor collates the reviewers' evaluations and sends them to or summarises them for the submitting author. Sometimes the feedback can be quite critical; however, even—perhaps, especially—when the feedback is highly critical, there is always something useful to learn from it and to improve in the revised version of the article, even if it is only to tighten the thesis or argument in response to the criticism or critique. Hence, two of the key qualities of a submitting author are openness or non-defensiveness to evaluation and feedback, and patience, as the process of two or even three rounds of submission, reviews and resubmissions can take a long time. If the submission is rejected, authors should be prepared to correspond with the editor about their submission, and to negotiate with the editor about the focus of a possible revised submission or resubmission.

FUTURE DIRECTIONS

The development of electronic media has had an impact on research itself which, for example, may now use data from online resources such as blogs, as well as on the publication of research which now may be published online in e-journals and e-books. While these forms of 'publication' have been discounted in some quarters as less than rigorous, there are now online publications that have standards of peer review equal to those of print publications. Also, as language is always changing, evolving and adapting to the needs of its users, developments which also include national variations such as Australian or New Zealand English, and variations of form as manifested in e-mails, texting, and so on, so the old 'rules' of writing and grammar are also changing. While aspects of this may be regrettable, such as the widespread use of the split infinitive ('To boldly go'), and the general demise of the adverb ('The boy done good'), the future holds the promise of the acceptance of greater diversity in research methodology and methods and in forms of writing and presentation.

SUMMARY

There are a number of stages or phases in seeing research through to publication: from reading and conducting the research itself, through writing and editing, to presentation and publication. All these phases require specific and distinct skills, and both creativity and discipline. As language and forms of presentation and publication develop and change, so too students, researchers and writers have to adapt and be open to presenting and publishing their research in ways that are accessible to professionals and the public.

REFLECTION POINTS

- What form of writing do you most read? Why, and what do you most learn from it?
- When talking, how much do you edit yourself?
- How comfortable are you speaking in public—or having something permanently in print?

STUDY QUESTIONS

1   What are the different ways in which you could present your research?
2   Why do you think writing style and grammar are changing?

ADDITIONAL READING

Bryson, B. (1997). *Troublesome words* (3rd ed.). London: Penguin.

Parkinson, J. (2007). *i before e (except after c): Old-school ways to remember stuff.* London: Michael O'Mara Books.

Trigg, G. (1979, 19 March). Grammar. *Physics Review Letters, 42*(12), 747–748.

Truss, L. (2003). *Eats shoots and leaves: The zero tolerance approach to punctuation.* London: Profile Books.

Wahlstrom, R. L. (2006). *The tao of writing.* Avon, MA: F&W Publications Co.

REFERENCES

Berne, E. (1966). *Principles of group treatment.* New York, NY: Grove Press.

Berne, E. (1975). *Transactional analysis in psychotherapy.* New York, NY: Souvenir Press. (Original work published 1961)

Gardner, H. (1983). *Frames of mind: The theory of multiple intelligences.* New York, NY: Basic Books.

King, S. (2000). *On writing: A memoir of the craft.* New York, NY: Scribner.

Leuzinger-Bohleber, M. (2006). What is conceptual research in psychoanalysis? *International Journal of Psychoanalysis, 87,* 1355–1386.

Orwell, G. (1946). Politics and the English language. *Horizon, 13*(76), 252–265.

Street, J., Baum, F., & Anderson, I. P. S. (2009). Is peer review useful in assessing research proposals in Indigenous health? A case study. *Health Research Policy and Systems, 7*(2).

Ware, M. (2008). *Peer review: Benefits, perceptions and alternatives.* London: Publishing Research Consortium.

Woolf, V. (1929). *A room of one's own.* London: Harcourt.

WEBSITES

American Psychological Association website:
   http://www.apastyle.org

PART 4

UNDERSTANDING RESEARCH IN PRACTICE

CHAPTER 16

EVIDENCE-BASED PRACTICE AND PRACTICE-BASED EVIDENCE

DAVID NICHOLLS

CHAPTER OVERVIEW

This chapter covers the following topics:

- Evidence
- Medicine
- Accounting for people
- Weighing the evidence
- Evidence-based practice and complexity
- Quantitative and qualitative research
- Making decisions

KEY TERMS

Biological

Cochrane Reviews

Fringe science

Hierarchy of evidence

Medical model

Placebo

Pseudo-scientific

When visiting a health professional, people want to trust that the practitioner knows what to do to help. They want to believe that the practitioner has been appropriately educated and that all those years of study have left them with a vast armoury of knowledge, skills and experience, so that walking in with problems can become walking out with solutions. Sometimes people want to be in total control of the process, and at other times they just want someone to make them feel better. Either way, there is an implicit relationship between the health-care worker and their client/patient—a relationship that relies on the health practitioner knowing what to do, and then doing it. In health care as much as anywhere else in society, there is an intimate link between what is known *of* in practice (evidence, knowledge and skills) and what is done *in* practice.

EVIDENCE

In a recent guest editorial in the *Scandinavian Journal of Caring Sciences*, Eriksson and Martinsen (2012) argued that the evidence used as the basis of practice 'is concerned with reality and truth' (p. 625), and that this search for truth relies on the ability to see the proof. They argued that often people trust only those treatments for which they have empirical evidence (or evidence that is based on, concerned with, or verifiable by observation or experience rather than theory or pure logic.) Unfortunately, it has long been known that human eyes can deceive—they are too easily fooled by optical illusions and tricks of the light. So what is this 'truth' that Eriksson and Martinsen speak of? What is real, standing at the end of the patient's bed listening to their story of a recent illness? What is the evidence upon which our practice should be based?

The question of how to know the truth about the world has long been a dilemma faced by science. How can we prove, beyond doubt, that what is seen is real? How can we be certain that this patient really has chronic back pain? How can we be sure that these cells are cancerous, or that this person has asthma? Throughout the history of modern medicine, health professionals have believed that the best way to find 'the truth' is through rigorous experimentation where all the potentially polluting variables are controlled, and what is subsequently seen relies on pure facts and is not dependent on bias and personal interpretations. Only in this way will health professionals be able to know the difference between good and bad science, real remedies and placebo, and effective and ineffective therapy.

There is an informal 'contract' between health professionals and clients/patients that is based on trust. Most of the trusting is done by the client/patient, and this places a responsibility upon health professionals to honour that trust and to try to find out what is right or wrong, effective and ineffective.

Placebo
An apparently inert intervention used in research as a control to test the effectiveness of an active intervention.

RESEARCH ALIVE 16.1
PLACEBO EFFECT

In randomised controlled trials the people who are in the control group and receive the placebo (as compared to the people in the intervention group who receive the real treatment that is being tested) can still perceive or experience changes in what is being measured (Finniss, Kaptchuk, Miller, & Bededetti, 2010). This can be due to research participants having *treatment expectations*, which in essence means if you think you are being treated you feel a bit better or different. For example, the placebo effect has been demonstrated in studies of perceived pain, drug addiction and anxiety (Finniss et al.). Accounting for the placebo effect in study design can challenge researchers in their efforts to separate out the actual evidence for effectiveness of a treatment.

CASE STUDY 16.1

MASSAGE AND LAVENDER OIL

I believe that massage with lavender oils can reduce muscle and joint pain, and so I think it ought to be used for people after they have had joint replacement surgery. I know this because I've used it myself and it has worked wonders. I can think of at least three people whom I have used it on and the results have been much better than anything else I've tried. But as a responsible health professional, I have to ask myself: is it sufficient, just because I think it is true, to say that it works? And was it the lavender, or the massage wax, or my hands, the massage itself or just my personal care that had the therapeutic effect?

Unfortunately, it is not simply the case that people only have to open a web page or take a book out of the library to find the truth. (If it were that simple, students wouldn't need to go through such a lengthy education because anyone could do it). The truth about what works and what doesn't is often highly elusive. In the case study above, for example, one could hypothesise that the patient's improvement after the massage with lavender oil could have just been natural healing, or something supernatural such as the alignment of the planet Venus in the sky. The problem is that absolute facts are often elusive in health care, and so the search is on, relentlessly, to find the truth—or as close as possible to it—behind all of those things in health care that are not known. Unfortunately, this lack of knowledge about what actually works means that a great deal of the money spent on health and well-being in the Western world goes on treatments that are no more proven than the lavender remedy for joint pain. (To explore some of the other myths and mistakes of health care, see Ben Goldacre's site http://www.badscience.net). So how does medicine—with all its dangerous procedures and drugs—manage this uncertainty and prove that its treatments are effective?

MEDICINE

Medicine has been trying to counter less than optimal science for more than 100 years, and it has done this by becoming increasingly reliant on properly conducted empirical studies. So, for example, if a practitioner really believed that lavender could improve people's pain after injury or surgery, a proper clinical trial should be conducted. The trial would be designed to make sure there was a large but specific population of people that could represent all of those who were recovering from, say, knee replacement surgery. All possible polluting variables would need to identified and controlled. For example, men might react differently to lavender than women, so the trial should only include one or the other, not both. The participants would need to be people of a particular age. They should all have had a knee replacement for osteoarthritis rather than for trauma, infection or other reasons, and only one joint should probably have been replaced. They could not be taking any medication, or if they were, they should have been taking it for a long time in a steady dose, because the question is about whether the lavender, not the drugs, works. And they should be moderately fit non-smokers.

This sample population should be randomly allocated to one of three groups. The first group would use the lavender, and it would be real lavender extract, produced very carefully and to a standard potency. The second group would use a placebo lavender— something that looks like lavender, smells like lavender and is in the same bottle, but is actually a fake. And the third group would get nothing. Everything would be controlled, from the way the lavender was applied to the fact that the person applying the lavender does so exactly the same way to everyone, and doesn't know which type of lavender they are using (they are 'blind' to the treatment and therefore can't influence people to think one treatment is better than the other). Dozens of doses would be applied over many weeks and months after the knee replacement, and rigorous measurements would be taken with standardised tools including pain scales, range of movement measurements, and tests of muscle strength and functional activity. Finally, the thousands of items of data would be analysed in a computer to establish via highly sophisticated statistical tests whether real lavender actually was a better therapy for pain after injury or surgery.

This kind of empirical research is conducted in thousands of hospital departments and university centres throughout the world today. It is a highly complex and expensive business and every undergraduate health science student needs to become familiar with it. Yet, despite the fact that medicine has provided a blueprint for how to prove something works, there is a lot to health care that does not fit within what is called the medical model.

ACCOUNTING FOR PEOPLE

The approach to research that has been favoured by medicine for the last century or more works best when all the variables of a problem can be identified, explained and understood. It also helps if the things being studied can be visualised. Empirical research relies on the ability to see things to confirm that they are true. So the medical model strongly emphasises research that is based on biology and chemistry, where physical properties can be seen to interact with one another. But it is harder to apply a medical model to aspects of health that cannot be seen, either because they are things that have no obvious physical basis, like feelings, or because they rely on mechanisms of action that cannot be observed (like 'life force' or Qi—pronounced 'chee'—common in many non-Western medical systems). There are many examples of these non-empirical concepts in health care that have, in the past, been dismissed as fringe science by Western doctors. In some cases, however, some of the things that cannot be easily explained by the biological or chemical sciences have become the basis for very well-established professions like psychology, which deals, in part, with the science of emotions (mental reactions) and feelings (the physical sensations of the body). Aspects of nursing that are concerned with caring science, and dimensions of occupational therapy that focus on people's engagement with meaningful activities, are important dimensions of health that do not sit easily with the quantitative medical model.

The emergence of qualitative research over the last half-century reflects a desire to find a scientific basis for the aspects of health care that cannot easily be measured. From the phenomenological interest in each person's experience of being healthy or ill, to ethnographic research into health cultures, and critical theorists' attacks on the power imbalances that exist in health care, qualitative research is generating a growing body of research that eschews 'traditional' science in favour of research that is more interested in studying people as a whole, not as a collection of biological or chemical processes.

WEIGHING THE EVIDENCE

The growth in complexity and sophistication of research in health, as well as the sheer volume of scientific knowledge now to hand, means that making a decision about what to believe in has become increasingly difficult for clients/patients *and* the people

Medical model
An approach to health care that privileges biological, mechanistic and reductive understandings of bodily structures and functions.

Fringe science
Knowledge or information considered not to be mainstream.

Biological
Pertaining to biology—the science of life.

Pseudo-scientific
Relating to information
which purports to
be scientific but is
not based on sound
principles or analysis.

who deliver health care. There are those who try to control what people believe by advocating that there are some types of research that are simply better than other types. There are some, for example, that argue that all medical research should be ignored because it fails to address people as 'wholes' and that it ignores, for instance, people's spirituality—those things that connect people with each other, the cosmos, ancestors or the environment. There are others who would dismiss this kind of talk as pseudo-scientific mumbo-jumbo.

Hierarchy of evidence
A tool for evaluating
research findings
according to the degree
of scientific rigour.

In health care the most widely used tool for distinguishing good knowledge from bad comes from what is called the hierarchy of evidence (Evans, 2013).

FIGURE 16.1   THE HIERARCHY OF EVIDENCE

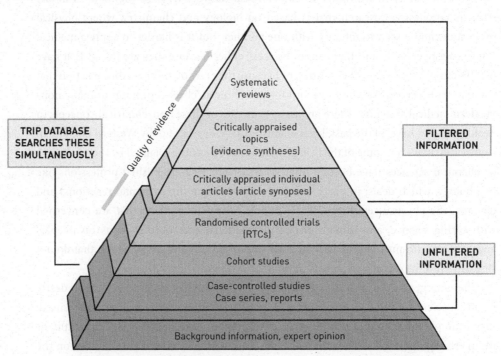

At the top of the pyramid are the forms of evidence that are believed to be the best because they are most reliable and trustworthy for showing causation. Evidence from a systematic review is considered by many to be the best evidence currently available about whether a treatment works. A systematic review involves a process of 'weighing up' all of the available evidence for a particular therapy, and is often performed by an expert panel of specialists who use strict criteria to evaluate the quality of individual research studies before making their pronouncements. The Cochrane Collaboration (http://www. cochrane.org) is the most well-known example of this process and Cochrane Reviews now cover most established health-care interventions.

Cochrane Reviews
Reviews produced
by the Cochrane
Collaboration.

Part of the problem with the hierarchy of evidence is that health care is immensely complex and involves aspects of health that are both visible and invisible to medical science. The hierarchy of evidence works well if the focus is biological and chemical, but does not really offer anything for the more qualitative or holistic aspects of health and well-being. Consequently, it has been criticised for promoting a highly mechanical, depersonalised view of health (Lupton, 2003; Redding, 1995).

EVIDENCE-BASED PRACTICE AND COMPLEXITY

Some years ago, David Sackett wrote about the concept of evidence-based practice as a way to manage some of the complexities of health care (Sackett, Rosenberg, Muir Gray, Haynes, & Richardson, 1996). Sackett and colleagues argued that evidence-based practice was a long-held principle in health care, going back to the nineteenth century and the birth of modern medicine. He argued that evidence-based practice involved 'the conscientious, explicit and judicious use of current best evidence in making decisions about the care of the individual patient' (Sackett et al., 1996, p. 71). Importantly, Sackett argued that proper evidence-based decision-making involved three things:

1   the clinical expertise of the individual (including skills, knowledge and experience);
2   the best available evidence from systematic research (see the Cochrane Reviews mentioned above, for example); and
3   the values and preferences of the client/patient.

Often in health care the last point gets lost, but it is a vital component of clinical decision-making. And when these three dimensions of decision-making are taken together, they reveal just how complex health-care decision-making can be.

CLINICAL REFLECTION 16.1: WHAT WOULD YOU DO?

Imagine standing at the end of the bed of a patient who has been admitted to hospital with an acute lung infection on top of a pre-existing chronic lung disease. She is conscious but in severe distress. Leads and lines are everywhere, running to machines which show her heart and lung functions. She is catheterised, and has intravenous fluids running into her arm and a nasogastric tube into her stomach to feed her. She hasn't eaten properly for 10 days because she can't breathe and chew at the same time; she hasn't been

[continued next page]

out of the house for a week. The closest family member is her daughter who lives overseas but is taking leave from her job to visit the hospital. The patient exists on a state pension. She has a host of secondary problems associated with her lung disease, including some right heart failure, swollen legs and fragile skin from years of steroid use, osteoporosis and some early stage renal failure.

Now imagine, as you stand there, that you are supposed to make a clinical decision about what to do to help this patient. You are, according to the evidence-based practice rhetoric, supposed to be able to weigh up all of the best available evidence—including the latest systematically appraised reviews of the treatment for all the conditions your patient presents with. Then you are supposed to draw on your own bank of knowledge, skills and experience to make a rational decision about what is best for the person right now, while always being ready to review your decision in an instant should your patient's clinical picture change. And then, after all that, you are supposed to offer your patient choices and understand something of her values, preferences, wants and desires. Clearly this is a hugely complex task that takes years to master.

While some people might find the complexity of this case study daunting, it is often true that it is the 'messiness' of cases like this that makes health care so interesting and rewarding as a career. There is an inbuilt 'undecidability'—as French philosopher Jacques Derrida called it—about health care: an extent, to which evidence-based recipes and formulas cannot provide the whole picture. Clients/patients need to be seen *as* people, in all their confounding unpredictability and beautiful complexity. Health care would be easy if practitioners only had to follow prewritten, evidence-based care plans that patients slotted into effortlessly and technicians administered without deviation or difficulty. But health care is not this easy and this is principally because every day, everywhere, people complicate it just by being themselves: by being human.

QUANTITATIVE AND QUALITATIVE RESEARCH

Over the last half-century, there have been two distinctly different approaches to the problem of the complexity in health care. The first has been followed by health professionals who favour the biological sciences. These largely quantitative sciences have sought to find rational and logical solutions, and evidence-based practice, randomised controlled trials and Cochrane Reviews are some of the products of very powerful lobbying in health care largely governed by the medical profession. An alternative approach has emerged in recent years from the qualitative sciences, and this approach, rather than trying to standardise and remove the bias inherent in individual personal beliefs and opinion, seeks to make a virtue out of it. Qualitative research puts the things that make us all unique at the centre of the decision-making process. It provides evidence for people's subjectivity, bias and partiality and champions the voices of individuals and groups who have, hitherto, been silenced by the biological sciences (Cheek, 2011; Morse, 2006).

Qualitative research takes many forms and provides many different kinds of evidence. It has become increasingly important in health care research to have a qualitative perspective when deciding what is the best approach to a particular problem, and there are now a growing number of research studies that use multiple or mixed methods of research, incorporating qualitative and quantitative approaches. Qualitative research is becoming increasingly important in supporting evidence-based decision-making, but these collaborations are in their infancy and these developments are not without their critics (Miles, Loughlin, & Polychronis, 2008).

CASE STUDY 16.2

QUANTITATIVE AND QUALITATIVE EVIDENCE TOGETHER IN A SYSTEMATIC REVIEW

The Joanna Briggs Institute (JBI) is an international, not-for-profit research and development arm of the School of Translational Science in the Faculty of Health Sciences at the University of Adelaide, South Australia. JBI provides a Database of Systematic Reviews and Implementation Reports that is designed to be used by clinicians to inform practice. Many JBI publications go beyond effectiveness to focus also on determining the feasibility, appropriateness and meaningfulness of evidence for practice (JBI, 2013).

Petriwskyj and colleagues (2013) provides an example of a JBI systematic review that includes both qualitative and quantitative research studies to summarise the state of knowledge on family involvement in decision-making for people with dementia living in residential aged care. People with dementia and living in assisted care situations are frequently not competent to make independent decisions due to deterioration in their cognitive abilities. Family involvement in care decision-making is important to ensure optimal outcomes. A series of questions about the experiences of caregivers; the barriers and facilitators for decision-making; the impact of decisions; and what processes and strategies families used guided the review and evaluation of 24 studies.

[continued next page]

Results indicate that family involvement in decision-making regarding their relative varies and that a range of factors positively and negatively influence experiences. In particular, the interpersonal interface between staff and family needs additional support as decision-making can be challenging for both care staff and families. As this review included both qualitative and quantitative studies, findings reflect a broader focus than would be obtained by including studies from one methodology.

RESEARCH ALIVE 16.2
QUESTIONING EVIDENCE

In recent years, a number of authors have argued that evidence-based practice is becoming increasingly misunderstood and misapplied in health care—that medical research, particularly, is taking precedence over clinical experience and the client/patient's preference in clinical decision-making. It is argued that evidence-based practice, driven by the funding of increasingly expensive clinical trials and systematic reviews, has become too one-sided.

Andrew Miles and colleagues (Miles, Loughlin, & Polychronis, 2008), in a lengthy editorial, argue that proponents of evidence-based medicine (EBM) had become dogmatic and almost 'cult-like' in the way they promoted certain truths about health care over others. In a stinging passage of criticism, Miles et al. (2008) argue that advocates of EBM are 'extraordinarily lacking in intellectual credibility, are profoundly revisionist and demonstrate that little has changed in terms of EBM's ideology or hubris with the exception of an increase in self-delusion and a refusal to accept that EBM is "finished" in scientific, philosophical and clinical terms' (Miles et al., p. 622).

Miles et al. (2008) go further to suggest that there is an inbuilt paradox in EBM: that it promotes the pursuit of rigorous evidence to prove that treatments work, but that there has been no effort to prove that EBM has done anything to improve people's lives.

This kind of passionate debate around evidence-based practice adds additional layers of complexity to the already complex work of health care.

CASE STUDY 16.3

FEVER IN CHILDREN: DRUG THERAPY AND CHILD OUTCOMES

Fever or temperature above the normal level is part of the body's immune response to an infection and is commonly observed when a child has a viral illness such as a cold, cough or sore throat. Fever makes a child feel unwell and distressed, and these symptoms worry parents and caregivers. Parents and health practitioners often use drug therapy to treat fever in children. Paracetamol and ibuprofen are two over-the-counter drug therapies with different mechanisms of action that can be used to lower temperature and resolve discomfort. According to Wong et al. (2013), parents or caregivers are often advised to try one drug first and, if the child's fever doesn't resolve, to try a further dose of the alternative. Another common recommendation is to give both drugs at once. Wong et al. conducted a systematic review of research into the use of combined or alternating paracetamol and ibuprofen therapy for children with a fever and concluded that using both drugs together was more effective at lowering mean measured temperature than a single dose (moderate quality evidence). However, what was remarkable about the review findings was that the main outcome reported was change in measured temperature level; child discomfort or distress was measured in only one small study. Any parent or clinician familiar with children will recognise that a child's distress and comfort, not numbers on the thermometer, is the most important outcome of drug therapy, and should be targeted for investigation. The review authors recommend that in future, research outcomes should focus on children's well-being. This research provides an example of the paradox referred to in Research Alive 16.2 and by Miles et al. (2008), where the focus on what is most important to the patient—in this case, resolving distress and discomfort caused by fever—has been missed.

MAKING DECISIONS

Ultimately, the evidence gleaned from research—whether it is quantitative, qualitative or both—is meant to be in service of practice. In other words, it should help practitioners make decisions when they need to figure out what to do. It should help with choosing between option A and option B, because knowing lots of things is useful in health care only when that knowledge is put to good use. The value of evidence is in helping practitioners and patients decide, when the sheer complexity of what confronts them scrambles their brains and defies the collective wisdom of our colleagues. Evidence helps people to understand what they do not know. Sometimes, turning to the evidence only seems to make the challenges all the greater. Sometimes practitioners have to distance themselves from the evidence and do the exact opposite of what is recommended because they trust their instinct for what is best for the patient at that moment in time, often presenting others with the evidence and empowering them to make the decisions, because rarely do people willingly relinquish all decisions about their health and well-being. More often than not, practitioners are responsible for knowing and interpreting the evidence and presenting it in a form that allows others to make their own decisions about what is right for them.

Health care is one of the most complex and challenging areas of human interaction, filled with all the human frailties, bureaucratic structures and age-old dogmas that exemplify life in the twenty-first century. More than ever, people are asking what helps and what hinders, what works and what is merely sham, who to trust and who to avoid. There are no easy answers to these questions, but in recent decades much more emphasis has fallen upon the systems used to make those decisions rather than simply trusting that 'doctor knows best'. Every health professional has a duty to enquire and to know the best evidence that exists for their practice, and to convey that in meaningful ways to their clients/patients. At times decisions made are so hard won that practitioners will question them for days or even weeks afterwards. But this is the nature of health care, and it is what helps it retain its allure and reminds practitioners of their fallibility when they get too comfortable and think they have finally worked out how to do it.

RESEARCH ALIVE 16.3
ELECTRONIC HEALTH RECORDS: CHANGING HOW EVIDENCE IS USED IN PRACTICE AND HOW PATIENTS ARE RECRUITED FOR RESEARCH

Many health agencies in the developed world have moved patient health-care records from hand written hard copy to computerised systems. The capacity to link datasets such as hospital records, disease registries and community general practitioner (GP) records electronically means that large data sets can be generated, and these enable low-cost, long-term follow up of major clinical outcomes to inform best practice (van Staa et al., 2012). A group in the United Kingdom (van Staa et al.) have recognised the potential of this change and have begun clinical feasibility studies. Patients are entered into treatment trials in real time in their GP's practice; outcomes are then followed up through electronic health records. Evidence-based prompts that support the GP's clinical decision-making are also built into the trial software. The group are investigating secondary stroke prevention (Dregan et al., 2012) and antibiotic prescribing (Gulliford et al., 2011). During your career as a practitioner, computerisation will advance and the way health evidence is generated, retrieved and used in practice will change exponentially.

SUMMARY

There are many complexities in health care and many ways that evidence-based practice operates to make sense of this complexity. Making decisions is implicit in health care, but making the right decisions is often much harder than it seems. Weighing the evidence to hand and balancing it against experience and the particular wishes of clients/patients lies at the heart of modern-day health professional practice.

REFLECTION POINTS

- Why do health professionals need to get involved in making decisions for, and with clients/patients?
- If clients/patients are free to make their own choices about what they want and need, and there is ample evidence to support or refute their decisions, why do clients/patients need us at all?
- Try to think about all the reasons why clients/patients might be either unable or unwilling to make their own choices when it comes to health care, and all the reasons why the decisions that need to be made are sometimes clouded in uncertainty.

STUDY QUESTIONS

1 List as many things as you know about health care that are absolutely, irrefutably true.
2 Think of a health problem you have experienced, and try to list those things that are measurable and those things that can only be explained in words.
3 Read David Sackett's original work on evidence-based practice so that you are familiar with its key concepts.
4 Using this book, try to identify five key differences between qualitative and quantitative research.

DAVID NICHOLLS

ADDITIONAL READING

Fink, A. (2013). *Evidence-based public health practice*. Los Angeles, CA: Sage Publications.

Hoffmann, T., Bennett, S. P., & Del Mar, C. (2009). *Evidence based practice across the health professions*. New York: Churchill Livingstone/Elsevier.

Melnyk, B. M., Fineout-Overholt, E., & Sigma Theta Tau, I. (2011). *Implementing evidence-based practice: real-life success stories*. Indianapolis, IN: Sigma Theta Tau International.

Newell, R., & Burnard, P. (2011). *Research for evidence-based practice in healthcare*. Ames, IA: Wiley-Blackwell.

Trinder, L., & Reynolds, S. (2000). *Evidence-based practice: a critical appraisal*. Malden, MA: Blackwell Science.

van Staa, T., Goldacre, B., Gulliford, M., Cassell, J., Pirohamed, M., & Taweel, A. et al. (2012). Pragmatic randomised trials using routine electronic health records: Putting them to the test. *British Medical Journal, 344*, e55.

REFERENCES

Cheek, J. (2011). Moving on: Researching, surviving, and thriving in the evidence-saturated world of health care. *Qualitative Health Research, 21*(5), 696–703.

Dregan, A., van Staa, T., Mcdermott, L., McCann, G., Ashworth, M., & Charlton, J. et al. (2012). Cluster randomised trial in the general practice research database: 2. Secondary prevention after first stroke (eCRT study): Study protocol for a randomised controlled trial. *Trials, 13*, 181.

Eriksson, K., & Martinsen, K. (2012). The hidden and forgotten evidence. *Scandinavian Journal of Caring Sciences, 26*(4), 625–626.

Evans, D. (2003). Hierarchy of evidence: a framework for ranking evidence evaluating healthcare interventions. *Journal of Clinical Nursing, 12*(1), 77–84.

Finniss, D., Kaptchuk, T., Miller, F., & Bededetti, F. (2010). Biological, clinical and ethical advances of placebo effects. *Lancet, 375* (Feb), 686–695.

Gulliford, M., van Staa, T., Mcdermott, L., Dregan, A., McCann, G., & Ashworth, M. et al. (2011). Cluster randomised trial in the general practice research database: 1. Electonic decision support to reduce antibiotic prescribing in primary care (eCRT study). *Trials, 12*, 115.

Joanna Briggs Institute (2013). Retrieved from http://joannabriggs.org

Lupton, D. (2003). *Medicine as culture: illness, disease and the body in western society.* London: Sage Publications.

Miles, A., Loughlin, M., & Polychronis, A. (2008). Evidence-based healthcare, clinical knowledge and the rise of personalised medicine. *Journal of Evaluation in Clinical Practice, 14,* 621–649.

Morse, J. (2006). Reconceptualizing qualitative evidence. *Qualitative Health Research, 16,* 415–422.

Petriwskyj, A., Parker, D., Robinson, A., Gibson, A., Andrews, S., & Banks, S. (2013). Family involvement in decision making for people with dementia in residential aged care: A systematic review of quantitative and qualitative evidence. *JBI Database of Systematic Reviews and Implementation Reports, 11*(7), 131–282.

Redding, P. (1995). Science, medicine and illness: rediscovering the patient as a person. In P. A. Komesaroff (Ed.), *Troubled bodies: Critical perspectives on postmodernism, medical ethics, and the body* (pp. 87–102). Durham, NC: Duke University Press.

Sackett, D. L., Rosenberg, W M.C., Muir Gray, J. A., Haynes, R. B., & Richardson, W. S. (1996). Evidence based medicine: what it is and what it isn't. *British Medical Journal, 312,* 71.

van Staa, T., Goldacre, B., Gulliford, M., Cassell, J., Pirohamed, M., & Taweel, A. et al. (2012). Pragmatic randonised trials using routine electronic health records: Putting them to the test. *British Medical Journal, 344,* e55.

Wong, T., Stang, A., Gashorn, H., Hartling, L., Maconochie, I. K., & Thomsen, A. N. et al. (2013). Combined and alternating paracetamol and ibuprofen therapy for febrile children. *Cochrane Database of Systematic Reviews, 10,* Art No. CD009572.

WEBSITES

Ben Goldacres's Bad Science website:
   http://www.badscience.net

Cochrane Collaboration:
   http://www.cochrane.org

Health Change Australia:
   http://www.healthchangeaustralia.com/health-coaching-au

Peter Ubel:
   http://www.peterubel.com

CHAPTER 17

LINKING RESEARCH AND PRACTICE

JOANNE RAMSBOTHAM

CHAPTER OVERVIEW

This chapter covers the following topics:

- Linking research and practice
- Evidence-based practice
- Research utilisation and practice change
- Locating relevant evidence to inform practice

KEY TERMS

Applied
Evidence-based practice
Expertise
Guidelines
PICO
Practitioner
Research utilisation

Understanding the key factors that influence the evidentiary basis for practice and using skills in retrieving evidence that informs practice change are essential to the development of a health professional's career, regardless of the discipline. This chapter focuses on the key links between research and practice, particularly how health professionals use various sources of evidence and new knowledge to inform and improve the effectiveness of their practice in order to benefit the health of clients. Evidence-based practice and research utilisation are two major global research/practice initiatives that form the basis for this chapter. Examples that illustrate the real-world application of these initiatives are included in the Research Alive and Case Study sections. How practice change can be facilitated within health organisations is also briefly introduced.

LINKING RESEARCH AND PRACTICE

People are complex, and, accordingly, resolving clinical problems in the dynamic health-care environment is a challenging task for clinicians. How a clinician goes about this task has changed in the last two decades and this has coincided with advances in the availability and accessibility of health information. These developments have improved clinician access to quality information that informs practice, while also increasing health consumers' information options and raising their expectations of health care. Concurrently, professional standards of responsibility and accountability have developed to include explicit expectations that health-care provision is based on scientific foundations. This means that, as students use research evidence and develop as practitioners, research and practice become strongly linked and the use of evidence to inform practice is an unavoidable reality.

The value of research is in how useful it is in informing health practice, specifically improving practice effectiveness and benefitting recipients' health-care outcomes. Within practice contexts, research and practice are most obviously linked in two major global health-care improvement initiatives: research utilisation and evidence-based practice. Research and practice can be thought of in these contexts as two inseparably linked elements in a continuous and evolving cycle. The problems a practitioner identifies in their practice prompt questions, and where there is no or little evidence to answer the questions, research studies that produce new knowledge ought to follow. The findings from these studies then inform practice change and innovation. Further questions may emerge, and so the process is cyclical. So important is the practice–research link that high-ranking academic journals commonly require authors to include explicit sections that detail the new knowledge gained and the contribution the study results make to current practice, be it recommending change, or reinforcing and extending existing practices.

Modern health care highly values client/patient safety and quality in care provision. Clinical decision-making that is based on evidence of what works best to achieve the

Evidence-based practice
Practice that is informed by the careful consideration and evaluation of relevant information, and client/patient and practitioner experience and preference.

Research utilisation
The process of using knowledge provided by research.

Practitioner
A person recognised by a professional group.

desired client outcomes makes a strong contribution to quality care. Different sources of research evidence suit the diversity of clinical decisions made by the various professional groups that work within health care; accordingly, no one research methodology has precedence over another (Esterman, Warland, & Deuter, 2010). It is not acceptable to base clinical decisions solely on ritual, tradition or personal experience. Conversely, it is also not possible to keep pace with every innovation by reading all the new research in a disciplinary field; nor is it feasible to constantly adjust practice to accommodate the results of each new published study. Rather, when an unfamiliar clinical problem arises or current approaches are not working, a clinician uses life-long learning skills to investigate the best approach for resolution. The evidence-based practice process provides relevant guidance.

EVIDENCE-BASED PRACTICE

A question that challenges all health-care professionals working in the practice environment every day is: 'What evidence will best inform my clinical decision in this particular situation, and benefit this person?' Finding the answers to such questions initiates a problem-solving process termed 'evidence-based practice' (EBP) whereby a clinician undertakes 'the conscientious, explicit, and judicious use of best evidence in making decisions about the care of [an] individual … incorporating … the client's values and clinicians' expertise' (Sackett, Straus, Richardson, Rosenberg, & Haynes, 2000). In simple terms, the aim of EBP is to improve client health outcomes by applying knowledge of what has been demonstrated to work best for the client.

Expertise
Expert skills and knowledge.

CLINICAL REFLECTION 17.1: IMPROVING PATIENTS' LIVES

It can be said that 'EBP should begin and end with the patient' (Nay & Fetherstonhaugh, 2007, p. 456). That is, the ultimate aim of research evidence should be to improve patients' lives. Look at the case studies in this chapter or recent evidence you have used in your studies: can you identify the nature of improvement from the patients' perspective?

EBP emerged in medicine in the 1980s and spread through the practice and education contexts of other health disciplines during the mid-1990s. In the twenty-first century EBP is an essential element of work readiness and health practitioner competence that makes an important contribution to achieving effective care and improving patient outcomes (Stevens, 2010). Dealing with the multidimensional aspects of people within the health-care environment requires clinicians to use their judgement to weigh up many factors and decide what the best course of action is. It has long been recognised that a clinician integrates considerations from four key sources of evidence to inform judgments

(Rycroft-Malone et al., 2004), as represented in Figure 17.1. These are professional knowledge and clinical experience; relevant research evidence that has accumulated on the topic; client preference; and local contextual factors such as available equipment or referral options. Drawing on considerations from all four elements, the clinician decides on the best course of action to resolve the problem and benefit the client. What results can be termed 'person- or patient- centred evidence-based care' (Rycroft-Malone et al., 2003). That is, health-care provision that accommodates the client's preferences relevant to their unique situation, has a scientific foundation and is implemented using the clinicians' particular professional skill set.

FIGURE 17.1   SOURCES OF EVIDENCE

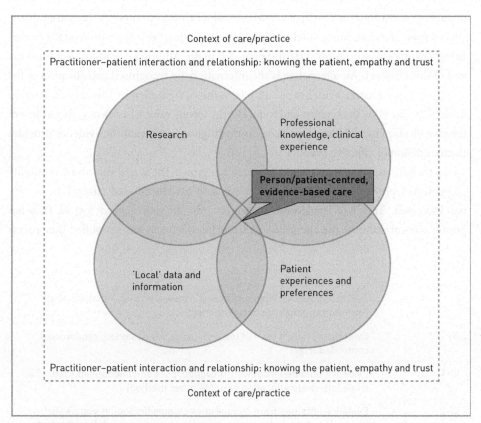

Source: Rycroft-Malone, J. et al., 2004, 87

The EBP process commonly follows five steps once the client has been clinically assessed and a health problem identified for treatment or intervention. The five steps are:

1   information needs are translated into clinical questions;
2   clinical evidence that answers the questions is efficiently tracked down from various sources;
3   the best available evidence is appraised for usefulness and value;

Applied
Put to practical use.

4 evidence is applied to the clinical situation; and

5 results are evaluated.

How to begin the EBP process and locate evidence that informs practice change (step 1) is addressed in a later section of this chapter and the next section in this book will help with the remaining steps (2–5).

A useful resource in the EBP process is the hierarchy or classification of evidence that provide guidance on the strength of available evidence. Such classification systems are particularly helpful in completing steps two and three of the EBP process. Organisations and discipline groups may employ somewhat different systems for classifying evidence, recognising that various methodologies provide evidence that is valuable in informing practice. For example, the Joanna Briggs Institute (2013) assigns evidence in four levels of value (one to four) across five criteria: feasibility, appropriateness, meaningfulness, effectiveness and economic evidence (FAME) (a link to further information on the Joanna Briggs Institute classification system is provided in the 'Additional reading' section at the end of this chapter). An alternative is the internationally recognised classification of the strength of quantitative evidence for an intervention, treatment or therapy, depicted in Table 17.1: one (I) is the highest and four (IV) the lowest value of evidence. Regardless of the classification used the main principle is that high-quality scientific evidence provides the foundation of effective practice.

Guidelines
Information providing
advice on how to
interpret policy or
procedure.

As the EBP movement and health research has grown, the availability and accessibility of published pre-appraised systematic reviews and evidence-based clinical guidelines has increased. This has transformed research into an information format that has greater clinical utility at the client-care practice interface and has simplified the process

TABLE 17.1 LEVELS OF EVIDENCE

I	Evidence obtained from a systematic review or meta-analysis of all relevant randomised controlled trials
II	Evidence obtained from at least one properly designed, randomised, controlled trial
III-1	Evidence obtained from well-designed, pseudo-randomised, controlled trials (alternate allocation or some other method)
III-2	Evidence obtained from comparative studies (including systematic reviews of such studies), with concurrent controls and allocation not randomised, cohort studies, case control studies, or interrupted time series with a control group
III-3	Evidence obtained from comparative studies with historical control, two or more single arm studies, or interrupted time series without a parallel control group
IV	Evidence obtained from case series, either post-test or pretest/post-test

Source: National Health and Medical Research Council, 2008

RESEARCH ALIVE 17.1
GET THE LATEST EVIDENCE ON A PRACTICE TOPIC EMAILED TO YOU

Many electronic databases have a function called a *search alert, news feed*, or something similar. This helps you set up an automated notification to your email of a new edition of a nominated journal, or of a journal article citing selected keywords. Many notification messages also have embedded internet links that take you straight to the online abstract or full article. Setting up a search alert or news feed is an efficient way to keep up with new research into topic areas that interest you.

of EBP in common practice contexts where health workers have easy access to online resources. As a beginning practitioner, referring to existing pre-appraised resources such as systematic reviews and clinical guidelines is a useful strategy, as most of searching, appraisal and synthesis (steps 2 and 3 of the EBP process) is already completed and clinical recommendations that inform practice implementation are also frequently included (step 4 of the EBP process). Several international collections offer high-quality multidisciplinary resources, for example the Australasian Cochrane Centre (http://acc.cochrane.org) and Joanna Briggs Institute (http://www.joannabriggs.edu.au/Home). Research Alive 17.2 contains an example of a Cochrane review of exercise-based rehabilitation for heart failure and practice links. A list of global and national organisation websites that make pre-appraised resources available is provided at the end of this chapter.

RESEARCH ALIVE 17.2
EXERCISE AND HEART FAILURE

Davies and colleagues (2010) undertook a systematic review of the evidence in relation to exercise-based rehabilitation for people with heart failure.

Clinical problem: Heart failure is a common complication of cardiovascular disease and is associated with a substantially increased risk of death. People who are affected experience difficulties in their activities of daily living and have reduced quality of life related to limited heart capacity. Symptoms can increase as fitness and ability to undertake exercise are reduced. Exercise training has a positive effect on exercise capacity, yet what is not known is the effect of exercise on health-related quality of life, mortality and hospital admissions.

[continued next page]

JOANNE RAMSBOTHAM

Results: The review determined that exercise training programmes improved health-related quality of life and reduced hospital admissions compared to usual care without exercise. It was concluded that exercise was not associated with a reduction or an increase in the risk of death in those with mild to moderate heart failure.

Practice link: This level I evidence (refer to Table 17.1) informs the practice of a range of clinicians, such as exercise physiologists, physiotherapists, doctors and nurses working with people who have heart failure, in the areas of referral, patient education and behaviour change coaching; in both acute and long term care situations.

RESEARCH UTILISATION AND PRACTICE CHANGE

Research utilisation (RU) has been described as the use of scientific research study findings to guide practice (Estabrooks, 2009), in contrast to the wider view of evidence sources used in EBP. RU may be characterised differently among various health disciplines (see Chapter 20). For example, practice development in nursing and midwifery contexts combines EBP with staff development and facilitated practice improvement to achieve local cultural reform and care improvement (Kent & McCormack, 2013). Alternately, knowledge translation is an active method of research utilisation and practice change used in health settings. Knowledge translation is defined as 'a dynamic and iterative process that includes synthesis, dissemination, exchange and ethically sound application of knowledge to improve health' (Canadian Institutes for Health Research, 2008, para 7). Regardless of the term used, the aim of research utilisation initiatives is to benefit clients through practice change based on the best available research findings.

CASE STUDY 17.1

PRESSURE INJURIES AND MEDICAL DEVICES USED IN INTENSIVE CARE

Patients in intensive care can get areas of skin injury and resulting ulceration caused by pressure and friction from medical devices. For example, the hard plastic tube that goes through the skin into a patient's vein so intravenous fluid can be infused can press on skin, which then erodes over a period of days, similar to how a blister can develop when you wear tight shoes. Coyer, Stotts and Blackman (2013) found that males over 60.5 years of age who were overweight were most at risk of skin injury, and that tubes used to support breathing and nutrition were the most common cause. This research can inform the practice of practitioners who manage these medical devices. A practitioner who reads the study by Coyer et al. might have seen similar pressure injuries during practice to those discussed in the research article. Concerned, the practitioner decides to observe the patient's skin more regularly and identify and relocate any medical devices that are exerting pressure, before the patient's skin is injured.

Research utilisation at the point of care has been widely acknowledged as a complex process of cultural change effected by multiple environmental and contextual factors, no matter what the discipline or practice context. Dissemination of new research and innovation does not automatically result in changes to practice or improvement. Despite a wealth of available published resources, gaps remain between evidence (what research demonstrates is best practice) and clinical practice (care that is actually provided to a person) (Courtney, Rickard, Vickerstaff, & Court, 2010). Facilitating health-care teams to develop their knowledge and skills, transform cultural expectations and implement practice improvement relies on substantial commitment to rigorous change and widespread organisational support (Kent & McCormack, 2013). This is illustrated in the case study example where McKinley and colleagues (2007) undertook a multidimensional research utilisation project in an acute-care hospital and involved a variety of health team disciplines in practice change to improve client safety.

LOCATING RELEVANT EVIDENCE TO INFORM PRACTICE

The first step in effectively solving a client problem or investigating a clinical topic is to conduct a literature search of relevant published research and other resources, such as clinical practice guidelines, to investigate if the answer to any clinical question is already available. Knowing how to efficiently access and retrieve the information required is a key skill for a research consumer in any health professional programme of study. Literature databases are primarily collections of scientific journal articles along with links to some other published resources, going back several decades. Health organisations often provide staff with database access through search portals such as PubMed or EBSCOhost, similar to what can be accessed through a university library. Some common databases used in health are CINAHL (nursing and allied health), Medline (medicine and bioscience), Embase (biomedical) and PsycINFO (psychology).

The PICO acronym is helpful when developing research questions (Chapter 10). These same four prompts will help in formulating a clinical question in response to a client problem or clinical issue and in identifying key words for an efficient database search for evidence. When designing a search for qualitative studies about persons' experiences, simply use the P and O. Case Study 17.2 provides an example of a clinical question and search strategy.

PICO
An acronym for developing research questions: Problem/Population; Intervention; Comparison/Control; Outcome.

CASE STUDY 17.2

THE PROBLEM OF FALLS

Falls are a leading cause of unintentional injury hospital care and can result in major functional loss for the individual and economic cost in increased length of stay in hospital (Australian Safety and Quality Council, 2009). A group of nurses in Western Australian identified the incidence of falls among hospitalised elderly clients as a frequent local clinical problem and undertook a multidisciplinary project to improve the issue (McKinley et al., 2007).

Locating evidence to inform practice: A simple clinical question from this problem is: 'Among elderly hospitalised people, do strategies such as risk assessment tools or bed rails reduce accidental injury or morbidity?' As part of the project planning the team searched for relevant evidence on how to reduce the rates of in-hospital falls. Using the PICO acronym some key words to start an efficient database search in Cinahl are easily identified.

PICO	KEYWORDS FOR DATABASE SEARCH
Patient/population/problem	elderly, falls in hospital
Intervention	falls prevention strategies
Comparison/control	risk assessment tool, bed rails
Outcome	injury, morbidity, length of stay

Evidence-based practice change: Research highlighted the fact that falls are reduced through the use of the following nursing practices: falls risk assessment tools, risk alert strategy such as 'at risk' colour-coded arm bands, adequate footwear to prevent slipping, and frequent supervision for hygiene and toileting. Ineffective nursing strategies include the use of bed rails and restraints. Interdisciplinary strategies were also located: pharmacist flags for people with potential risk of falls related to drug interactions or commencement of new drugs—for example, opioids or hypnotics. Environmental changes like the use of low-gloss floors and high-colour-contrast furniture and bathroom equipment also contribute to prevention. Combining this evidence with their professional expertise and local knowledge, McKinley and colleagues (2007) were able to plan a multidisciplinary, multidimensional programme, implement change and monitor its effectiveness in terms of ongoing falls rates.

SUMMARY

Research and practice can be thought of as two inseparably linked elements in a continuous and evolving cycle. Health-care professionals need to be able to understand the ways in which various types of evidence inform their professional judgment and professional decision-making in a practice context. Skills in locating and applying new knowledge to enhance interventional effectiveness and benefit the client in some way are an essential area of competence for all health professionals.

REFLECTION POINTS

- Recall your most recent practice experience, and professional practice you either observed or in which you were supervised.
- Referring to Figure 17.1, consider what sources of evidence were employed to inform the decision.
- Were all four sources of evidence employed equally, or did one or two dominate?

STUDY QUESTIONS

1   What is the central focus of links between research and practice?
2   Identify what databases, information portals and pre-appraised resource libraries are available through the university where you are studying and which ones primarily publish research relevant to your practice discipline.
3   Which databases would you access to locate information on the following practice topics or problems? Rephrase each into a practice question and make a list of key words to use that will assist in conducting an efficient and targeted search.
    a   Caring for a partner with dementia at home;
    b   The experience of pain in chronic migraine and work absence.

ADDITIONAL READING

Brown, T., Tseng, M., Casey, J., McDonald, R., & Lyons, C. (2010). Predictors of research utilization among pediatric occupational therapists. *Otjr-Occupation Participation and Health, 30*(4), 172–183.

Joanna Briggs Institute (2013) *Levels of evidence FAME.* Retrieved February 6, 2013, from http://www.joannabriggs.edu.au/Levels%20of%20Evidence%20%20FAME

McCormack, B., Dewing, J., Breslin, L., Coyne-Nevin, A., Kennedy, K., Manning, M., Peelo-Kilroe, L. and Tobin, C. (2009) Practice development: realising active learning for sustainable change, *Contemporary Nurse, 32*(1–2), 92–104.

Weller, C. and Evan, S. (2012) Venous leg ulcer management in general practice— practice nurses and evidence based guidelines *Australian Family Physician, 41*(5), 331–336.

REFERENCES

Australian Safety and Quality Council. (2009). *Preventing falls and harm from falls in older people.* Retrieved February 6, 2013, from http://www.activeandhealthy.nsw.gov.au/assets/pdf/RACF_Guidelines.pdf

Canadian Institutes for Health Research. (2008). *About knowledge translation.* Retrieved February 7, 2013, from http://www.cihr-irsc.gc.ca/e/29418.html

Courtney, M., Rickard, C., Vickerstaff, J. and Court, A. (2010). Evidence-based nursing practice. In M. Courtney, & H. McCutcheon (Eds.), *Using evidence to guide nursing practice* (pp. 3–19). Sydney: Elsevier.

Coyer, F., Stotts, N., & Blackman, V. (2013). A prospective window into medical device-related pressure ulcers in intensive care. *International Wound Journal.* (In Press) Retrieved from http://eprints.qut.edu.au/58281

Davies, E., Moxham, T., Rees, K., Singh, S., Coats, A., Ebrahim, S., et al. (2010). Evidence based rehabilitation for heart failure. *Cochrane Database of Systematic Reviews, 4*, 1–3.

Estabrooks, C. (2009). Mapping the research utilization field in nursing. *Canadian Journal of Nursing Research, 41*(1), 219–235.

Esterman, A., Warland, J., & Deuter, K. (2010). Using the right type of evidence to answer clinical questions, In M. Courtney and H. McCutcheon (Eds.), *Using evidence to guide nursing practice* (pp. 27–41). Sydney: Elsevier.

Joanna Briggs Institute. (2013). *Levels of evidence FAME.* Retrieved February 6, 2013, from http://www.joannabriggs.edu.au/Levels%20of%20Evidence%20%20FAME

Kent, B., & McCormack, B. (2013). Applying research knowledge: evidence-based practice, practice development and knowledge translation. In Z. Schneider, D. Whitehead, G. LoBiondo-Wood, & J. Faber (Eds.), *Nursing and midwifery research* (pp. 317–331). Sydney: Elsevier.

National Health and Medical Research Council. (2008). *NHMRC additional levels of evidence and grades for recommendations for developers of guidelines*. Stage 2 Consultation 2008–2010. Canberra: Commonwealth of Australia.

Nay, R. & Fetherstonhaugh, D. (2007). Evidence-based practice limitations and successful implementation. *Annals of the New York Academy of Sciences, 1114*, 456–463.

McKinley, C., Fletcher, A., Biggins, A., McMurray, A., Birtwhistle, S., Gardiner, L., et al. (2007). Evidence-based management practice: reducing falls in hospital. *Collegian, 14*(2), 20–25.

Rycroft-Malone, J., Seers, K., Titchen, A., Harvey, G., Kitson, A., & McCormack, B. (2004). What counts as evidence in evidence based practice, *Journal of Advanced Nursing, 47*(1), 81–90.

Sackett, D., Straus, S., Richardson, W., Rosenberg, W., & Haynes, R. (2000). *Evidence based medicine: how to practice and teach EBM* (2nd ed.). London: Churchill Livingstone.

Stevens, K. (2010). Evidence-based practice: Destination or journey? *Nursing Outlook, 58*, 273–275.

WEBSITES

Accident Compensation Corporation (New Zealand):
http://www.acc.co.nz/for-providers/clinical-best-practice/index.htm

Guidelines International Network (GIN):
http://www.g-i-n.net/library/health-topics-collection/

Joanna Briggs Institute:
http://joannabriggs.org

National Health and Medical Research Council (NHMRC) clinical practice guidelines development:
http://www.nhmrc.gov.au/publications/synopses/cp30syn.htm

National Institute for Health and Care Excellence (NICE):
http://www.nice.org.uk

Cochrane Collaboration:
http://www.cochrane.org

CHAPTER 18

TOOLS FOR REVIEW

PAULA KERSTEN AND PETER LARMER

CHAPTER OVERVIEW

This chapter covers the following topics:

- Critical appraisal
- Critical appraisal tools for quantitative research
- Critical appraisal tools for qualitative research
- Critical appraisal tools for mixed methods research
- Critical appraisal tools for clinical guidelines

KEY TERMS

Bias	Interpretation
Blinding	Limitations
Cochrane Collaboration	Objective
Critical appraisal	Randomisation
Delphi	Reliability
Grey literature	Sampling

There are vast amounts of information available to practitioners and it is essential to understand tools that help with judging the quality and usefulness of it.

CRITICAL APPRAISAL

It is important to search the literature systematically to be sure that you have found all relevant information about a topic. After finding this information it can be tempting to simply summarise the authors' bottom line results of each study—and why not? Surely authors can be trusted to summarise their study well? Well, no; for example, there are authors who report on ill-designed studies, or studies with limited data or poor quality data, or those who overstate their conclusions. Even when authors report on perfectly designed studies, there will be limitations to their work. There is also evidence that studies with positive outcomes are more likely to be published (and faster) than those with negative results, and are also more likely to demonstrate greater effects than those in the 'grey literature' (Song et al., 2010). For these reasons publications are peer reviewed. Peers are subject experts who are supposed to be experts at the same level as the author of the source to be evaluated (Hjørland, 2012). Journals that do not use peer review or other non-peer reviewed resources are usually excluded from systematic reviews because they have not been scrutinised in this manner. However, peer review is not failsafe for judging research quality. One study showed that agreement between independent reviewers of articles submitted to a prestigious journal was no greater than would be expected by chance (Rothwell & Martyn, 2000). Therefore, it is important that students and practitioners have the skills to undertake their own reviews of any article, using critical appraisal skills. Critical appraisal is the assessment of evidence by systematically reviewing its relevance, validity and results to specific situations (Chambers Boath, & Rogers, 2004) and this is not restricted to systematic reviews of clinical trials (Crowe & Sheppard, 2011).

There are a number of tools, outlined below, to assist with critical appraisal, essentially by asking questions about the following:

1 the validity of the study design;
2 the robustness of the study results; and
3 the applicability of the findings to a clinical situation.

Critical appraisal tools can be designed using open questions, closed questions or with statements (Crowe & Sheppard, 2011); each has its own advantages and disadvantages. Confusingly, there are many different appraisal tools. For example, one systematic review of critical appraisal tools identified 121 different ones (Katrak et al., 2004). Of these tools some had been developed for primary research (78%), some were research design specific (87%) and others (9%) were suitable for any research design. A range of tools is outlined

Limitations
Restrictions on applicability or consequences.

Grey literature
Published information which is not peer reviewed.

Critical appraisal
A process of considering information from a perspective of critique.

below. The tools have been grouped according to types of study design, for example quantitative, qualitative, mixed methods, and guideline studies. Tools for reviewing systematic reviews have been described in Chapter 19 and will not be discussed in any more detail.

No judgments are made about any strengths and challenges of particular research designs, and there are no assumptions about the value of evidence from various approaches—for example, that the most valuable evidence comes from randomised controlled trials (RCTs). Different designs contribute different sorts of evidence, which may be more or less useful depending on the research question.

CRITICAL APPRAISAL TOOLS FOR QUANTITATIVE RESEARCH

There are many critical appraisal tools for quantitative studies in the literature and more for qualitative or mixed methods studies (Katrak et al., 2004; Crowe & Sheppard, 2011).

CRITICAL APPRAISAL TOOLS FOR RCTs

Cochrane Collaboration
An organisation which acts as a repository for evidence-based practice in health-care practice.

Bias
The preference of one particular response over another one.

Carrying out a review of the evidence of effectiveness of an intervention should include searching for RCTs. The Cochrane Collaboration is the most established organisation for the review of trials. Methods for systematic reviews can be found in its online handbook (Higgins & Green, 2011). This includes the requirement of only including RCTs, which should be assessed for their internal validity or their risk of bias using a domain-based evaluation (Higgins & Green, 2011). This tool includes the explicit assessment of the following types of bias:

• *selection bias:* bias due to inadequate generation of a randomised sequence or inadequate concealment of allocations prior to assignment;
• *performance bias:* bias due to knowledge of the allocated interventions by participants and personnel during the study;
• *detection bias:* bias due to knowledge of the allocated interventions by outcome assessors;
• *attrition bias:* bias due to amount, nature or handling of incomplete outcome data;
• *reporting bias:* bias due to selective outcome reporting; and
• *other bias:* bias due to problems not covered elsewhere in the table.

The assessment of bias results in a categorisation of each study into low risk, unclear risk or high risk of bias. The online Cochrane handbook (see the list of websites at the end of this chapter) is extremely useful for developing a search question, deciding on relevance of studies, how to assess other aspects of study quality and how to pool data from included studies with satisfactory quality.

In physiotherapy a commonly used critical appraisal tool is the PEDro scale (Maher et al., 2003). Its reliability has been examined and found to be fair to good when scored by more than one reviewer (Maher et al., 2003) and has been shown to be valid when summed into a total score (De Morton, 2009). The first item (eligibility criteria were specified) is not scored or added into the total score. The remaining 10 items are scored either as zero (criterion not met) or 1 (criterion met). The items include assessments of:

1 random allocation;
2 concealed allocation;
3 similarity of groups at baseline regarding the most important prognostic indicators;
4 blinding of all subjects;
5 blinding of all therapists who administered the therapy;
6 blinding of all assessors who measured at least one key outcome;
7 measures of at least one key outcome from more than 85% of the subjects initially allocated to groups;
8 intention to treat analysis;
9 between-group statistical comparisons reported for at least one key outcome; and
10 point measures and measures of variability for at least one key outcome provided.

The PEDro website provides an explanation of each of the criteria and tutorials. In addition, the site provides reviews of evidence for therapy using the PEDro tool.

Other tools for RCTs include the Downs and Black tool (1998) and the Consort statement (Wang et al., 2010).

CRITICAL APPRAISAL TOOLS FOR OBSERVATIONAL STUDIES

A relatively recent systematic review of critical appraisal tools for observational studies identified 86 tools, including simple checklists (48%), checklists with summary judgments (14%) and scales (38%) (Sanderson et al., 2007). It concluded that none of the tools could be recommended for use but suggested that the STROBE statement should provide a suitable starting point for development of a quality assessment tool. The STROBE tool (STrengthening the Reporting of OBservational studies in Epidemiology) was developed by an international interdisciplinary group with the aim of improving the reporting of observational studies (Von Elm et al., 2007). Its website lists an impressive range of journals that have endorsed STROBE. Three STROBE tools are available for cohort, case-control and cross-sectional studies each including 22 items that should be reported, under six headings:

1 Title and abstract;
2 Introduction: background/rationale, objectives;
3 Methods: study design, setting, participants, variables, data sources/measurement, bias, study design, quantitative variables and statistical methods;

Reliability
The extent to which the same results are elicited when an investigation is repeated.

Blinding
A research process that maintains anonymity, such as preventing research participants and/or researchers from identifying key details.

4   Results: participants, descriptive data, outcome data, main results and other analyses;

5   Discussion: key results, limitations, interpretation, generalisability; and

6   Other information: funding.

When using the STROBE tool, it is also wise to consult the explanatory paper on the tool (Vandenbroucke et al., 2007), which assists in undertaking a systematic appraisal.

Interpretation
Adapting or explaining information in a meaningful and relevant way.

CRITICAL APPRAISAL TOOLS FOR OUTCOME MEASUREMENT STUDIES

The COSMIN initiative (COnsensus-based Standards for the selection of health Measurement Instruments) aims to support researchers to evaluate the evidence of psychometric properties of health outcome measures (Mokkink, Terwee, et al., 2010; Angst, 2011). It has developed a checklist by means of Delphi approach. This is the first time a checklist for health measures has been developed by means of an international study. Although it is quite a new checklist, numerous studies that have used this approach are already published (Granger, McDonald, Parry, Oliveira, & Denehy, 2013; Mijnarends et al., 2013; Mutsaers, Peters, Pool-Goudzwaard, Koes, & Verhagen, 2012).

Delphi
A process for gathering data that involves layers of collection.

It is also helpful for students learning about outcome measurement studies. The COSMIN website includes the checklist, the scoring system and guidelines on searching for evidence (Terwee et al., 2009). It is recommended that the user undertakes some training to ensure the reliability of their scoring (Mokkink, Mokkink, et al., 2010). Essentially, the COSMIN takes the reviewer through four distinct steps with detailed questions in 12 boxes:

1   Determine which measurement properties are evaluated in the article.

2   Determine if the statistical method used in the article is based on classical test theory or item response theory.

3   Determine if a study meets the standards for good methodological quality. To make this assessment the checklist provides detailed questions in 12 boxes (which are completed only for those measurement properties evaluated in the article): an assessment of the methodological quality of the study, including internal consistency, reliability, measurement error, content validity, structural validity, hypotheses testing, cross-cultural validity, criterion validity, responsiveness and interpretability.

4   Determine the generalisability of the results.

CRITICAL APPRAISAL TOOLS FOR QUALITATIVE RESEARCH

There is debate within the academic literature as to the appropriateness of critical appraisal of qualitative research (Tate & Douglas, 2011). As in quantitative research, many argue that qualitative research can be of good as well as poor quality (Walsh &

Downe, 2006) and that the use of appraisal tools is therefore appropriate. Others contend that knowledge is constructed and therefore not as stable or as objective as quantitative research (Crotty, 1998) and not appropriate for critical appraisal (see Cohen & Crabtree, 2008, for a discussion on these issues). Tate and Douglas (2011) conclude that evidence from qualitative studies can make an important contribution to systematic reviews across healthcare practice. Cohen and Crabtree (2008) conducted a systematic review of qualitative evaluation tools and identified seven common evaluative criteria but not all were accepted by researchers. In particular, there was extensive debate on the importance of reflexivity or attending to researcher bias, the importance of establishing validity or credibility, and the importance of verification or reliability. Walsh and Downe (2006) undertook a review of qualitative research appraisal tools and identified eight checklists: six which were interpretative, one positivist and one unstated. They used their findings to develop a new tool for the appraisal of qualitative studies. This tool includes prompts for essential criteria, which they grouped into eight stages:

Objective
An approach that implies a completely external or detached view of an object or phenomenon.

1 scope and purpose;
2 design;
3 sampling strategy;
4 analysis;
5 interpretation;
6 reflexivity;
7 ethical dimensions; and
8 relevance and transferability.

Another recommended tool, developed by Malterud (2001), includes guidelines for the aim of the study, reflexivity, methods and design, data collection and sampling, theoretical frameworks, analysis, findings and discussion.

Sampling
The process of identifying participants for a study.

CASE STUDY 18.1

MONITORING BLOOD GLUCOSE

Janet is a nurse clinical specialist working with diabetes patients. She has noticed that many of her patients don't regularly monitor their blood glucose, despite most of them promising they will when they attend clinic. She has been reading the literature around adherence and is aware that there are many reasons why patients do not monitor their symptoms consistently. One of her

[continued next page]

regular patients, Joe, will be attending clinic on Monday and she knows he is one of those patients that monitors his glucose levels very inconsistently. She is keen to check the literature for an approach that may help Joe to improve on this. Janet's colleague has mentioned that the development of implementation intentions may help Joe to set some goals around self-monitoring of his blood glucose, but also to set some plans that specifically describe when, where and what he might do to meet these goals. She has found an interesting article describing this approach (Nadkarni et al., 2010). As Janet recently attended a professional development workshop on critiquing research evidence she has decided to use the PEDro tool (Maher et al., 2003) to critique this randomised controlled trial.

In this study the intervention group is asked to complete a questionnaire, designed to induce participants to form self-monitoring of blood glucose (SMBG) implementation plans:

- Participants were asked a series of questions to get them to start thinking about their self-monitoring behaviour such as questions regarding their glucometer.
- They were instructed to form their plans using the instructions and table illustrated in the paper, writing down when, where and whether someone else would assist them in performing SMBG.
- Participants were told to close their eyes for a moment and to think about the plans they made.
- They were then asked how committed they were to following through with their SMBG plans.

The intervention was written at the eighth grade level and piloted using cognitive interviewing. Janet's review of the study are summarised in Table 18.1.

TABLE 18.1   USING PEDro TO CRITIQUE RESEARCH

METHODS QUALITY (PEDRO SCALE)	DESCRIPTION (HTTP://WWW.PEDRO.ORG.AU/ENGLISH/DOWNLOADS/PEDRO-SCALE)	SCORING AND COMMENTS
Eligibility criteria were specified.	1 This criterion is satisfied if the report describes the source of subjects and a list of criteria used to determine who was eligible to participate in the study.	☑

METHODS QUALITY (PEDRO SCALE)	DESCRIPTION (HTTP://WWW.PEDRO.ORG.AU/ ENGLISH/DOWNLOADS/PEDRO-SCALE)	SCORING AND COMMENTS
Subjects were randomly allocated to groups (in a cross-over study, subjects were randomly allocated an order in which treatments were received).	2 A study is considered to have used random allocation if the report states that allocation was random. The precise method of randomisation need not be specified. Procedures such as coin-tossing and dice-rolling should be considered random. Quasi-randomised allocation procedures such as allocation by hospital record number or birth date, or alternation, do not satisfy this criterion. Score 1 for yes and 0 for no	1
Allocation was concealed.	3 *Concealed allocation* means that the person who determined if a subject was eligible for inclusion in the trial was unaware, when this decision was made, of which group the subject would be allocated to. A point is awarded for this criterion, even if it is not stated that allocation was concealed, when the report states that allocation was by sealed opaque envelopes or that allocation involved contacting the holder of the allocation schedule who was 'off-site'. Score 1 for yes and 0 for no	*No face–to-face intervention, so not really relevant. The researcher has to know which group so as to send the right pack.* 1
The groups were similar at baseline regarding the most important prognostic indicators.	4 At a minimum, in studies of therapeutic interventions, the report must describe at least one measure of the severity of the condition being treated and at least one (different) key outcome measure at baseline. The rater must be satisfied that the groups' outcomes would not be expected to differ, on the basis of baseline differences in prognostic variables alone, by a clinically significant amount. This criterion is satisfied even if only baseline data of study completers are presented. Score 1 for yes and 0 for no	1
There was blinding of all subjects.	5 *Blinding* means the person in question (subject) did not know which group the subject had been allocated to. In addition, subjects are considered to be 'blind' only if it could be expected that they would have been unable to distinguish between the treatments applied to different groups. Score 1 for yes and 0 for no	*Probably but not clearly stated* 0

[continued next page]

PAULA KERSTEN AND PETER LARMER

TABLE 18.1   USING PEDro TO CRITIQUE RESEARCH (*continued*)

METHODS QUALITY (PEDRO SCALE)	DESCRIPTION (HTTP://WWW.PEDRO.ORG.AU/ ENGLISH/DOWNLOADS/PEDRO-SCALE)	SCORING AND COMMENTS
There was blinding of all therapists who administered the therapy.	6 *Blinding* means the person in question (therapist) did not know which group the subject had been allocated to. In addition, therapists are considered to be 'blind' only if it could be expected that they would have been unable to distinguish between the treatments applied to different groups. Score 1 for yes and 0 for no	*Not really relevant as intervention delivered by post* 1
There was blinding of all assessors who measured at least one key outcome.	7 *Blinding* means the person in question (assessor) did not know which group the subject had been allocated to. In trials in which key outcomes are self-reported (e.g. visual analogue scale, pain diary), the assessor is considered to be blind if the subject was blind. Score 1 for yes and 0 for no	*If subject was blinded then yes, but that wasn't clear.* 0
Measures of at least one key outcome were obtained from more than 85% of the subjects initially allocated to groups.	8 This criterion is satisfied only if the report explicitly states *both* the number of subjects initially allocated to groups *and* the number of subjects from whom key outcome measures were obtained. In trials in which outcomes are measured at several points in time, a key outcome must have been measured in more than 85% of subjects at one of those points in time. Score 1 for yes and 0 for no	*Not known how many questionnaires sent to each group or how many returned but not included in the analysis.* 0
All subjects for whom outcome measures were available received the treatment or control condition as allocated or, where this was not the case, data for at least one key outcome were analysed by 'intention to treat'.	9 An *intention to treat* analysis means that, where subjects did not receive treatment (or the control condition) as allocated and where measures of outcomes were available, the analysis was performed as if subjects received the treatment (or control condition) they were allocated to. This criterion is satisfied, even if there is no mention of analysis by intention to treat, if the report explicitly states that all subjects received treatment or control conditions as allocated. Score 1 for yes and 0 for no	1

The results of between-group statistical comparisons were reported for at least one key outcome.	10 A *between-group* statistical comparison involves statistical comparison of one group with another. Depending on the design of the study, this may involve comparison of two or more treatments, or comparison of treatment with a control condition. The analysis may be a simple comparison of outcomes measured after the treatment was administered, or a comparison of the change in one group with the change in another (when a factorial analysis of variance has been used to analyse the data, the latter is often reported as a group × time interaction). The comparison may be in the form of hypothesis testing (which provides a *p*-value, describing the probability that the groups differed only by chance) or in the form of an estimate (e.g. the mean or median difference, or a difference in proportions, or number needed to treat, or a relative risk or hazard ratio) and its confidence interval. Score 1 for yes and 0 for no	1
The study provided both point measures and measures of variability for at least one key outcome.	11 A *point measure* is a measure of the size of the treatment effect. The treatment effect may be described as a difference in group outcomes, or as the outcome in (each of) all groups. *Measures of variability* include standard deviations, standard errors, confidence intervals, interquartile ranges (or other quartile ranges), and ranges. Point measures and/or measures of variability may be provided graphically (for example, standard deviations may be given as error bars in a figure) as long as it is clear what is being graphed (e.g. as long as it is clear whether error bars represent standard deviations or standard errors). Where outcomes are categorical, this criterion is considered to have been met if the number of subjects in each category is given for each group. Score 1 for yes and 0 for no	0
Total PEDro score	Sum of PEDro criteria.	6

[continued next page]

PAULA KERSTEN AND PETER LARMER

Based on her critique of this trial Janet comes to the conclusion that the trial has some limitations (for example, it wasn't clear if the subject in the intervention group and the study researchers were blinded, she couldn't determine from the paper if 85% of the subjects had been included in the data analysis and the study didn't provide both point measures and measures of variability for at least one key outcome. However, other aspects of the study had been well conducted, the intervention group had fared better than the control groups and, importantly, there were no adverse effects in the intervention group. On balance, she therefore decides to go ahead and try this novel approach with Joe when he comes in on Monday.

CRITICAL APPRAISAL TOOLS FOR MIXED METHODS RESEARCH

Reviews of mixed method studies are able to bring together the strengths of qualitative and quantitative methods and combine in-depth descriptions of qualitative findings with statistical generalisability of the quantitative results (Pace et al., 2012). Dixon-Woods et al. (2006) conducted a study exploring the inclusion of qualitative research in (quantitative) systematic reviews. They found a large number of qualitative appraisal tools (more than 100), with very few making distinctions between different study designs or theoretical approaches. A consensus tool for mixed methods studies has therefore been called for (Bouchard, Dubuisson, Simard, & Dorval, 2011). A recently developed tool for mixed method studies is the Mixed Methods Appraisal Tool (MMAT), including a scoring system (Pluye et al., 2009). The MMAT was developed following an extensive literature review, with acceptable reliability (Pace et al., 2012). It includes 15 methodological quality criteria under four headings:

1 *qualitative:* qualitative objective or question, appropriate qualitative approach or design or method, description of the context, description of participants and justification of sampling, description of qualitative data collection and analysis, discussion of researchers' reflexivity;

2 *quantitative experimental:* appropriate sequence generation and/or randomisation, allocation concealment and/or blinding, complete outcome data and/or low withdrawal or drop-out;

Randomisation
The process of allocating research participants or elements to different parts of an experiment (such as control group or active treatment group).

3   *quantitative observational:* appropriate sampling and sample, justification of measurements (validity and standards), control of confounding variables; and

4   *mixed methods:* justification of the mixed methods design, combination of qualitative and quantitative data collection and analysis techniques or procedures, and integration of qualitative and quantitative data or results.

CRITICAL APPRAISAL TOOLS FOR CLINICAL GUIDELINES

Clinical guidelines are incredibly useful for clinicians and ensure an evidence-based approach to interventions. However, not all guidelines have been developed using robust research and it is therefore important to critically appraise the evidence for them. A well-established tool for the review of guidelines is the AGREE instrument (Appraisal of Guidelines for Research & Evaluation) (Cluzeau et al., 2003), which has recently been revamped into the AGREE II instrument. This instrument includes 23 items in six domains, each scored on a scale ranging from 1 (strongly disagree) to 7 (strongly agree):

1   *scope and purpose:* objectives of the guideline, health questions covered and target population;

2   *stakeholder involvement:* constitution of the development group, views of the target population, and target users defined;

3   *rigour of development:* systematic search methods, criteria for selecting the evidence; strengths and limitations of the body of evidence; methods for formulating the recommendations; health benefits, side effects and risks considered; an explicit link between the recommendations and the supporting evidence; an external review before publication, and a procedure for updating the guideline;

4   *clarity of presentation:* specific and unambiguous recommendations, clear presentation of different options for management of the condition or health issue, and key recommendations easily identifiable;

5   *applicability:* facilitators and barriers to its application, advice and/or tools on how the recommendations can be put into practice, potential resource implications, and monitoring and/or auditing criteria; and

6   *editorial independence:* views of the funding body have not influenced the content of the guideline; competing interests have been recorded and addressed.

RESEARCH ALIVE 18.1
TRAUMATIC BRAIN INJURY

Recently, a review of the literature was undertaken to explore approaches that may help people after a traumatic brain injury (TBI) achieve better participation, defined as 'involvement in a life situation' (World Health Organization, 2001). The reseachers were interested whether mentoring for people with a recent TBI by others who had sustained a TBI was useful. Three articles were identified, then critically appraised (Hibbard et al., 2002; Struchen et al., 2011; Hanks, Rapport et al., 2012). The first study showed that peer mentoring can result in positive findings on knowledge, quality of life, general outlook and ability to cope with depression post-TBI (Hibbard et al., 2002). However, a key limitation of this study was that it didn't include a control group so it was not possible to work out whether the outcomes could have arisen because people received attention from someone, or through the specific intervention. Another study didn't find significant improvements in social activity level or social network size, but showed a trend toward increased satisfaction with social life (Struchen et al., 2011). Criticisms included the fact that there was a large drop-out of trained mentors and of randomised mentees, a range of validated and unvalidated outcome measures were used in the study, the set intervention dosage (number of outings) was not met in all cases, and the sample size was small. The third study (Hanks et al., 2012) found significant differences between groups (in favour of those with TBI who were mentored) for behavioural control, less chaos in the living environment, lower alcohol use, less emotion-focused and avoidance coping, and better quality of life (physical subscale) and community integration. However, the frequency of social outings and mentor contact was lower than planned and there were few participants from more rural areas in this study.

In summary, the three studies showed some encouraging findings and no adverse events. However, their methodological limitations and the fact they were all carried out in the United States of America, which may not be comparable to the context of Aotearoa New Zealand or Australia, meant the findings were not directly transferable. This led to the development of a research protocol, for which a funding application was submitted.

SUMMARY

Critical appraisal of research is important and provides superior evaluation compared to unstructured reviews. There is no consensus on the best critical appraisal tool.

The choice of a critical appraisal tool should be based on how relevant it is to the research design and on the rigour with which the tool was developed. This is a fast-changing research area and students and practitioners need to regularly update themselves about new tools.

REFLECTION POINTS

- What stands out for you after reading this chapter?
- How confident are you in looking for a critical appraisal tool? Why?
- How confident are you in choosing an appropriate critical appraisal tool?
- What skills do you need to gain to build your confidence using a critical appraisal tool?
- How might you go about this?

STUDY QUESTIONS

1   Choose an article of interest in your field of practice.
2   Read the article.
3   Summarise your views on the article without using a critical appraisal tool.
4   Choose an appropriate critical appraisal tool and use this to evaluate the paper.
5   Compare the review you did with and without the critical appraisal tool—what stands out to you? For example, is your conclusion the same or not, and why might this be?

ADDITIONAL READING

Gosall, N., & Gosall, G. (2012) *The doctor's guide to critical appraisal* (3rd ed.). Knutsford: PasTest.

Nayar, S., & Stanley, M. (Eds). (in press) *Talking qualitative research*. London: Routledge.

Rose-Grippa, K., Haber, J., Berry, C., & Yost, J. (2010) *Study guide for nursing research: Methods and critical appraisal for evidence-based practice* (7th ed.). Pageburst e-book on VitalSource.

Sackett, D. L., &. Rosenberg, W. M., Gray, J. A., Haynes, R. B., & Richardson, W. S. (1996). Evidence based medicine: what it is and what it isn't. *BMJ (Clinical Research Ed.) 312*(7023), 71–72.

REFERENCES

Angst, F. (2011). The new COSMIN guidelines confront traditional concepts of responsiveness. *BMC Medical Research Methodology, 11*, 152.

Bouchard, K., Dubuisson, W., Simard, J., & Dorval, M. (2011). Systematic mixed-methods reviews are not ready to be assessed with the available tools. *Journal of Clinical Epidemiology, 64*(8), 926–928.

Chambers, R., Boath, E., & Rogers, D. (2004). *Clinical effectiveness and clinical governance made easy.* Abingdon: Radcliffe Medical Press Ltd.

Cluzeau, F., & Burgers, J., et al. (2003). Development and validation of an international appraisal instrument for assessing the quality of clinical practice guidelines: The AGREE project. *Quality and Safety in Health Care, 12*(1), 18–23.

Cohen, D. J., & Crabtree, B. F. (2008). Evaluative criteria for qualitative research in health care: Controversies and recommendations. *Annals of Family Medicine, 6*(4), 331–339.

Crotty, M. (1998). *The foundations of social research: meaning and perspective in the research process.* London, Sage Publications.

Crowe, M., & Sheppard, L. (2011). A review of critical appraisal tools show they lack rigor: Alternative tool structure is proposed. *Journal of Clinical Epidemiology, 64*(1), 79–89.

De Morton, N. A. (2009). The PEDro scale is a valid measure of the methodological quality of clinical trials: a demographic study. *Australian Journal of Physiotherapy, 55*(2), 129–133.

Dixon-Woods, M., Bonas, S., Booth, A., Jones, D. R., Miller, T., Sutton, A. J., et al. (2006). How can systematic reviews incorporate qualitative research? A critical perspective. *Qualitative Research, 6*(1), 27–44.

Downs, S. H., & Black, N. (1998). The feasibility of creating a checklist for the assessment of the methodological quality both of randomised and non-randomised studies of health care interventions. *Journal of Epidemiology and Community Health, 52*(6), 377–384.

Granger, C. L., McDonald, C. F., Parry, S. M., Oliveira, C. C., & Denehy, L. (2013). Functional capacity, physical activity and muscle strength assessment of individuals with non-small cell lung cancer: a systematic review of instruments and their measurement properties. *BMC Cancer, 13*, 135–135.

Hanks, R.A., & Rapport, L. J. et al. (2012). Randomized controlled trial of peer mentoring for individuals with traumatic brain injury and their significant others. *Archives of Physical Medicine & Rehabilitation, 93*(a8), 1297–1304.

Hibbard, M. R., Cantor, J., Charatz, H. J., Rosenthal, R., Ashman, T. A., Gundersen, N., et al. (2002). Peer support in the community: initial findings of a mentoring program for individuals with traumatic brain injury and their families. *Journal of Head Trauma Rehabilitation, 17*(2), 112–131.

Higgins, J. P. T., & Green, S. (Eds.). (2011). *Cochrane handbook for systematic reviews of interventions.* Version 5.1.0 (updated March 2011). Available from http://www.cochrane-handbook.org.

Hjørland, B. (2012). Methods for evaluating information sources: An annotated catalogue. *Journal of Information Science 38*(3), 258–268.

Katrak, P., Bialocerkowski, A. E., Massy-Westropp, N., Kumar, V. S., Grimmer, K. (2004). A systematic review of the content of critical appraisal tools. *BMC Medical Research Methodology, 4*(1), 22.

Maher, C. G., Sherrington, C., Herbert, R. D., Moseley, A. M., & Elkins, M. (2003). Reliability of the PEDro scale for rating quality of randomized controlled trials. *Physical Therapy, 83*(8), 713–721.

Malterud, K. (2001). Qualitative research: Standards, challenges, and guidelines. *The Lancet, 358*(9280), 483–488.

Mijnarends, D. M., Meijers, J. M. M., Halfens, R. J. G., ter Borg, S., Luiking, Y. C., et al. (2013). Validity and reliability of tools to measure muscle mass, strength, and physical performance in community-dwelling older people: A systematic review. *Journal of the American Medical Directors Association, 14*(3), 170–178.

Mokkink, L. B., Terwee, C. B., Gibbons, E., Stratford, P. W., Alonso, J., Patrick, D. L., et al. (2010). Inter-rater agreement and reliability of the COSMIN (COnsensus-based Standards for the selection of health status Measurement Instruments) Checklist. *BMC Medical Research Methodology, 10*(1), 82.

Mokkink, L. B., Mokkink, L., Terwee, C., Knol, D., Stratford, P., Alonso, J., et al. (2010). The COSMIN checklist for evaluating the methodological quality of studies on measurement properties: a clarification of its content. *BMC Medical Research Methodology, 10*, 22.

Mutsaers, J. H. A. M., Peters, R., Pool-Goudzwaard, A. L., Koes, B. W., & Verhagen, A. P. (2012). Psychometric properties of the pain attitudes and beliefs scale for physiotherapists: A systematic review. *Manual Therapy, 17*(3), 213–218.

Nadkarni, A., Kucukarslan, S. N., Bagozzi, R. P., Yates, J. F., & Erickson, S. R. (2010). A simple and promising tool to improve self-monitoring of blood glucose in patients with diabetes. *Diabetes Research and Clinical Practice, 89*(1), 30–37.

Pace, R., Pluye, P., Bartlett, G., Macaulay, A. C., Salsberg, J., Jagosh, J., et al. (2012). Testing the reliability and efficiency of the pilot Mixed Methods Appraisal Tool (MMAT) for systematic mixed studies review. *International Journal of Nursing Studies, 49*(1), 47–53.

Pluye, P., & Gagnon, M. P., Griffiths, F., & Johnson-Lafleur, J. (2009). A scoring system for appraising mixed methods research, and concomitantly appraising qualitative, quantitative and mixed methods primary studies in mixed studies reviews. *International Journal of Nursing Studies, 46*(4), 529–546.

Rothwell, P. M., & Martyn C. N. (2000). Reproducibility of peer review in clinical neuroscience: Is agreement between reviewers any greater than would be expected by chance alone? *Brain, 123*(9), 1964–1969.

Sanderson, S., Tatt, I. D., & Higgins, J. P. (2007). Tools for assessing quality and susceptibility to bias in observational studies in epidemiology: A systematic review and annotated bibliography. *International Journal of Epidemiology, 36*(3), 666–676.

Song, F., Parekh, S., Hooper, L., Loke, Y. K., Ryder, J., Sutton, A. J., et al. (2010). Dissemination and publication of research findings: An updated review of related biases. *Health Technology Assessment, 14*(8), 1–220.

Struchen, M. A., Davis, L. C., Bogaards, J. A., Hudler-Hull, T., Clark, A. N., Mazzei, D. M., et al. (2011). Making connections after brain injury: development and evaluation of a social peer-mentoring program for persons with traumatic brain injury. *Journal of Head Trauma Rehabilitation, 26*(1), 4–19.

Tate, R. L., & Douglas, J. (2011). Use of reporting guidelines in scientific writing: PRISMA, CONSORT, STROBE, STARD and other resources. *Brain Impairment, 12*(1), 2–21.

Terwee, C.B., Jansma, E. P., Riphagen, I. I., & de Vet, H.C.W. (2009). Development of a methodological PubMed search filter for finding studies on measurement properties of measurement instruments. *Quality of Life Research, 18*(8), 1115–1123.

Vandenbroucke, J. P., Von Elm, E., Altman, D. G., Gøtzsche, P. C., Mulrow, C. D., Pocock, S. J., et al. (2007). Strengthening the Reporting of Observational Studies in Epidemiology (STROBE): Explanation and elaboration. *PLoS Medicine, 4*(10), 1628–1654.

Von Elm, E., Altman, D. G., Egger, M., Pocock, S. J., Gøtzsche, P. C., & Vandenbroucke J. P. (2007). The Strengthening of the Reporting of Observational Studies in Epidemiology (STROBE) statement: Guidelines for reporting observational studies. *Annals of Internal Medicine, 147*(8), 573–577.

Walsh, D., & Downe, S. (2006). Appraising the quality of qualitative research. *Midwifery, 22*(2), 108–119.

Wang, C. Y., Lee, C. S., Lin, Y. C., Chen, L. Y., Fang, Z. R., Tsai1, Y. C. et al. (2010). An evidence-based guide and assessment tool for reports of randomized controlled trials-CONSORT statement 2010. *Journal of Internal Medicine of Taiwan, 21*(6), 408–418.

World Health Organization. (2001). *International classification of functioning, disability and health: ICF*. Geneva: Author.

WEBSITES

Agree Enterprise:
http://www.agreetrust.org

Resources for the review of guidelines, such as on line tutorials, on line recording of the review and links to the Appraisal of Guidelines for Research & Evaluation Instrument (AGREE II).

CONSORT Group:
http://www.consort-statement.org

Resources for the Consolidated Standards of Reporting Trials (CONSORT), an evidence-based, minimum set of recommendations for reporting RCTs.

COSMIN initiative:
http://www.cosmin.nl

Resources for the evaluation of the methodological quality of studies on the measurement properties of health measurement instruments: COnsensus-based Standards for the selection of health Measurement Instruments (COSMIN).

Critical Appraisal Skills Programme (CASP):
http://www.casp-uk.net

Resources for the critical appraisal of a range of study designs, including quantiative and qualitative studies.

Grading of Recommendations Assessment, Development and Evaluation (GRADE) Working Group:
http://www.gradeworkinggroup.org/index.htm

GRADE working provides resources for grading quality of evidence and strength of recommendations (quantitative research).

McGill University:

   mixedmethodsappraisaltoolpublic.pbworks.com/f/MMAT 202011
   20criteriaandtutorial2011-06-29.pdf

Resources for the Mixed Methods Appraisal Tool (MMAT) Version 2011. This critical
   appraisal tool is still in development.

McMaster University, Centre for Evidence-Based Medicine (CEBM):

   fhswedge.csu.mcmaster.ca/cepftp/qasite/CriticalAppraisal.html

Resources on evidence-based medicine, with links to descriptions of study designs,
   levels of evidence and critical appraisal tools for quantitative research studies.

McMasters University:

   http://www.srs-mcmaster.ca/Portals/20/pdf/ebp/qualreview_version2.0.pdf

A critical appraisal tool for qualitative studies.

CHAPTER 19

UNDERSTANDING SYSTEMATIC REVIEWS

PETER LARMER AND PAULA KERSTEN

CHAPTER OVERVIEW

This chapter covers the following topics:

- What is a systematic review?
- What is involved in a systematic review?
- Meta-analysis
- The Cochrane Collaboration
- Reviews of qualitative studies

KEY TERMS

Control
Hierarchy of evidence
Interpretative
Library databases
Meta-analysis
PICO
Power
Theory

Within the field of health-care practice there are some highly developed and recognised tools for considering research. Systematic reviews provide high quality and useful information, which contributes to current practice and practice development.

WHAT IS A SYSTEMATIC REVIEW?

Systematic reviews of both qualitative and quantitative research provide highly valuable research for practice and therefore influence the outcomes of patients and service users. Undertaking a systematic review is a complex task which normally involves a group of colleagues working together over an extended period of time to follow a carefully designed protocol. The process of undertaking a systematic review is complex and beyond the scope of this chapter. However, it is important to appreciate the process of this type of research.

Systematic reviews are a very specific approach to research. They provide a framework for bringing together and analysing a number of studies that have considered similar questions (such as exercise and osteoarthritis, or nursing and hand washing). In an attempt to understand and critique all the papers that may contribute to a systematic review, academics and clinicians have often collected similar research articles and summarised the findings, referring to the outcome as a review article. In the past, review articles were essentially a 'cut and paste' of the conclusions of the original articles. Often, these reviewers would not separate the good research from the poor research, so there is always a need to be cautious about taking useful information from such reviews.

The process of review has now been refined into what are referred to as a 'systematic review'. It involves systematically (hence the name) and thoroughly searching all the relevant and related research, which is then critiqued and quality rated before providing evidence-based conclusions. These systematic reviews first started appearing around the 1970s, but have become much more rigorous in how findings are presented. A number of authors have written extensively on this topic (Guyatt, Sackett, & Cook, 1993; Guyatt et al., 1995; Haynes, Sackett, Gray, Cook, & Guyatt, 1997; Muir Gray, Haynes, Sackett, Cook, & Guyatt, 1997; Oxman, Sackett, & Guyatt, 1993).

WHAT IS INVOLVED IN A SYSTEMATIC REVIEW?

Undertaking a systematic review can be considered original research in its own right. This may seem contradictory as it involves the research of others. However, the process of collecting data, analysing them and reaching a finding is the foundation of research, and systematic reviews are fundamentally involved with collecting data (albeit those of others), analysing the information and then reaching a conclusion.

THE QUESTION

As with all research processes, systematic reviews begin with a question. The more detailed or precise the question, the easier it will be to identify relevant studies. Spending time thinking and refining the question will make things easier as the project progresses. Below are examples of two general questions and then more refined questions. Refining the questions helps to reduce the number of relevant articles identified.

CASE STUDY 19.1

THE DEVELOPMENT OF A QUESTION

Example 1: Arthritis Question

- How effective is exercise for osteoarthritis? (2433 articles found)
- How effective is isometric strengthening exercise for knee osteoarthritis in adults? (15 articles found)

Example 2: Hand-Washing Question

- Hand hygiene in hospitals (892 articles found)
- How effective is nurses' hand hygiene in an intensive care unit? (23 articles found)

It is recommended that search questions follow a PICO format (see Chapter 17) wherever possible, containing information about the Population of interest, the Intervention being researched, which Control it is being compared with, and the Outcome of interest. The more refined and specific the question, the smaller the number of articles there are to retrieve from the library databases, as shown in the examples above. The skills used to carry out a literature search (such as what terms to use) are very useful when undertaking systematic views and it is advisable to have the support of an experienced librarian to assist with the search strategy (such as with the search terms, keywords and databases to use).

PICO
An acronym for developing research questions: Problem/Population; Intervention; Comparison/Control; Outcome.

Control
A research cohort not treated in an active way to provide a point of comparison.

Library databases
Tools for cataloguing information that enable many sources to be searched.

INCLUSION AND EXCLUSION CRITERIA

Once the search on databases has been completed and the articles have been summarised (synopsis) it is necessary to identify which are relevant to the question. Even though specific terms will have been searched some articles that contain the words or terms may be of little or no relevance to the research question or context. They may be completely unhelpful in answering the question and so need to be discarded. Ideally, the search will result in a manageable number of studies to read. If there are too many articles to be practical there may be a need to refine the question even further. In formulating the question some other points that may be too detailed to include in the search strategy will have been considered. These points are referred to as the inclusion and exclusion criteria: the essential research characteristics to determine which articles are included for review and which articles are to be discarded and not reviewed. It is useful to note these criteria down before starting to search the literature. Articles can then be scanned to make sure they meet the inclusion criteria and those that fall into the exclusion criteria can be discarded. It is always important to note down the number of articles originally found, the number discarded and the number included.

CASE STUDY 19.2

EXCLUSION AND INCLUSION

Example 1: Arthritis Inclusion and Exclusion Criteria

Inclusion:
* Only studies that included men over 60 years of age with osteoarthritis
* Only randomised controlled studies

Exclusion:
* Studies that included men who have had polio or other forms of arthritis

Example 2: Hand Washing Inclusion and Exclusion Criteria

Inclusion:
* Only studies that investigated nurse's compliance with hand hygiene

Exclusion:
* Studies that included rural hospitals

Once you are sure you have all the articles that have looked at areas similar to your original question, you then need to read them and extract the relevant information (or data) from them. Normally you would put this information into a table. Examples of column headings in such tables can be seen in tables 19.1 and 19.2.

TABLE 19.1   SUMMARY OF STUDIES COMPARING ISOMETRIC
STRENGTHENING EXERCISE IN MEN WITH KNEE
OSTEOARTHRITIS

AUTHOR YEAR	STUDY DESIGN	PARTICIPANT DEMOGRAPHICS	INTERVENTION		OUTCOME MEASURES	RESULTS
			EXERCISE	CONTROL		

TABLE 19.2   SUMMARY OF TRIALS COMPARING THE ANTIMICROBIAL
EFFICACY OF HAND HYGIENE USAGE

AUTHOR YEAR	STUDY DESIGN	INTERVENTION: MEDICATED OR PLAIN SOAP	MONITORING	OUTCOME

QUALITY RATING

After identifying the included articles, the next challenge is to decide which articles provide the best information or evidence. Depending on the question there may be a number of different types of studies, both quantitative and qualitative. Quantitative studies may include a range of approaches such as randomised controlled trials (RCTs), cohort studies or case studies, all of which provide varying levels of information. A case study may provide good information if the question relates exactly to the case that is described. Unfortunately this rarely occurs (particularly for patients, as no two patients are ever the same). At other times an RCT may provide better information as these studies can include a range of participants that may have attributes related to the question. Particularly in quantitative research when different types of studies are grouped together, they can be ranked according to their risk of bias, often called 'levels of evidence' or the hierarchy of evidence (Table 19.3). Different levels of evidence vary in their ability to predict an outcome. The higher the ranking of the study the more confidence the reader or consumer of research, can have that the outcome results of the study can be applied.

Hierarchy of evidence
A tool for evaluating research findings according to the degree of scientific rigour.

TABLE 19.3 LEVELS OF EVIDENCE OF RESEARCH STUDIES

PREDICTABILITY OF OUTCOME	STUDY DESIGN
Greater predictability	Double-blind randomised control trial
	Single-blind randomised control trial
	Randomised control trial
	Cohort study
	Case control
	Case study
Least predictability	Expert opinion

It might come as a surprise that expert opinion is the least predictable form of evidence when undertaking a systematic review. This is said to occur because an 'expert' will have their own particular bias as to what they think will work. In addition to the levels of evidence, each study should be critiqued. All types of studies will have some form of bias or weakness. That is an accepted fact. Readers and consumers of research need to understand where that bias may be found through critiquing any research article. So how do we critique studies?

RESEARCH ALIVE 19.1
OSTEOARTHRITIS

There is a lot of information about the management for osteoarthritis. We wanted to collect all the information that would help us provide useful information for people with arthritis. In the recent past if someone was told they had arthritis they were told to rest and not to exercise. However, many researchers did not believe this was best and conducted studies to investigate how exercise affected people with arthritis. After a few years many studies were repeated with slightly different exercise interventions. Then people started to undertake systematic reviews on this subject. The individual studies were collected up and conclusions were made from the evidence. The next progression from the systematic review is to develop a 'guideline' which puts the information from the systematic review into a practical clinical setting. We found a number of guidelines that looked at the management of osteoarthritis. We found that there was very strong evidence from all the guidelines that in fact exercise is very beneficial for you if you have arthritis.

Chapter 18 describes tools that assist with critiquing and scoring an individual study. In a systematic review a tool is used to critique the strength of every study. After critiquing and scoring every study and ranking the studies according to the level of evidence, there is a need to put this all together to arrive at some meaningful statements or recommendations that make sense. It is likely that some of the studies identified will find a positive result and some will show that there is no difference using the intervention. This is why using a tool to critique is so important. Based on the critique some value judgments can be made.

CASE STUDY 19.3

JUDGING EVIDENCE

Let us suppose that you found six studies that looked at an intervention. Now, if we say three of the studies were randomised controlled trials, had all scored highly using your critiquing tool and all showed a positive result, and the other three studies were case-controlled studies, had scored poorly with your critiquing tool and all three showed no difference in the intervention, then you could be fairly confident to suggest that the intervention would be worth recommending. This is where having at least another 'author' assisting you in the review is so important. You can then talk about your results and how you evaluate the results to see if you agree with each other.

META-ANALYSIS

The term meta-analysis is often used when a lot of studies have been considered together. Sometimes researchers will call their paper something like 'A meta-analysis of the effect of [a particular intervention]'. A meta-analysis is really a part of a systematic review. The meta-analysis refers to the 'pooling' of the data from all the individual studies that have been found. So these researchers will combine the raw data of the individual studies they have found and put them together if appropriate. This can be a powerful way to study large numbers of people using a particular intervention when each individual study has only small numbers of participants.

Meta-analysis
The process of undertaking a quantitative analysis of similar research studies.

CASE STUDY 19.4

EXAMPLE OF A META-ANALYSIS

Power
A judgment about the
importance or weight of
a statistic.

Suppose you have five studies: study 1 has 50 people ($N = 50$), study 2 has 40 ($N = 40$), study 3 has 45 ($N = 45$), study 4 has 25 ($N = 25$), and study 5 has 20 ($N = 20$). By themselves each of these studies may not have enough power to achieve a significant result, but by combining the data from these studies (doing a meta-analysis) you have 180 participants and you might be able to show that the intervention was or was not effective from a statistical point of view.

You need to be careful when you are reading a meta-analysis to ensure that each individual study is comparing exactly the same intervention and has a very similar study method.

THE COCHRANE COLLABORATION

To save a lot of time when looking for evidence to a question there is a group of researchers who have volunteered to join together, called the Cochrane Collaboration (http://www .cochrane.org); this group undertakes and publishes systematic reviews. Anyone can join, but to get a systematic review published on the Cochrane website, you need to follow a very strict protocol. The reviews are very thorough and before considering undertaking a systematic review it is important to check that the Cochrane Collaboration has not already published a review about the question. The Cochrane Group continually reviews and updates its published reviews.

CASE STUDY 19.5

SEEKING INFORMATION

Perhaps you have a history of back pain and you have heard from newspaper articles and advertising that Pilates is very good at helping this condition. So you decide to have a look if any scientific studies have been written about this. You go to the library databases and start your search. This may be a simple search and you could start with the terms 'Pilates' and 'low back pain'.

This brings up about 25–40 articles depending on which databases you use. However, if you add the term 'systematic review' you get only one article, called 'Effectiveness of Pilates exercise in treating people with chronic low back pain: A systematic review of systematic reviews' (Wells et al., 2013). This is a good example of a systematic review and will provide you with some information that will allow you to judge whether you will spend your money on this activity or try something else.

REVIEWS OF QUALITATIVE STUDIES

Qualitative studies provide different types of evidence to that found in quantitative studies. However, this can be very important information that can inform practice. Using a systematic approach to review these sorts of data is helpful for making sense of the body of information in the literature. Relevant articles on a topic can be found by searching a specific question. These searches should include key qualitative words and concepts such as 'experiences' and/or 'perceptions'. The inclusion criteria for the studies should also reflect the type of information obtained from qualitative studies. The specific formulation of the question is key. For example, a poorly phrased question is: 'experiences of rehabilitation'. A more specific question would yield more relevant papers. An example is: 'What are the experiences of sports rehabilitation for athletes who have sustained an Achilles tendon tear?'

Before searching for articles it is wise to have developed a plan for their review. There is some controversy in the literature about this. It has been suggested that qualitative research is sometimes regarded as 'soft' research (Boulton, Fitzpatrick, & Swinburn, 1996). The analysis of qualitative data is considered to be so interpretative that it is difficult to critically appraise. This view is based on the argument that two different researchers could be obtaining different accounts from the same research participants even when they use the same methodology, simply because they may be using different interview prompts, have different interviewing styles and so forth. In addition, two researchers analysing the same data (for example, a transcript of an interview) may arrive at different conclusions. However, others argue that while qualitative data analysis is interpretive it is important to review the robustness of qualitative studies. A helpful discussion of these arguments can be found in the paper by Dixon-Woods et al. (2006). There is now increasing acknowledgement that the synthesis of qualitative data can produce new insights and conceptual developments over and above what could be achieved from a single study (Pope & Mays, 2009). Two broad views of qualitative reviews can

Interpretative
Interpreting in order to explain or make sense.

be identified. These are aggregative synthesis and interpretative synthesis (Dixon-Woods et al., 2006). Dixon-Woods et al. defined these as follows:

- Aggregative syntheses focuses on summarising data, where the concepts (categories or variables) under which data are to be summarised are assumed to be largely secure and well specified.
- Interpretive synthesis is concerned with the development of concepts, and with the development and specification of theories that integrate those concepts.

There are different review methods of qualitative data. Dixon-Woods et al. (2005) identified 10 methods although some are used more frequently and are more established than others. For example, the meta-ethnography (Noblit & Hare, 1988) and realist synthesis (Pawson, 2002) are now regularly found in health-related literature. Meta-ethnography is systematic and has the potential for preserving the interpretative properties of the primary data. Realist synthesis, by contrast, starts off with a theory and then seeks evidence from a range of sources, including, for example, research and media.

Theory
An explanation of a phenomenon.

SUMMARY

A systematic review is an efficient way of gaining a broad understanding of the evidence and effectiveness for an intervention. Just as in reading any literature you need to be aware of the strengths and weaknesses of the systematic review. This chapter has not set out to teach you how to undertake a systematic review, but rather to understand how systematic reviews are constructed so that they can assist you to find a lot of information and the best evidence in a short time.

REFLECTION POINTS

- What stands out for you after reading this chapter?
- How confident are you in looking for a critical appraisal tool? Why?
- How confident are you in choosing an appropriate critical appraisal tool?
- What skills do you need to gain to build your confidence using a critical appraisal tool?
- How might you go about this?

STUDY QUESTIONS

1 Choose an article of interest in your field of practice.
2 Read the article.
3 Summarise your views on the article without using a critical appraisal tool.

4   Choose an appropriate critical appraisal tool and use this to evaluate the paper.
5   Compare the reviews you did with and without the critical appraisal tool. What stands
    out to you? For example, is your conclusion the same or not, and why might this be?

ADDITIONAL READING

Gough, D., Oliver, S., & Thomas, J. (2012). *An introduction to systematic reviews.*
    London: Sage Publications.

REFERENCES

Boulton, M., Fitzpatrick, R., & Swinburn, C. (1996). Qualitative research in health care:
    II. A structured review and evaluation of studies. *Journal of Evaluation in Clinical
    Practice, 2*(3), 171–179. Retrieved from http://eu.wiley.com/WileyCDA/WileyTitle/
    productCd-JEP.html

Dixon-Woods, M., Agarwal, S., Jones, D., Young, B., & Sutton, A. (2005). Synthesising
    qualitative and quantitative evidence: A review of possible methods. *Journal of
    Health Services Research and Policy, 10*(1), 45–53.

Dixon-Woods, M., Bonas, S., Booth, A., Jones, D. R., Miller, T., Sutton, A. J., et al.
    (2006). How can systematic reviews incorporate qualitative research? A critical
    perspective. *Qualitative Research, 6*(1), 27–44.

Guyatt, G. H., Sackett, D. L., & Cook, D. J. (1993). Users' guide to the medical literature.
    II. How to use an article about therapy and prevention: A. Are the results of the
    study valid? *Journal of the American Medical Association, 270*(21), 2598–2601.
    Retrieved from http://jama.ama-assn.org/

Guyatt, G. H., Sackett, D. L., Sinclair, J. C., Hayward, R., Cook, D. J., & Cook, R. J.
    (1995). Users' guides to the medical literature: IX. A method for grading health
    care recommendations. *Journal of the American Medical Association, 274*(22),
    1800–1804. Retrieved from http://jama.ama-assn.org/

Haynes, R. B., Sackett, D. L., Gray, J. A., Cook, D. L., & Guyatt, G. H. (1997).
    Transferring evidence from research into practice: 2. Getting the evidence straight.
    ACP Journal Club, 126(1), A14–A16.

Muir Gray, J. A., Haynes, R. B., Sackett, D. L., Cook, D. J., & Guyatt, G. H. (1997).
    Transferring evidence from research into practice: 3. Developing evidence-based
    clinical policy. *ACP Journal Club, 126*(2), A14–A16.

Noblit, G. W., & Hare, R. D. (1988). *Meta-ethnography: Synthesising qualitative studies.*
    Newbury Park, CA: Sage Publications.

Oxman, A. D., Sackett, D. L., & Guyatt, G. H. (1993). Users' guides to the medical literature: l. How to get started. *Journal of the American Medical Association, 270*(17), 2093–2095. Retrieved from http://jama.ama-assn.org/

Pawson, R. (2002). Evidence-based policy: The promise of 'Realist Synthesis'. *Evaluation, 8*(3), 340–358.

Pope, C., & Mays, N. (2009). Critical reflections on the rise of qualitative research. *BMJ, 339*(7723), 737–739.

Wells, C., Kolt, G. S., Marshall, P., Hill, B., & Bialocerkowski, A. (2013). Effectiveness of Pilates exercise in treating people with chronic low back pain: A systematic review of systematic reviews. *BMC Medical Research Methodology, 13,* 7.

WEBSITES

Physiotherapy Evidence Database (PEDro):
http://www.pedro.org.au

Robert Wood Johnson Foundation—the qualitative research guidelines project:
http://www.qualres.org

Scottish Intercollegiate Guideline Network—appraisal tools for quantitative research:
http://www.sign.ac.uk/guidelines/fulltext/50/annexc.html

STROBE Group—tools for reviewing observational research:
http://www.strobe-statement.org/index.php?id=strobe-home

CHAPTER 20

SUPPORTING PRACTITIONERS TO ENGAGE WITH RESEARCH

SANDY RUTHERFORD AND FELICITY BRIGHT

CHAPTER OVERVIEW

This chapter covers the following topics:

- Why engage with research?
- Levels of research engagement
- Strategies for engaging with research

KEY TERMS

Best practice
Evidence-based practice
Interprofessional
Philosophy
Reflection
Research–practice gap
Treaty of Waitangi

Research–practice gap
The gap between what is known about practice and when or how it changes to reflect that knowledge.

Reflection
The process of considering action.

Evidence-based practice
Practice that is informed by the careful consideration and evaluation of relevant information, and client/ patient and practitioner experience and preference.

Sometimes when new graduates first enter practice they encounter a research–practice gap, when the realities of practice do not always match the ideal envisaged during their education. Theoretical knowledge may be at a fairly high level at this time, with practical skills requiring further development. Senior clinicians, on the other hand, may appear to have a high level of practical skill or setting-based knowledge, but their theoretical knowledge and ability to access research literature may have faded or lost currency (Krom, Batten, & Bautista, 2010). Therefore, new practitioners may find that, in a busy practice setting, things are done in the same way that they have always been done with little review or reflection around whether assessments, treatments, guidelines and policies are still current and appropriate. Clinicians can also sometimes perceive change as difficult and time-consuming, and they may lack the skills for implementing evidence-based practice (Bennett et al., 2003).

CLINICAL REFLECTION 20.1: DON'T HESITATE TO ASK QUESTIONS AND ADOPT A CRITICAL PERSPECTIVE

As a beginning practitioner you don't have the same set of assumptions as your more experienced colleagues, so you're well placed to ask questions about the evidence for practice when you're undertaking your clinical experience elements of your study—in fact you are expected to do so. This is a great opportunity to initiate a discussion about the evidentiary basis for care or practice decisions. Your mentors may not have all the answers but most will guide you by explaining their decision making. You may be surprised where there are evidence gaps for clinical care, and your questions may create a literature search and learning opportunity.

WHY ENGAGE WITH RESEARCH?

There are a number of benefits to embracing research in practice. Working in entrenched and outdated ways of practice can feel uncomfortable. Engaging in and with research can increase practical skills and theoretical knowledge, and result in greater levels of satisfaction. Work becomes more enjoyable and confidence in clinical decision-making increases when research and new information are accessed and considered. There are also benefits to patients in that intervention outcomes are maximised (Fink, Thompson, & Bonnes, 2005).

Engaging with research has benefits for students and practitioners as they meet individual professional goals and the requirements for demonstrating ongoing competence and registration for practice. But this activity can also link to team goals and enable contribution to the wider environment, department and organisation. Being able to access literature and apply research findings critically also provides evidence to support the need for change (Gerrish et al., 2011) and enables people to make the most of the resources available to patients (Kagee, 2012). Reviewing practice can also mean that practitioners can better manage their workload and are working smarter, not harder, to achieve good outcomes for patients. Evidence-based practice is an important part of developing as a practitioner, and assists the journey from novice to expert.

LEVELS OF RESEARCH ENGAGEMENT

There are a number of ways that clinicians can engage with research, from being passive readers and knowers, to being active users and implementers to being active researchers (Spring, 2007).

CASE STUDY 20.1

REALLY MAKING A DIFFERENCE

A multidisciplinary prosthetic rehabilitation team working with people following lower limb amputation (van Twillert, Postema, Geertzen, Hemminga, & Lettinga, 2009) were concerned that their older patients experienced a decline in function after discharge.

When the team reviewed the amputee rehabilitation literature they found that it focused on impairment and was underpinned by biomedical and biomechanical theories. This explained, to an extent, what they needed to cover in their programme, but they found little about why recommended practices and treatments were carried out and how they worked. When they looked at stroke rehabilitation and self-management literature, they realised that they needed to think more about how they were delivering treatment and engaging their patients in the rehabilitation process.

When reviewing the literature and their programme they formulated questions such as:

- *What?* What does each member of the team need to do? What is this treatment based on?
- *How?* How does it produce change in the patient? How is the content of the programme delivered?
- *Why?* Why do we do it this way?

[continued next page]

Subsequently, the team designed a project to improve their programme in terms of content and to examine and make explicit the underlying theory and treatment models, rather than increasing knowledge of pathology or impairment. From this, van Twillert et al. (2009) outlined a five-stage process for using evidence to improve and update practice starting with a clinical question or problem. The translation process, from evidence to practice, involved:

1   documenting the content and theoretical underpinnings of their existing programme and identifying gaps;

2   an initial search of the literature targeting prosthetic rehabilitation, reflecting on the type of knowledge found, and identifying areas for further searches;

3   conducting a broad literature search targeting rehabilitation processes, models and theories that could be applied in their setting;

4   documenting the clinicians' knowledge and asking patients about the problems they encounter once they get home; and

5   synthesising this knowledge to develop new parts of the programme based on the literature and clinician and patient knowledge.

This is a good example of practitioners reflecting on clinical questions and concerns and taking action in a systematic way to address these concerns. Regularly reviewing how you work, as knowledge and circumstances change, is good practice. It is important to acknowledge that it is not possible to know everything. This case study also highlights what is often not talked about—that going to the literature (particularly that condition-specific) alone does not always answer clinical questions. What is often required is an interactive process whereby practitioners translate research findings and recommendations into the practice setting. This involves taking account of the context, the resources, the patient population, the clinicians' experiences and knowledge, and the team's expertise.

PASSIVELY USING RESEARCH

The 'easiest' way to engage with research may simply be regularly accessing it through journal articles and credible blogs, or attending special interest group meetings (SIGs) or journal clubs. Such opportunities are commonly offered in workplaces or through professional organisations. In this way, clinicians may not be *actively* seeking specific defined knowledge; it may come from scheduled professional development events.

ACTIVELY USING AND IMPLEMENTING RESEARCH KNOWLEDGE IN DIRECT CLINICAL CARE

It is widely accepted that evidence-based practice is essential in today's health-care environment, with some arguing that clinicians have an ethical obligation to ensure practice is informed by, and is reflective of, best practice (Christiansen & Lou, 2001). It is not enough to simply 'read' literature or passively access research if you seek to both develop clinical skills and offer evidence-based interventions. Critically reviewing the literature and integrating it into clinical practice (see Chapters 14 and 18) are key steps in working in this way. This process may involve reflecting on practice, gaps in knowledge, questions about the service users and developing as a clinician, and identifying priorities for change and growth. This form of research engagement is likely to be centred around specific patient-related questions such as 'What's the most effective treatment for a spastic upper limb?', 'How does this medication impact on this client's cognitive function?' or 'How does this treatment work to reduce stuttering?'.

Best practice
An approach to practice that has been investigated and has been acknowledged as enabling optimum outcomes.

ACTIVELY DEVELOPING PRACTICE PHILOSOPHY AND PROFESSIONAL SELF

The early days of professional practice can be challenging for any professional. Implementing knowledge gained at university and new knowledge from practice is challenging. An additional challenge comes when developing a professional identity and philosophy, a way of working and reflecting. Opie (1998), Paterson (2001) and Wilding and Whiteford (2009) challenge clinicians to move from *knowing about* concepts to *practising* these concepts. Practitioners (including student practitioners) need to reflect on their practice, what and how they prioritise different aspects of practice and the variables that influence practice. It is often scary giving voice to what creates discomfort. Do not be afraid to ask questions. Only through reflecting and asking questions about what is happening, as well as exploring values and practice philosophies held to be important, can practitioners move towards truly client-centred care (Bright, Boland, Rutherford, Kayes, & McPherson, 2012). Having a practice philosophy assists with reflecting on the literature, identifying what is relevant or consistent within the practice setting, and what should be attended to or disregarded.

Philosophy
The study of thought, meaning and existence.

ACTIVELY PARTICIPATING IN RESEARCH

While practitioners, especially those new to practice, may think 'I can't be involved in research; I don't know enough', they already have a lot to offer to the research process. An active relationship between clinicians and research findings is critical for knowledge translation such as translating findings of research studies into clinical practice (Baumbusch et al., 2008; Sudsawad, 2007). Internationally, funding bodies are requiring researchers to demonstrate how they plan to translate their findings into practice. Being an active research participant may be as simple as volunteering to participate in studies when the opportunity arises, or helping researchers identify potential participants. Participation may involve suggesting research topics to colleagues, managers and university staff, or through a research team or professional leader. The questions that practitioners have often significantly contribute to research directions. Conducting research is also possible, perhaps as a research assistant, a summer studentship and later on as part of postgraduate study or contribution to a clinical audit process, or through studies done in conjunction with established research teams.

STRATEGIES FOR ENGAGING WITH RESEARCH

Actively engaging with research and using it to inform practice is not a quick, one-off activity. It requires intentional effort and a range of strategies, and it requires time. Evidence-based practice requires specific attitudes, values and a commitment to life-long learning (McCluskey & Cusick, 2002). Engaging with research, particularly when seeking to answer practice questions or critically reflect on practice, is not a one-way process of simply going to the literature and finding the one article that answers a question.

CASE STUDY 20.2

ENGAGING WITH THE LITERATURE

There are many ways that practitioners can engage with the literature. The following table summarises a number of strategies that can be used, from passive use of the literature through to active research participation. It is generally most effective to use a combination of strategies (Gira, Kessler, & Poertner, 2004)—only attending journal clubs or only using supervision is unlikely to provide a comprehensive and critical approach to evidence-based practice given the complexity of the population.

LEVEL OF ENGAGEMENT	STRATEGIES/EXAMPLES
Passively using research	Read blogs.
	Get RSS feeds with journal tables of contents.
	Attend journal clubs and Special Interest Group (SIG) meetings.
	Read professional development material from your professional body.
	Shadow expert clinicians to observe their practice.
	Access training through your workplace. This often focuses on broader professional issues such as applying the Treaty of Waitangi in clinical practice, managing challenging behaviours, how to be a supervisee or supervisor.
	Subscribe to reviews such as *Spotlight on Occupation*, the *NZSP Bulletin*, *Communication Matters*, *Kai Tiaki* and others.
	Make sure that you take the time to do it!Timetable professional development into your weekly schedule .
Actively using and implementing research knowledge	Use your librarian—they can support you with literature searches.
	Reflect on your practice. Ask questions of what you're doing, what you're thinking and how you're feeling. What is causing discontent or frustration? What's working well and what's not working so well? What would help you feel more confident? Why are you doing this but not that?
	Actively contribute to SIGs and journal clubs. Use these as opportunities to reflect on cases and on your professional practice.
	Use supervision to reflect on what you're doing, how you're doing it, how you're feeling when you're providing services, what is challenging you.
	Actively incorporate research engagement into your professional development plan. Get input from expert clinicians—have them follow you and give feedback about your practice.
	Let your manager know what you're doing and learning so that they can support changes in practice.
	Take students on placement once you graduate.
	Consider postgraduate study.
Actively developing practice philosophy and professional self	Use supervision to reflect on your philosophy of practice or professional values—what drives you as a clinician? How congruent are your current practice and your philosophy of practice?
	Critically reflect on your practice—why are you working in this way? How does this fit with different models of care?
	Read literature and consider how it applies to your practice (e.g. how you value and implement the CMOP-E in practice; whether the 'body-as-machine' (Nicholls & Gibson, 2010) philosophy is evident and/or appropriate in your practice).

Treaty of Waitangi
The founding document of Aotearoa New Zealand signed between indigenous Māori and the British Crown in 1840.

[continued next page]

LEVEL OF ENGAGEMENT	STRATEGIES/EXAMPLES
Actively participating in research	Become familiar with your organisation's research policies and procedures.
	Support research that others are doing. Help with participant recruitment and consider being a participant yourself.
	Make contributions to existing research. Make links with university or work-based researchers and suggest research ideas. Consider supporting final-year research students.
	Do your own research. Consider presenting in work-based poster competitions and at conferences. Work with existing research teams or your clinical teams to develop research questions and conduct the research. Conduct clinical audits to critically evaluate existing practice and improve future service delivery.
	Explore what scholarships and grants are available in your workplace.

The articles may be few and far between and often hard to find, if they even exist. Instead, it requires both broad and focused searching (for example, searching for literature on amputation but also on broader rehabilitation principles as in the case study above), synthesis of the findings and then critical reflection on how those findings relate to the setting, the patients, the team, and the practitioner's practice philosophy. It can also involve sharing synthesis with the team. Practitioners often work in interdisciplinary or interprofessional teams; this means that if any member of the team changes their practice it affects the rest of the team and the clients receiving services from that team. Sharing questions and knowledge and thinking through implications for practice *together* are more likely to facilitate meaningful engagement with, and uptake of, the literature.

Interprofessional
Relating to the interaction between two or more professionals.

RESEARCH ALIVE 20.1
A PRACTITIONER AND RESEARCH

Felicity was a speech-language therapist and previously worked in a rehabilitation centre in a district health board. She had approximately seven years' postgraduate clinical experience and had completed a postgraduate diploma in rehabilitation. Through her clinical experience and her study, she had become more aware of how she worked and was somewhat dissatisfied with her current way of working. She found that she often focused on the impairments patients presented with instead of focusing at more of a functional level, addressing what was important to the patient and their everyday interactions. Although she had observed other experienced clinicians and drew on supervision to reflect on her clinical practice, she struggled to make significant changes to how she worked.

One strategy Felicity used was to regularly review new literature relevant to rehabilitation and speech-language therapy, having subscribed to journal alerts through the library at her work. An alert from the journal *Aphasiology* identified a new paper entitled 'The piano lesson: An autoethnography about changing clinical paradigms in aphasia practice' (Hinckley, 2005). The autoethnography was a focused study of the clinician, how they worked and why they worked in this way; it challenged dominant approaches to clinical practice. It explored how different ways of working might better respond to the client and what they need from therapy. The paper was written in a very different style to most that she had read and it engaged her from the start. It helped her realise that it addressed some of the clinical challenges she faced and that it considered the issue of philosophy of practice, a concept that she hadn't been overly conscious of before. Reflecting on both her desired philosophy of practice (wanting to be client-centred, addressing what was important to the client, considering function) and her current dominant way of working (often impairment-focused, sessions only offered in her clinic but not in the community or other places meaningful to clients, service structures determined by the service management rather than the clients' needs) helped reveal the source of her dissatisfaction with how she worked. The autoethnographic study put into words some of the skills and ways of working that she had observed in expert clinicians that she admired. However, implementing this reflection into practice wasn't easy. Like most research publications, it was not a prescription of how to do practice. Instead, it required her to reflect on the key points, reflect on her own practice and mindfully consider how and where she could make changes. Utilising supervision sessions helped her think through her ways of working, how these might influence clinical practice and how she could work differently with her clients.

Felicity's role required her to organise professional development for other clinicians and to develop service-wide quality initiatives. Her increased awareness of the impact of ways of working saw her introduce a broader range of papers to journal club—articles that didn't just focus on impairments and therapeutic techniques, but on the role of the clinician, different models of practice and on the patient experience. Qualitative articles become more prominent as these captured patient experiences and perspectives which appeared to be crucial when reflecting on practice. She also started to become

[continued next page]

an active researcher, not just a research reader and user. She led a clinical audit of patient satisfaction with rehabilitation services. She later conducted her own autoethnographic study with colleagues, exploring how they worked with patients with traumatic brain injury to facilitate a client-centred approach to rehabilitation practice (Bright et al., 2012). By this time, Felicity could say that her philosophy of practice and her way of working were (mostly) in unison. There were still times of tension, for example when working within systems and structures that did not prioritise a client-centred approach. However, her ongoing reflection about how she was working, and what might be influencing this, helped her think critically about how she could best work within the services and structures around her and her client, to ensure that she still worked in a client-centred way.

Felicity's key strategies for engaging with research:

- accessing a variety of literature on a regular basis;
- ensuring that she had time to read and reflect on the literature;
- utilising supervision to think through the question, 'What does this mean for my clinical practice?';
- focusing on both direct patient service delivery ('What do I do?') and broader issues of philosophy of practice ('How do I do it? Why do I do it? Who am I as a clinician?');
- providing opportunities for staff to explore different forms of literature; and
- taking opportunities to engage in research in order to develop knowledge and inform clinical practice.

CLINICAL REFLECTION 20.2: KEEPING UP TO DATE

Most health professions have practice standards that require you keep up to date with new evidence and changes in practice norms. For example, as part of health registration processes you may need to make an annual declaration that you have undertaken informal and formal professional development activities that maintain the currency of your knowledge. As a student you are immersed in learning, frequently locating and using evidence in preparing assessments, but once you finish university your priorities change. How will you value and engage with new research once you qualify and workplace priorities take over? As a first step, what IT-based applications will assist you to efficiently access evidence within your practice environment?

Knowledge is not static and evidence changes constantly (Keenan & Redmond, 2002). Finding practical, doable ways to regularly engage with research enables practitioners to stay current and relevant, and also connected to the bigger picture. Knowing about different types of research and good ways to search the literature alerts practitioners to the importance of looking outside their own profession's literature. Searching beyond the practice setting and patients' diagnoses to find evidence from other fields can assist in answering practice questions.

SUMMARY

Engaging with research in an active and reflective way can have benefits for patients, practitioners and organisations that are offering care and support. There are a number of ways to access and engage with evidence. A clear question, a combination of strategies and a framework can make integrating research into practice possible and worth doing. Evidence-based practice is an interactive and ongoing process which involves asking not only what should or could be done, but how and why. It is worth the effort.

REFLECTION POINTS

- What research is relevant to my practice?
- How have I engaged with research to date?
- What do I need to think about when searching the literature?
- What am I uncomfortable about in relation to engaging with research?

STUDY QUESTIONS

1 What are some of the challenges that the clinicians in the case study encountered in answering their practice question and how did they address them?
2 Think of your own clinical question or concern; this could be from class discussions, case studies, lectures or your observations of practice. Formulate 'what', 'how' and 'why' questions to ask of the evidence.

ADDITIONAL READING

Nutley, S., Walter, I., & Davies, H. T. O. (2003). From knowing to doing: a framework for understanding the evidence-into-practice agenda. *Evaluation*, 9(2): 125–148.

Spring, B. (2007). Evidence-based practice in clinical psychology: What it is, why it matters; what you need to know. *Journal of Clinical Psychology*, 63(7): 611–631.

Thurin, J.-M. M. N. (2012). Does participation in research lead to changes in attitudes among clinicians? Report on a survey of those involved in a French practice research network. *Counselling & Psychotherapy Research, 12*(3): 187–193.

REFERENCES

Baumbusch, J. L., Kirkham, S. R., Khan, K. B., McDonald, H., Semeniuk, P., Tan, E., & Anderson, J. M. (2008). Pursuing common agendas: A collaborative model for knowledge translation between research and practice in clinical settings. *Research in Nursing & Health, 31*(2), 130–140.

Bennett, S., Tooth, L., McKenna, K., Rodger, S., Strong, J., Ziviani, J., et al. (2003). Perceptions of evidence-based practice: a survey of Australian occupational therapists. *Australian Occupational Therapy Journal, 50*(1), 13–22.

Bright, F. A. S., Boland, P., Rutherford, S. J., Kayes, N. M., & McPherson, K. M. (2012). Implementing a client-centred approach in rehabilitation: an autoethnography. *Disability and Rehabilitation, 34*(12), 997–1004.

Christiansen, C., & Lou, J. Q. (2001). Ethical considerations related to evidence-based practice. *The American Journal of Occupational Therapy, 55*(3), 345–349.

Fink, R., Thompson, C. J., & Bonnes, D. (2005). Overcoming barriers and promoting the use of research in practice. *Journal of Nursing Administration, 35*(3), 121–129.

Gerrish, K., McDonnell, A., Nolan, M., Guillaume, L., Kirshbaum, M., & Tod, A. (2011). The role of advanced practice nurses in knowledge brokering as a means of promoting evidence-based practice among clinical nurses. *Journal of Advanced Nursing, 67*(9), 2004–2014.

Gira, E. C., Kessler, M. L., & Poertner, J. (2004). Influencing social workers to use research evidence in practice: Lessons from medicine and the allied health professions. *Research on Social Work Practice, 14*(2), 68–79.

Hinckley, J. (2005). The piano lesson: An autoethnography about changing clinical paradigms in aphasia practice. *Aphasiology, 19*(8), 765–779.

Kagee, A. C. (2012). Psychology training directors' reflections on evidence-based practice in South Africa. *South African Journal of Psychology, 42*(1), 103–113.

Keenan, A.-M., & Redmond, A. C. (2002). Integrating research into the clinic: What evidence based practice means to the practising podiatrist. *Journal of the American Podiatric Medical Association, 92*(2), 115–122.

Krom, Z. R. M. R. C., Batten, J. M. A., & Bautista, C. P. R. N. C. (2010). A unique collaborative nursing evidence-based practice initiative using the Iowa model: A clinical nurse specialist, a health science librarian, and a staff nurse's success story. *Clinical Nurse Specialist March/April*, *24*(2), 54–59.

McCluskey, A., & Cusick, A. (2002). Strategies for introducing evidence-based practice and changing clinician behaviour: A manager's toolbox. *Australian Occupational Therapy Journal*, *49*(2), 63–70.

Nicholls, D. A., & Gibson, B. E. (2010). The body and physiotherapy. *Physiotherapy Theory and Practice*, *26*(8), 497–509.

Opie, A. (1998). 'Nobody's asked me for my view': Users' empowerment by multidisciplinary health teams. *Qualitative Health Research*, *8*(2), 188–206.

Paterson, B. (2001). Myth of empowerment in chronic illness. *Journal of Advanced Nursing*, *34*(5), 574–581.

Spring, B. (2007). Evidence-based practice in clinical psychology: What it is, why it matters; what you need to know. *Journal of Clinical Psychology*, *63*(7), 611–631.

Sudsawad, P. (2007). Knowledge translation: Introduction to models, strategies and measures. Retrieved from http://www.ncddr.org/kt/products/ktintro

van Twillert, S., Postema, K., Geertzen, J. H. B., Hemminga, T., & Lettinga, A. T. (2009). Improving rehabilitation treatment in a local setting: a case study of prosthetic rehabilitation. *Clinical Rehabilitation*, *23*(10), 938–947.

Wilding, C., & Whiteford, G. (2009). From practice to praxis: reconnecting moral vision with philosophical underpinnings. *British Journal of Occupational Therapy*, *72*(10), 434–441.

WEBSITES

Smith College School for Social Work: evidence-based practice:
http://sophia.smith.edu/~jdrisko/evidence_based_practice.htm

American Speech-Language-Hearing Association:
http://www.asha.org/members/ebp

Speech and language therapy using social media to participate in EBP:
http://therapyideas.org

Giving birth based on best evidence:
http://evidencebasedbirth.com

PART 5

PRACTICE
AND PRACTITIONERS

CHAPTER 21

NURSING

JANET LARKMAN, ANITA BAMFORD-WADE AND DEB SPENCE

CHAPTER OVERVIEW

This chapter covers the following topics:

- Why is EBP important for nursing?
- What constitutes evidence?
- Patients' preferences, choices and experience
- The complex world of patients and nurses
- What are the challenges for EBP?

KEY TERMS

Clinical trial
Design
Humanism
Measurement
Power
Rigour

The aim of evidence-based practice (EBP) is to ensure that nursing practice provides nursing care that is efficient, effective, to the best possible standard, doing the least harm, and is based on the most up-to-date evidence (Craig & Stevens, 2012). This means using scientific inquiry as the basis of nursing practice (Holmes, Perron, & O'Byrne, 2006). Funders and policy-makers are also keenly interested in evidence-based practice as they seek to minimise costs that do not directly benefit the quality of patient outcomes, thereby freeing resources for other uses (Goode & Piedalue, 1999). It is the responsibility of health professionals, funders and policy-makers to ensure that every health dollar is maximised for the quality of health outcomes.

Humanism
The belief that people are fundamentally good and that reasoning can prevail to address problems.

Nursing as a profession is informed by philosophies of science and humanism. Best practice draws on available research but also requires reflective practice, professional dialogue and practical wisdom. Concerns about evidence-based practice centre on the fact that not all questions are answered by research that adheres to a model that prioritises quantitative research, particularly the systematic review of randomised controlled clinical trials (RCTs). Practising in a cultural safe manner, for example, presents nurses with challenges for which there are no straightforward solutions (Evans, 2005). It has been questioned whether the interpreted meanings of different cultural groups can be measured and/or reduced statistically (Kearns & Dyck, 2005)?

Clinical trial
A formally structured approach to research that includes standards and processes for identifying the problem and investigating it.

WHY IS EBP IMPORTANT FOR NURSING?

The need for quality patient outcomes and cost-effective nursing care is not new (Edwards & Chapman, 2002). In the Crimean War, Florence Nightingale collected and analysed data that reduced the mortality rates for soldiers. Her research changed military practices with regard to the medical care of soldiers, the cleanliness and overcrowding within the hospital environment, patients' nutritional needs and infection control (Burns & Grove, 2003). Many of these are still important issues and continue to need attention today. Effective hand washing is one such example. It is recognised that effective hand washing is one of the best means of infection control. The following case study of hand hygiene is one such example where evidence-based practice informs nursing policy development.

However, changing culture among health-care professionals with respect to hand hygiene practice is an ongoing challenge (Freeman, et al., 2012). Studies show that consistent promotion is required to maintain compliance (Pittet, et al., 2000). Posters used to promote hand hygiene can be placed at the entrance to clinical areas, beside alcohol-dispensing units and basins in clinical areas. Role modelling by senior leaders is necessary to improve hand hygiene compliance, especially among the senior doctors. The lowest compliance rates were observed among medical staff (52%) (Freeman, et al., 2012). Nurses play a pivotal role in maintaining safe, high-quality care environments for patients.

CASE STUDY 21.1

HAND HYGIENE POLICY IN AOTEAROA NEW ZEALAND

Globally, hospital-acquired infections continue to cause a great deal of concern. Up to 10% of patients admitted to modern hospitals get one or more hospital acquired infections (*Hand Hygiene NZ Guidelines*, 2012). Hand hygiene is one of the most effective means of reducing health-care-associated infections. In 2003, the overall cost of health-care-associated infections to the NZ health-care system was estimated at $140 million NZ dollars. In one study, it was concluded that every time an individual health-care worker fails to perform hand hygiene at an 'appropriate moment' during patient care, the cost to the New Zealand health care is somewhere between US$2 and US$50 (Freeman, et al., 2012).

A comprehensive research project led to the development of a globally-targeted *Hand Hygiene Guideline* (WHO, 2005). Subsequently, the '5 moments' (before patient contact, before nursing procedure, after the procedure or body fluid exposure risk, after patient contact, and after contact with patient surroundings) (WHO, 2009) of hand hygiene were taken up in New Zealand nursing practice policy.

There needs to more evidence of best practice in nursing, based on research, to improve patient outcomes. At present there is still a culture of following process because 'that was what I was taught', or the 'way we do it here' or 'I had a hunch that it would work' (Boswell & Cannon, 2007). Nurses today have more options available for care, such as the range of wound-care dressings; this increases the need for the use of research to support their decisions.

Nursing practice is constantly evolving, becoming increasingly more specialised, acute and complicated (Craig & Stevens, 2012), not to mention more expensive (Xiaoshi, 2008). There is also an exponential increase in knowledge, which textbooks cannot hope to keep abreast with (Valiga, 2006). It is important for student nurses to learn how to use evidence as the basis of their nursing practice to ensure they can meet their patients' needs and the requirements of the health system. The New Zealand Nursing Council Competence (4.4) requires registered nurses (RNs) to base their care and advice on the best available evidence to ensure they do 'more good than harm' and to improve their patients' experiences with health care (Nursing Council of New Zealand, 2012). Nurses are accountable to the government, the Nursing Council of New Zealand, their employers and their patients and their families to ensure quality nursing care (McSherry, Simmons & Pearce, 2002). Evidence based on research is an important element of quality nursing care and nurses are required to articulate and defend care decisions.

WHAT CONSTITUTES EVIDENCE?

Valuing a range of evidence, including quantitative and qualitative research, increases the usefulness of research when nurses make clinical decisions (Levin, 2006). The methodologies are complementary as they inform each other (Burnard, Morrison & Gluyas, 2011) and bring a range of different perspectives to the same topic.

Quantitative research is important for finding out how often events occur, such as the rates of pain relief for postoperative patients; the relationship between concepts, such as the rates of cancer and smoking; and to determine the effectiveness of treatments, such as relaxation techniques for sleeping (Burns & Grove, 2003). Multiple authors argue that this ranking has meant that there has been a strong focus on the strength of quantitative research, and critique the authenticity of this ranking for nursing decision-making (Fisher & Happell, 2009; Leeman & Sandelowski, 2012; Winters & Echeverri, 2012). One critique argues that most of the nursing research available has used a quantitative methodology, which oversimplifies the complex reality of nursing practice to enable measurement or observations (Holmes, Perron, & O'Byrne, 2006). Quantitative research is very important as the basis for nursing practice and so are other forms of evidence.

Measurement
The process of measuring the size or amount of something; also, the size or amount itself.

Qualitative research endeavours to tell stories or make sense of events from the perspective of the people who participate in the study. Qualitative methodologies may be more suited to answer the types of questions which guide nurses and which focus on the patient's story: for example, why a patient had a particular reaction to an event, to understand their 'lived experience', or how they felt about events they experienced (Abbott, 2002). Fisher and Happell (2009) argue that best evidence must incorporate patient-centred, clinically relevant information and is based on patient feedback and clinicians' observations and experiences. They suggest that clinical judgments and decisions are enhanced by integrating research with nurses' perceptions, practices and the context within which it is taking place. Evidence from both quantitative and qualitative research is best when combined with the patients' perspectives and clinical expertise (Leeman & Sandelowski, 2012).

CASE STUDY 21.2

CLINICAL EXPERTISE

A nurse in the ward suggests that in recent years manuka honey has been found to have antibiotic effects which improve rates of wound healing. A search of currently available research undertaken by a nurse found that manuka honey lowers the pH of wounds, and thus increases healing (Gethin, Cowman & Conroy, 2008). Subsequently, a meta-analysis of 43 randomised controlled trails, with a total of 3556 participants, confirmed improved healing times for many types of wounds (Molan, 2011). The honey-treated wounds were found to have reduced infection rates and inflammation, and greater cellular growth. Based on this evidence, the nurses decided to trial the use of manuka honey dressings on their ward.

This is a good example of how a quantitative approach to evidence provided by randomised trials can inform nursing practice.

PATIENTS' PREFERENCES, CHOICES AND EXPERIENCE

Patients' values and preferences are pivotal within the evidence for decision-making for patient-centred care (Fisher & Happell, 2009). Hearing patients' voices regarding their experiences and their understanding of their condition or illness is vital within this process (Jutel, 2008). In Aotearoa New Zealand, there is an expectation that nursing practice will involve patients (and their relatives) in the development of guidelines for patient care (Code of Health and Disability Services Consumers' Rights, 2012).

CASE STUDY 21.3

PATIENT PERSPECTIVE AND EXPERIENCE

In 2006, there was a review of the clinical evidence regarding what is best to use when dressing wounds (Joanna Briggs Institute, 2006). It found that tap water, or podded water, was the solution of choice for lacerations and postoperative wounds. Showering was recommended for such wounds, and it was suggested that not only did it work as well as saline, but it might also contribute positively to the patient's feeling of well-being.

JANET LARKMAN, ANITA BAMFORD-WADE AND DEB SPENCE

THE COMPLEX WORLD
OF PATIENTS AND NURSES

Power
The exercise of
strength or control.

Cultural safety recognises the essential place of power in the construction of knowledge and its implementation in practice. The development of cultural safety in Aotearoa New Zealand has been significantly influenced by the Treaty of Waitangi and biculturalism (Ramsden, 1990) and guidelines for education and practice have been implemented by the Nursing Council of New Zealand (Nursing Council of New Zealand 1992, 1996).

Because the experience of cultural safety is dependent on context, it will always be variable. When nursing a person from another culture, 'getting it right' (Spence, 2004) is predominantly learned and evaluated in a clinical environment that is constantly in flux. Achieving cultural safety relies more on the creation and substance of environments that enable the surfacing of prejudices and the collaborative exploration of possibilities for change than it does on defining, measuring and searching for truth. This is an example of a complex element of nursing practice that is best served by a qualitative or mixed approach to research as it involves human experiences, responses and interpretations.

WHAT ARE THE CHALLENGES FOR EBP?

It has previously been noted that nurses in Aotearoa New Zealand tend to rely on experience-based knowledge rather than using research findings to inform their clinical decision-making, despite the increase in research outputs (Xiaoshi, 2008). Any lack of education about or emphasis on evidence for nursing in clinical settings means nurses are likely to lack the skills to seek evidence or to carry out research. A further complexity is that service-based research tends to publish its findings 'in-house', rather than in journals (Leeman & Sandelowsi, 2012). This may be related to the limited breadth and depth of research outputs based on clinical practice (Abbott, 2002). This 'grey literature', or written work that is not commercially published, is not widely available. Problems identified include the time it takes to find relevant research, the necessary understanding of research, and a lack of clinically credible research to ensure clinical, informed decision-making (Abbott, 2002; Jutel, 2008). It may be useful to visualise the components of clinical decision-making as a four-legged stool. The seat at the top of the stool represents the clinical decision-making, and is supported by equal weighting on each of the legs to the stool (see Figure 21.1).

Evidence from qualitative research, quantitative research, clinical experience and expertise, and the patients' values, experience and preferences needs to be collected and integrated to support the actions taken by nurses (Craig & Stevens, 2012; Leeman & Sandelowski, 2012).

FIGURE 21.1   EVIDENCE FOR CLINICAL DECISION-MAKING SHOULD BE DRAWN FROM MULTIPLE SOURCES

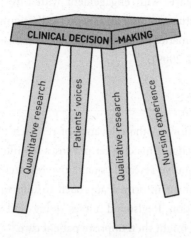

Source: Model developed by J. Larkman (2013).

RESEARCH ALIVE 21.1
NURSING GRADUATES AND RESEARCH

One of the challenges for practitioners is that they are surrounded by information. It is important to develop skills for evaluating and responding to evidence and below are some suggestions for how to engage with research and link it to practice:

- Analyse relevance of specific research articles to practice and to assess the **rigour** of both the **design** and the method (Craig & Stevens, 2012; Valiga, 2006).
- Question the appropriateness of the methodology to the clinical context, and the consistency of the findings of similar studies (Fisher & Happell, 2009, Jutel, 2008).
- Evaluate research findings against clinical experience (Craig & Stevens, 2012).
- Ask how similar their patient's situation is to the participants in the study and how feasible the recommendations are to their context (Haddock, 2002).
- Analyse the possible risks and benefits, and check this against their patient's preferences and values (Haddock, 2002).
- Consider the feasibility and the cost of implementation, along with the impact on the health-care system (Craig & Stevens, 2012).

Rigour
The degree to which research process and findings stand up to challenge.

Design
The process of planning and creating a solution to a problem.

The aim is for nurses to be able to defend their practice (Haddock, 2002) and to be informed sceptics of research, not accepting any results at face value (Edwards & Chapman, 2002). This starts with engagement with EBP as a student, through the integration of research within practice and theoretical assignments (Haddock, 2002) and the development of informatics skills to enable effective searching of relevant research articles (Fisher & Happell, 2009).

SUMMARY

Open and robust discussion on the relevance of research findings is required for the growth of nursing knowledge. This chapter proposes the integration of each of the four types of evidence (quantitative research, qualitative research, clinical expertise and the patients' perspectives) for an informed approach to inform clinical decision-making, based on shared information. Registered nurses 'doing' and implementing contextually relevant nursing research might then improve patient care.

REFLECTION POINTS

Think of a time you felt you had an occasion when the patient's voice, perspective and preferences were valued during a nursing care encounter. If you have not had this experience, perhaps a relative or friend has.

- How important was this to you or your relative or friend?
- How did this affect your or their experience or recovery?

STUDY QUESTIONS

In relation to Case Study 21.2, what would be good questions to ask:

- before having the honey applied?
- during the trial?
- after the trial?

ADDITIONAL READING

Davidson, C., & Tolich, M. (Eds.). (2001). *Social science research in New Zealand: Many paths to understanding*. Auckland: Pearson Education NZ Ltd.

Grove, S.K., Burns, N., & Gray, J. (2013) *The practice nursing research: appraisal, synthesis and generation of evidence*. St Louis, MO: Elsevier/Saunders.

Hughes, F., & Calder, S. (2007). *Have your say: Influencing public policy in New Zealand*. Wellington: Dunmore Publishing Ltd.

McSherry, R., Simmons, M., & Abbott, P. (Eds.). (2002).*Evidence-informed nursing: A guide for clinical nurses* (pp. 1–13). London: Routledge.

REFERENCES

Abbott, P. (2002). Implementing evidence-informed nursing; Research awareness. In R. McSheery, M. Simmons, & P. Abbott (Eds.), *Evidence-informed nursing: A guide for clinical nurses* (pp.14–40). London, UK: Routledge.

Boswell, C., & Cannon, S. (Eds). (2007). *Introduction to nursing research incorporating evidence-based practice.* Sudbury, MA: Jones and Bartlett Publishers.

Burnard, P., Morrison P., & Gluyas, H. (2011). *Nursing research in action: Exploring, understanding and developing skills* (3rd ed.). Hampshire: MacMillan Publishers.

Burns, N., & Grove, S.K. (2003). *Understanding nursing research* (3rd ed.). Philadelphia, PA: Saunders.

Code of Health and Disability Services Consumers' Rights. (2012). Retrieved from http://www.healthpoint.co.nz/useful-information/patient-rights/code-of-rights

Craig, J.V. & Stevens, K.R. (2012). Evidence-based practice in nursing. In J.V. Craig, & R.L. Smyth (Eds.), *The evidence-based practice manual for nurses* (3rd ed., pp. 3–32). London: Elsevier.

Edwards, H., & Chapman, H. (2002). Utilization of research evidence by nurses. *Nursing and Health Sciences, 4,* 89–95.

Evans, D. (2005). Ethical considerations in health care when working crossculturally. In D. Wepa (Ed.). *Cultural safety in Aotearoa New Zealand* (pp. 79–88). Auckland: Pearson Education.

Fisher, J. E. & Happell, B. (2009). Implications of evidence-based practice for mental health nursing. *International Journal of Mental Health Nursing 18,* 179–185.

Freeman, J., Sieczkowski, C., Anderson, T., Morris, A. J., Keenan, A., & Roberts, S. A. (2012). Improving hand hygiene in New Zealand hospitals to increase patient safety and reduce costs: Results from the first hand hygiene national compliance audit for 2012. *New Zealand Medical Journal, 125*(1357), 178.

Gethin, G. T., Cowman, S., & Conroy, R. M. (2008). The impact of Manuka honey dressings on the surface pH of chronic wounds. *International Wound Journal, 5*(2), 185–194.

Goode, C. J., & Piedalue, F. (1999). Evidence based clinical practice. *Journal of Nursing Administration, 29*(6), 15–21.

Hand Hygiene New Zealand Guidelines (2012). Retrieved from http://www.handhygiene.org.nz

Haddock, J. (2002). Reflective practice and decision-making related to research implementation. In R. McSheery, M. Simmons, & P. Abbott (Eds.), *Evidence-informed nursing: A guide for clinical nurses* (pp. 78–97). London: Routledge.

Holmes, D., Perron, A., & O'Byrne, P. (2006). Evidence, virulence, and the disappearance of nursing knowledge: A critique of the evidence-based dogma. *Worldviews on Evidence-Based Nursing, 3*(3), 95–102.

Joanna Briggs Institute (2006). Solutions, techniques and pressure in wound cleansing. *Best Practice, 10*(2), 1–4. Retrieved from http://www.connect.jbiconnectplus.org/ViewSourceFile.aspx?0=4341

Jutel, A. (2008). Beyond evidence-based nursing: tools for practice. *Journal of Nursing Management, 16*, 417–421.

Leeman, J. & Sandelowski, M. (2012). Practice-based evidence and qualitative inquiry. *Journal of Nursing Scholarship, 44*(2), 171–179.

Levin, R.F. (2006). Evidence-based practice nursing: What is it? In R. F. Levin, & H. R. Feldman (Eds). *Teaching evidence-based practice in nursing: A guide for academic and clinical settings* (pp. 5–13). New York, NY: Springer Publishing.

Kearns & Dyck (2005). Culturally safe research. In D. Wepa (Ed.), *Cultural safety in Aotearoa New Zealand* (pp. 68–78). Auckland: Pearson Education.

McSherry, R., Simmons, M., & Pearce, P., (2002). An introduction to evidence-informed nursing. In R. McSherry, M. Simmons, & P. Abbott (Eds), *Evidence-informed nursing: A guide for clinical nurses* (pp. 1–13). London: Routledge.

Molan, P.C. (2011). The evidence and the rationale for the use of honey as a wound dressing. *Wound Practice and Research, 19*(4), 204–220.

Nursing Council of New Zealand (1992). *Kawa Whakaruruhau: Guidelines for nursing and midwifery education*. Wellington: Author.

Nursing Council of New Zealand (1996). *Guidelines for cultural safety in nursing and midwifery education*. Wellington: Author.

Nursing Council of New Zealand (2012). *Nursing Council Competencies*. Retrieved from http://www.nursingcouncil.org.nz/index.cfm/1,55,html/Competencies

Pittet, D., Hugonnet, S., Harbath, S., Mourouga, P., Sauvan, V., Touveneau, S., & Perneger, T. (2000). Effectiveness of a hospital-wide programme to improve compliance with hand hygiene. *The Lancet, 356*, 1307–1312.

Ramsden, I. (1990). Cultural safety. *New Zealand Nursing Journal, 83*, 18–19.

Spence, D. (2004). Prejudice, paradox and possibility: the experience of nursing people from cultures other than one's own, pp. 140–180. In H. Kavanagh and V. Knowlden (Eds.), *Many voices: towards caring culture in health care and healing*. Madison: University of Wisconsin Press.

Valiga, T. M., (2006). Why we need evidence-based teaching practices. In R. F. Levin, & H. R. Feldman (Eds.). *Teaching evidence-based practice in nursing: A guide for academic and clinical settings* (pp. 261–271). New York, NY: Springer Publishing.

World Health Organization (WHO). (2005). *WHO launches global patient safety challenge; issues guidelines on hand hygiene in health care.* Retrieved from http://www.who.int/mediacentre/news/releases/2005/pr50/en

World Health Organization (WHO). (2009). *Guidelines on hand hygiene health care.* Retrieved from http://www.who.int/patientsafety/en

Winters, C. A., & Echeverri, R. (2012). Teaching strategies to support evidence-based practice. *Critical Care Nurse, 32*(3), 49–54.

Xiaoshi, L. (2008). Evidence-based practice in nursing: What is it and what is the impact of leadership and management practices on implementation? *Nursing Journal: Tai Tokerau Wanga, 12*, 6–12.

WEBSITES

Hand Hygiene New Zealand:
http://www.handhygiene.org.nz

CHAPTER 22

OCCUPATIONAL THERAPY AND OCCUPATIONAL SCIENCE

HELEEN REID AND KIRK REED

CHAPTER OVERVIEW

This chapter covers the following topics:

- Historical drivers of occupational therapy research
- Research in occupational therapy
- The future of occupational therapy research
- Occupational science

KEY TERMS

Clinical trial

Engagement

Evidence-based practice

Medical model

Occupation

Paradigm shift

Rigour

Scholarly

Treatment

There are a number of drivers behind research in occupational therapy. These range from providing evidence for practice to better understanding the notion of occupation, defined here as including 'all the things that people do in their everyday lives' (Sundkvist & Zingmark, 2003, p. 40). This diverse research agenda demands that occupational therapy is not bound by one method; it is strongly embedded in exploratory, descriptive and experimental methods, across qualitative, quantitative and critical research paradigms.

Occupation
An activity that people engage in.

HISTORICAL DRIVERS OF OCCUPATIONAL THERAPY RESEARCH

Despite the term evidence-based practice (EBP) being coined in the 1990s (Ilott, 2012; Law, Pollock, & Stewart, 2004), practice based on sound evidence has been around since the inception of occupational therapy. Occupational therapy emerged from a shared belief in the healing potential of occupation held by a group of American health professionals shortly after the turn of the twentieth century. From early on, the evidence used by champions of the profession to determine *what practice was best* was their own observations, outcomes from discussion with other professionals, and measuring the effects of occupation on the patients themselves (Schwartz, 2003). Much of the early evidence for the profession's value came from classical and Renaissance medicine, which valued occupation for health. In particular, scholarly physicians Adolph Meyer and William Dunton published on, lectured on and advocated the specific 'method of training the sick or injured by means of instruction and employment in productive occupation' (American Occupational Therapy Association, 1925, p. 280). Thus, measurement of treatment outcomes remained based on systematic observation and illness mechanics adopted from the medical profession, rather than on empirical methodologies or patient experience (Hoffmann, Bennett, & Del Mar, 2010).

Historically, as outlined in Figure 22.1, many shifts and changes that pushed the profession both away from and back to its original roots have occurred (Kielhofner, 1997; Wilcock, 2001). One significant change came around the 1940s with war veterans rehabilitated back into society. This period saw a rapid growth in the technical, anatomical and physiologically focused professional knowledge (Turner, Foster, & Johnson, 2002). Occupational therapy became increasingly mechanistic under the influence of an ever specialising medical profession (Kielhofner, 1997; Wilcock, 2001). Research was being published on subjects more favourably funded, such as remediation following amputation, adaptive and compensatory strategies for arthritis (Roberts, Kurfuest, & Low, 2008) or occupational therapy intervention for tuberculosis (Peloquin, 1989). However, this came from other 'scientific' sources rather than research initiated by occupational

Evidence-based practice
Practice that is informed by the careful consideration and evaluation of relevant information, and client/patient and practitioner experience and preference.

Scholarly
Relating to rigorously exploring, sharing and developing knowledge.

Treatment
The act of carrying out an intervention for the purpose of alleviating or curing a problem.

Medical model
An approach to health care that privileges biological, mechanistic and reductive understandings of bodily structures and functions.

Paradigm shift
A change in the theoretical framework or perspective from which information and knowledge has been viewed.

therapists. Occupational therapists applied or extrapolated such scientific knowledge to their own clinical domain to increase credibility. The occupation-focused constructs that the founders had established were eroded and occupational therapy's failure to fit the medical model meant professional identity and confidence were lacking. This lack of confidence was noticed by some leaders in the profession, most notably Mary Reilly and Elizabeth Yerxa, who called for the profession to reorientate itself to the original vision and establish a body of knowledge based on the central tenet of occupation (Reilly, 1962). This significant paradigm shift took some time to take hold. All these changes led to the eventual development in the 1980s of occupational science, which had the promise of being able to inform occupational therapy practice.

FIGURE 22.1   PARADIGM SHIFTS THAT HAVE INFLUENCED AND SHAPED OCCUPATIONAL THERAPY PRACTICE

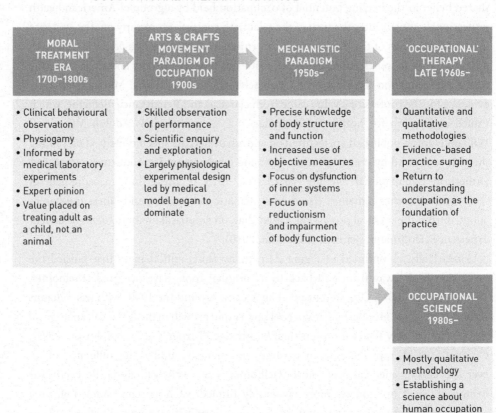

RESEARCH IN OCCUPATIONAL THERAPY

Over the course of time, occupational therapy progressed and occupational therapists challenged the focus of practice, taking a fresh look at occupation as a basis for health and well-being. What emerged is a strengthening discipline that is forging its own research path and using methodologies that align with the profession's values. Occupational therapists are concerned with enabling people to engage in occupation within their environment. A profession that traverses the complexities of any person engaging in meaningful and mundane occupations (Blijlevens, Hocking, & Paddy, 2009; Polatajko et al., 2007; Reed, Hocking, & Smythe, 2010; see also Research Alive 22.1) needs to draw on and generate many types of evidence to inform practice. Research about the person, occupation and/or the environment is showing that the outcome of occupational therapy supports well-being, but more can be done to enhance the evidence base (Pierce, 2012).

RESEARCH ALIVE 22.1
UNDERSTANDINGS OF OCCUPATION INFORMING PRACTICE

It is critical for effective and authentic occupational therapy practice that the meaning of occupation is understood and is the focus of practice. A hermeneutic phenomenological study reported in the *Journal of Occupational Science* (Reed, Hocking, & Smythe, 2010) explored the meaning of occupation. Twelve New Zealand adults who experienced a disruption to their occupations were interviewed. The findings suggest that the meaning of occupation is complex and tends to remain hidden, but reveals itself in the call to occupation—what it is we care about or what concerns us. Being-with others while engaging in an occupation creates a bond and mood; the meaning changes depending on who the occupation is done with or without. The meaning of occupation also shows itself in the possibilities that are opened up or closed down. The findings of this study have implications for practice in that while meaningful occupation is the hallmark of occupational therapy practice it is complex and not well understood. This study provided insights into what gives occupation meaning and suggests that therapists need to take the time to explore the meaning of occupation for their clients by looking beyond the individual to the wider context, in particular to how relationships and connections with others contribute to the meaning of occupation.

Contemporary occupational therapy researchers have a richer repertoire of tools and methodologies at their fingertips than were available in previous decades. Systematic reviews and meta-analyses have become more common as the research base expands; quantitative research testing of occupational therapy assessments and interventions is becoming more frequent, and qualitative research exploring participants' experiences are also increasing. Some of these topics and methodologies may also sit within an occupational science arena. The richness of occupational therapy's research and its impact on practice has been captured by some examples in Table 22.1.

TABLE 22.1 OVERVIEW OF OCCUPATIONAL THERAPY RESEARCH TOPICS AND METHODS

RESEARCH TOPIC	RESEARCH METHOD	TYPICAL RESEARCH QUESTION	RESEARCH FINDINGS	IMPLICATIONS FOR INFORMING PRACTICE
Effect of occupation- and activity-based interventions on the instrumental activities of daily living performance among community dwelling older adults (Orellano, Colon, & Arbesman, 2012)	Systematic review of 38 studies, 31 at Level I	Varied types of clinical question	Strong evidence from two RCT's that multicomponent interventions (provided by more than one discipline) targeting a number of outcomes improve and maintain activities of daily living performance in community dwelling older adults. No evidence exists that home modification and assistive devices improve activities of daily living.	Provides practitioners and educators with evidence on where there is strong, moderate and no evidence for effectiveness of interventions. Identifies a need to develop further evidence on assistive technologies.
A cross-diagnostic validation of an instrument measuring participation in everyday occupations: the Occupational Gaps Questionnaire (OGQ) (Eriksson, Tham, & Kottorp, 2012)	Cross-diagnostic validation using Rasch analysis	Diagnostic validity of assessments	The results provided evidence that the OGQ is a valid measure across different diagnostic groups. A generic version of the OGQ can separate at least two levels of perceived occupational gaps.	The OGQ may have relevance as a tool for identifying gaps as a basis for planning interventions, as an introduction to the Canadian Occupational Performance Measure, and for prioritising clients to occupational therapy services.

RESEARCH TOPIC	RESEARCH METHOD	TYPICAL RESEARCH QUESTION	RESEARCH FINDINGS	IMPLICATIONS FOR INFORMING PRACTICE
Ageing with traumatic brain injury (TBI): follow-up of people receiving inpatient rehabilitation over more than three decades (Sendroy-Terrill, Whiteneck, & Brooks, 2010)	Cross-sectional follow-up with 243 people	Prognosis of long-term consequences of TBI	Both age post-injury and age at injury are predictive of several outcomes after TBI. Improvement occurred between injury and five years post-injury.	Evidence provides a better understanding of the process of ageing with TBI and what barriers may exist for those who experienced a TBI.
Understanding family routines in families dealing with adolescent mental illness (Koome, Hocking, & Sutton, 2013)	Qualitative descriptive study of four adolescents aged between 13 and 18 years and their mothers	What routines mean to families and adolescents with mental illness	Routines were similar to those of other studies examining family routines. Differences were that routines in this study were found to be far more complex and explicit in their intent, helped gauge mental state and re-engagement in daily life.	Understanding the role of routine in families can assist practitioners in measuring and developing healthy routines for the benefit of all members of the family.

THE FUTURE OF OCCUPATIONAL THERAPY RESEARCH

Despite the growth in research, there is still limited quality evidence to comfortably support EBP in *all* domains of occupational therapy (Dirette, Rozich, & Viau, 2009). To address the need for evidence to support practice, the Canadian and American Occupational Therapy Association statements about research concerns (American Occupational Therapy Foundation, 2007; Canadian and American Occupational Therapists, 2009) identified that research should involve collaborative research to examine:

- assessment and intervention outcomes and cost-effectiveness, especially in mental health;
- occupational performance and community integration; and
- translation of research results into evidence-based practice guidelines.

Within the context of Aotearoa New Zealand, this would equally fit with occupation-focused health issues in society related to obesity, poverty and deprivation. These concerns can be related to occupational engagement issues such as occupational balance, lifestyle design, and to occupational justice issues such as equitable access to everyday occupations. Research and funding are closely aligned with national health agendas. In Aotearoa New Zealand there are high numbers of people with cardiovascular conditions, diabetes, mental health disorders, dementia, asthma, arthritis and chronic pain, and childhood obesity, along with the unmet health needs of Māori and Pacific Island children (Ministry of Health, 2012). All of these have an impact on the person's ability to engage and participate in the things they want or need to do in their daily lives. O'Sullivan's work (see Research Alive 22.2), is one example of how occupational therapy research can inform the overall care of people with dementia and how it has the potential to change government policy.

Engagement
Meaningful interaction.

CASE STUDY 22.1

SENSORY STIMULATION IS EFFECTIVE IN IMPROVING BEHAVIOURAL PROBLEMS AMONG PEOPLE WITH DEMENTIA: RESULTS OF A SYSTEMATIC REVIEW

In developed countries the population is aging, people are living longer and as part of this change the incidence of people living with dementia is increasing. Depending on family choice and resources, people with dementia may be cared for at home or in residential aged care. Within this context occupational therapists may intervene to assist the person with dementia to enhance or maintain their ability to perform activities of daily living, or assist them to participate in social activities that improve their depression symptoms and quality of life and that ease the burden on carers (Kim, Yoo, Jung, Park, & Park, 2012). Kim et al. conducted a systematic review and meta-analysis of the effects of occupational therapy for persons with dementia. This review found that the use of sensory stimulation based interventions (e.g. light effects or meditative music) was effective and improved peoples' behavioural problems such as wandering or agitation. However, reviewers (Kim et al.) identified that the number of studies in the review was small and that further research into the evidence for interventions in people with dementia was needed, particularly in the area of environment modification and functional task activity. This review gives clear direction to future research investigations that will inform occupational therapist practice in the dementia care setting.

RESEARCH ALIVE 22.2
RESEARCH INFORMING THE CARE OF OLDER ADULTS

Grace O'Sullivan, a New Zealand occupational therapist, undertook an action research study exploring how people who live with dementia in the community can be supported to engage in daily activities (O'Sullivan, 2011). She engaged 11 people with mild to moderate dementia and 11 family/whānau members in dialogue with herself and with each other in focus groups, and supported them to engage in their own action. Three interacting themes emerged from the data analysis:

1 the nature of being in the world with dementia;
2 difference;
3 prejudice and power.

People with dementia and their family/whānau were found to be keen to challenge the disease process and show that they can and do problem-solve and use their initiative. The findings revealed a constant tension between ways of living with dementia, political strategies, the social environment, and opportunities for occupational engagement. Implications for primary health-care providers and policy-makers highlighted the need to change the ways in which dementia is perceived and how care is delivered. The central argument arising from the findings is the significance of attitudes, in particular the personal attitudes of people with dementia. Implications for primary health-care providers and policy-makers highlight the need to change the ways in which dementia is perceived, as the pursuit of positive attitudes may help to change histories and enable people with dementia to live well. O'Sullivan's work has received many accolades and has been instrumental in the development of dementia care guidelines by the Ministry of Health.

AUSTRALIAN CONTEXT

Also within the dementia care practice area but from the health professional perspective, an Australia study (Bennett, Shand, & Liddle, 2011) surveyed occupational therapists working with people with dementia to describe practice and to understand the current work role within the aged care sector. 134 occupational therapists responded, and their opinions were collected in four areas: referral processes; assessments and interventions; barriers to delivery of interventions; and education needs. Results revealed the most common area of practice was in environment modification and prescription of assistive equipment for the person with dementia, and the major barriers

[continued next page]

HELEEN REID AND KIRK REED

in practice were time and organisational role restrictions. The research also identified these occupational therapists' training needs specific to the dementia and aged care setting. The authors conclude that time is a major barrier to an occupational therapist fulfilling their role, and recommend change. This study provides evidence that could be used with other research to improve care for people with dementia.

Population-based studies similar to the occupational component in the New Zealand Life and Living in Advanced Age (LiLAC) study (Hayman et al., 2012) are one future direction for occupational therapy research. Individual level research with occupation-focused interventions geared toward client participation is another way. For this kind of evidence to be developed, larger quantitative and/or mixed method studies are needed to show the cost-effectiveness of occupational therapy and the effect on client health and well-being outcomes. The evidence gathered from one single study cannot change practice. It often requires large scale, longitudinal research and/or multiple research projects. One example is the Well Elderly Study (see Research Alive 22.3), which gained professional acclaim and recognition for its rigour and shows how occupational science can inform occupational therapy practice.

Rigour
The degree to which research process and findings stand up to challenge.

RESEARCH ALIVE 22.3
OCCUPATIONAL SCIENCE INFORMING PRACTICE

In 1997, the Well Elderly Study (Clark, 1997) received international publicity as the largest occupational therapy outcomes study ever conducted and the first occupationally-based research to be published in the prestigious *Journal of the American Medical Association*. The treatment in this clinical trial study was based on the application of occupational science theory and supported the profession's emphasis on occupation influencing health and well-being. The first study was followed up recently by a second randomised controlled trial (Clark et al., 2011). The aim of this follow-up study was to determine the effectiveness and cost-effectiveness of a preventive, lifestyle-based, occupational therapy intervention. This was administered in a variety of community sites, and was highly effective in improving mental and physical well-being and cognitive functioning in ethnically diverse older people. Because the intervention is cost-effective and is applicable on a wide-scale basis, it is helping reduce health decline, and promoting well-being in older

Clinical trial
A formally structured approach to research which includes standards and processes for identifying the problem and investigating it.

people. In New Zealand this research still needs to be formally replicated. Although not explicit, this research has shed light on what is possible in aged care and supports the practice of occupational therapists in these settings in Aotearoa New Zealand.

OCCUPATIONAL SCIENCE

Occupational science is relatively new. While it emerged from occupational therapy it has diversified to involve other disciplines and its researchers continue to openly discuss and consider its future. Until now it has focused more on understanding the concept of occupation, using a range of research methods to answer a plethora of questions related to occupation. As occupational science continues to evolve there are many questions that still need to be explored. These include developing knowledge of how occupation is experienced and notions such as co-occupation and occupational potential, which are questions that suit qualitative methods. In addition there is a need to generate evidence to identify positive or negative outcomes of engagement in occupation. Quantitative methods, such as randomised control trials and other methods using statistical analysis, will assist in showing the relationship between occupation and health or well-being.

As described in the Research Alive 22.3 above, the University of Southern California has conducted empirical studies to establish the influence that occupation has on health (Clark, Jackson & Carlson, 2004; Clark et al., 2011). Such large empirical studies are important, but are rare and more are needed. The findings from these studies have the potential to inform health practice in the broadest sense and raise questions about the importance of prevention, the use of non-pharmacological interventions, and the provision of services that allow people to stay engaged in all aspects of life.

CASE STUDY 22.2

A PHENOMENOLOGICAL STUDY

An example of how occupational science research can inform occupational therapy practice can be captured in the phenomenological study conducted in New Zealand by Sutton, Hocking, and Smythe (2012). The aim of the study was to explore the experience and meaning of occupation of 13 people living in the community and who were recovering from mental illness. The study

[continued next page]

HELEEN REID AND KIRK REED

revealed that mental illness can create a continuum of disengagement, partial engagement, everyday engagement and full engagement. Everyday activity was found to be an important medium for change as well as an indicator of recovery. In particular, the study highlights the dynamics at play in different modes of doing and the way in which carers can influence the experience and meaning of activity. Many of the findings in this study are echoed in the Mental Health Foundation's 'five ways to well-being' where the occupations and activities aligned with connecting, giving, taking notice, learning and being active are seen as five ways to a positive state of mental, physical and spiritual existence (Mental Health Foundation, n.d.). From an occupational science perspective, this study showed how people dwell in a range of occupational states of engagement in the course of their recovery. It informs occupational therapy practice by showing that all forms of occupational engagement can be meaningful in the recovery process. What Sutton et al. do call for is more research on strategies people can or do use to navigate between the states of disengagement to engagement. This research can stem from qualitative but also quantitative methodologies to increase rigour and generalisability. This is in addition to gaining a deeper understanding of the perspectives of the people who support those recovering from mental illness.

SUMMARY

Occupational therapy research foci have shifted and changed over time. Its origins under the umbrella of medicine has created challenges that the profession has questioned and answered by drawing research back to what the profession is really about: human occupation. Occupational therapists must draw on evidence from multiple sources— from qualitative, quantitative and mixed methods research to inform everyday practice. The future for occupational science and occupational therapy research lies in keeping true to the underlying notion of both disciplines and that of occupation, and by ensuring that rigorous, quality research is conducted. Occupational therapy's research mandate, increasingly informed by occupational science research, is to answer questions about the relationship between participation in an occupation and health and well-being with larger scale, robust studies that can be translated into practice.

REFLECTION POINTS

- What research methods has occupational therapy research tended to focus on and why?
- What are the key differences between the research that occupational science and occupational therapy are focused on?
- What kind of research can best answer the question, 'How does engaging in everyday activities contribute to health and well-being for people and communities?'

STUDY QUESTIONS

1 What knowledge is important to translate into practice?
2 What new research should be generated to inform practice?
3 How would you use current occupational therapy evidence to guide your clinical practice?
4 Which sort of methodology is best suited to answer your practice-based research questions?
5 Which methodologies are likely to be more widely used in occupational therapy research in the future?
6 How does engaging in everyday activities contribute to health and well-being for people and communities?

ADDITIONAL READING

Laliberte Rudman, D., Dennhardt, S., Fok, D., Huot, S., Molke, D., Park, A., et al. (2008). A vision for occupational science: Reflecting on our disciplinary culture. *Journal of Occupational Science, 15*(3), 136–146.

Shaw, J., & Shaw, D. (2011). Evidence and ethics in occupational therapy. *British Journal of Occupational Therapy, 74*(5), 254–256.

Townsend, E., Wicks, A., van Bruggen, H., & Wright-St. Clair. V. (2012). Imagining occupational therapy. *British Journal of Occupational Therapy, 75*(1), 42–44.

Wright-St Clair, V. A., & Hocking, C. (2013). Occupational science: The study of occupation. In B. A. Boyt Schell, G. Gillen, & M. E. Scaffa (Eds.), *Willard & Spackman's occupational therapy* (12th ed., pp. 82–94). Baltimore, MD: Lippincott, Williams & Wilkins.

REFERENCES

American Occupational Therapy Association. (1925). An outline of lectures on occupational therapy to medical students and physicians. *Occupational Therapy and Rehabilitation, 4*(4), 15.

American Occupational Therapy Foundation. (2007). Occupational therapy research agenda. *American Journal of Occupational Therapy, 65*(Suppl), S4–S7.

Bennet, S., Shand, S., & Liddle, J. (2011). Occupational therapy practice in Australia with people with dementia: A profile in need of change. *Australian Occupational Therapy Journal, 58,* 155–163.

Blijlevens, H., Hocking, C., & Paddy, A. (2009). Rehabilitation of adults with dyspraxia: Health professionals learning from patients. *Disability and Rehabilitation, 31*(6), 466–475.

Canadian and American Occupational Therapists. (2009). *CAOT position statement: Research in occupational therapy.* Ottawa: Author.

Clark, F. (1997). Occupational therapy for independent-living older adults. A randomized controlled trial. *Journal of the American Medical Association, 278*(16), 1321–1326.

Clark, F. A., Jackson, J. M., & Carlson, M. E. (2004). Occupational science, occupational therapy and evidence-based practice: What the Well Elderly Study has taught us. In M. Molineux (Ed.), Occupation for occupational therapists (pp. 200–218). Oxford: Blackwell Publishing.

Clark, F., Jackson, J., Carlson, M., Chou, C-P., Cherry, B. J., Jordan-Marsh, M., et al. (2011). Effectiveness of a lifestyle intervention in promoting the well-being of independently living older people: Results of the Well Elderly 2 Randomised Controlled Trial. *Journal of Epidemiology and Community Health, 66,* 326–336.

Dirette, D., Rozich, A., & Viau, S. (2009). Is there enough evidence for evidence-based practice in occupational therapy? *American Journal of Occupational Therapy, 63*(6), 782–786.

Eriksson, G., Tham, K., & Kottorp, A. (2013). A cross-diagnostic validation of an instrument measuring participation in everyday occupations: The Occupational Gaps Questionnaire (OGQ). *Scandinavian Journal of Occupational Therapy, 20*(2), 152–160.

Hayman, K. J., Kerse, N., Dyall, L., Kepa, M., Teh, R., Wham, C., et al. (2012). Life and living in advanced age: A cohort study in New Zealand—te puawaitanga o nga tapuwae kia ora tonu, LiLACS NZ: Study protocol. *Bio Medical Central Journals-Geriatrics, 12*(33).

Hoffmann, T., Bennett, S., & Del Mar, C. (Eds.). (2010). *Introduction to evidence-based practice.* Chatswood: Elsevier.

Ilott, I. (2012). Evidence-based pratice: A critical appraisal. *Occupational Therapy International, 19,* 1–6.

Kielhofner, G. (1997). *Conceptual foundations of occupational therapy* (2nd ed.). Philadelphia, PA: F. A. Davis.

Kim, S., Yoo, E., Jung, M., Park, S., & Park, J. (2012). A systematic review of the effects of occupational therapy for persons with dementia: A meta-analysis of randomised controlled trials. *NeuroRehabilitation, 31*, 107–115.

Koome, F., Hocking, C., & Sutton, D. (2013). Why routines matter: The nature and meaning of family routines in the context of adolescent mental illness. *Journal of Occupational Science, 19*(4), 312–325.

Law, M., Pollock, N., & Stewart, D. (2004). Evidence-based occupational therapy: Concepts and strategies. *New Zealand Journal of Occupational Therapy, 51*(1), 14–22.

Mental Health Foundation. (n.d.). *Five ways to well-being*. Retrieved April 12, 2013, from http://www.mentalhealth.org.nz/page/1180-5-ways-to-well-being

Ministry of Health. (2012). *The health of New Zealand Adults 2011/12: Key findings of the New Zealand Health Survey*. Wellington: Ministry of Health. Retrieved from http://www.health.govt.nz.

O'Sullivan, G. (2011). *Living with dementia in New Zealand: An action research study*. Unpublished doctoral dissertation, AUT University, Auckland, New Zealand.

Orellano, E., Colon, W. I., & Arbesman, M. (2012). Effect of occupation- and activity-based interventions on instrumental activities of daily living performance among community-dwelling older adults: A systematic review. *American Journal of Occupational Therapy, 66*(3), 292–300.

Peloquin, S. (1989). Moral treatment: Contexts considered. *American Journal of Occupational Therapy, 43*(8), 537–544.

Pierce, D. (2012). Promise: The 2011 Ruth Zemke Lecture in Occupational Science. *Journal of Occupational Science, 19*(4), 298–311.

Polatajko, H. J., Backman, C., Baptiste, S., Davis, J., Eftekhar, P., Harvey, A., et al. (2007). *Human occupation in context*. Ottawa: CAOT Publications ACE.

Reed, K., Hocking, C., & Smythe, L. (2010). The interconnected meaning of occupation: The call, being-with, possibilities. *Journal of Occupational Science, 17*(3), 140–149.

Reilly, M. (1962). Eleanor Clarke Slagle Lecture: Occupational therapy can be one of the great ideas of 20th century medicine. *American Journal of Occupational Therapy, 16*, 1–9.

Roberts, P., Kurfuest, S., & Low, J. F. (2008). Historical and social foundations for practice. In M. Vining Radomski, & C. A. Trombly Latham (Eds.), *Occupational therapy for physical dysfunction* (6th ed., pp. 21–39). Baltimore, MD: Lippincott, Williams & Wilkins.

Sendroy-Terrill, M., Whiteneck, G. G., & Brooks, C. A. (2010). Aging with traumatic brain injury: Cross-sectional follow-up of people receiving inpatient rehabilitation more than 3 decades. *Archives of Physical Medicine Rehabilitation, 91*(3), 489–497. doi:10.1016/j.apmr.2009.11.011.

Schwartz, K. B. (2003). History of occupation. *Perspectives in human occupation: Participation in life* (pp. 18–31). Baltimore: Lippincott Williams & Wilkins.

Sundkvist, Y., & Zingmark, K. (2003). Leading from intermediary positions: First-line administrators' experiences of their occupational role situation. *Scandinavian Journal of Occupational Therapy, 10*, 40–46.

Sutton, D., Hocking, C., & Smythe, L. (2012). A phenomenological study of occupational engagement in recovery from mental illness. *Canadian Occupational Therapy Journal, 79*(3), 142–150.

Turner, A., Foster, M., & Johnson, S. (Ed.). (2002). *History and philosophy of occupational therapy* (5th ed.). Edinburgh: Churchill Livingstone.

Wilcock, A. (2001). Occupational science: The key to broadening horizons. *British Journal of Occupational Therapy, 64*(8), 412–417.

WEBSITES

Journal of Occupational Science:
http://www.tandfonline.com/toc/rocc20/current

OT Seeker:
http://otseeker.com

OTCATS (Occupational Therapy Critically Appraised Topics):
http://www.otcats.com

Joanna Briggs Institute:
http://www.joannabriggs.edu.au

New Zealand Guidelines Group:
http://www.nzgg.org.nz

New Zealand Association of Occupational Therapists:
http://www.nzaot.com

McMaster University, Occupational Therapy Evidence-Based Practice research Group:
http://www.srs-mcmaster.ca/Default.aspx?tabid=630

OTDBASE, occupational therapy journal literature database service:
http://www.otdbase.org

CHAPTER 23

PARAMEDICINE

BRENDA COSTA-SCORSE AND GRAHAM HOWIE

CHAPTER OVERVIEW

This chapter covers the following topics:

- A quiet revolution
- Clinical guidelines and international consensus
- Research literacy
- Evidence-based paramedic practice

KEY TERMS

Consensus

Guidelines

Hierarchy of evidence

Hypothesis

Placebo

Pragmatism

Reliability

Trial and error

Writing

Research is at the heart of academic endeavour. Research has value in its own right, for the richness that it can bring to society, and because research informs and supports the professional practice of paramedics. To date, paramedics have been active consumers of research, but less involved than primary researchers. In the past, research within this discipline was largely undertaken by others (predominantly from medicine), with paramedics as subjects or in the role of data collectors.

A QUIET REVOLUTION

The twentieth century was dominated by industry-based apprenticeship style education. Most education occurred in ambulance 'training schools'—and the word 'training' reflected the fact that technical skills and knowledge used to be the key focus of education, with little room for more abstract forms of inquiry. The cultural shift to paramedic-led research has occurred in tandem with the move to a tertiary education model. University-based degree education for paramedics commenced in Aotearoa New Zealand at the Auckland University of Technology in 2002 and some states of Australia made the move to paramedic tertiary education in the mid-1990s. Locating the education of health professionals within universities and other tertiary education settings has raised the profile of and opportunities for research within the paramedic community.

CASE STUDY 23.1

OXYGEN IS A NATURAL SUBSTANCE AND CAN DO NO HARM—OR CAN IT?

Noeline is 81 years old, plays 18 holes of golf each week to keep her healthy handicap of 24, and mows the lawns regularly to within a centimetre of their life. She is fitter than many folk 30 years her junior. However, this autumn morning Noeline complains of chest pain at the ninth hole. It looks like a heart attack: substernal crushing pain that came on at rest, radiating to the left arm. She is cool to touch and her capillary refill time (CRT) is three seconds. ECG changes with ST-elevation confirm the diagnosis. One of the time-honoured emergency treatments for acute myocardial infarction (AMI) is high-flow oxygen. After all, blocked coronary arteries and myocardial tissue starved of oxygen underpin the very definition of ischemic pain and infarction. Besides, oxygen is unquestionably 'natural'—it's in the air, and everyone needs it to survive! So why not administer a bit more of it when the heart is damaged and the patient is pale, diaphoretic, in tachycardia and in obvious pain?

When you locate at the golf club rooms the local responders are administering 8 litres/min of oxygen through an acute re-breather mask. The responders are pleased when the pulse oximeter shows a SpO_2 of 100%, but they are not at all impressed when you turn the oxygen off and remove the mask. Noeline is also not impressed, given her many years of nursing; clearly some diplomatic explanation is needed.

Oxygen therapy seems so obvious that it has rarely been questioned, possibly because it is the most widely used drug in medicine, considered safe because it is in the air around us. There have not been many randomised controlled trials (RCTs) concerning the use of oxygen. Indeed, we only have to look back to 1976 to find a (small, underpowered) study which compared AMI patients receiving oxygen with those who simply received air. Those on oxygen did get worse, although the figures did not reach statistical significance (Rawles & Kenmure, 1976). The modern consensus is towards less oxygen—see Iscoe, Beasley & Fisher (2011). The evidence is not yet entirely in for AMI patients, but oxygen can certainly be detrimental in stroke—see Ronning and Guldvog (1999). In the ambulance setting we now need good clinical reasons to administer oxygen to patients—they must be hypoxemic, and it is not just given to everyone as a 'blanket treatment'. Noeline is likely to do better without the oxygen.

Noeline goes on to make a full and speedy recovery. She returns to playing golf within three months of the acute cardiac event. By her lead she encourages all of us to keep active.

Consensus
A general agreement on any given issue.

CLINICAL GUIDELINES AND INTERNATIONAL CONSENSUS

An example of the move towards a research-led culture has been the change in the development and the application of clinical procedures. Traditionally the care that paramedics could provide to patients was rigidly encoded in 'procedures' determined by ambulance service medical directors. Rote procedural care was entrenched in ambulance service culture. Some of the rationale for procedures was standardisation of care; however, written instructions could not cover every possible condition that a paramedic might encounter in the field. Gaps between the procedures tended to be bridged by pragmatism and trial-and-error—but trial and error based approaches increase clinical risk. Snowden (2002) stressed that in complex situations there is a 'phenomenon of retrospective coherence … [that is,] the current state of affairs always makes logical sense,

Pragmatism
The demonstration of logical and practical responses to problems.

Trial and error
The process of developing practice by trying various approaches and deciding what seems to be most effective.

but only when we look backwards' (p. 106). By contrast, the questioning and inquiry that underpins clinical research looks to the future, by asking whether or not better ways exist to serve patients who call for ambulance services. With degree education the old attitude of 'just follow the procedures' is being replaced by an emphasis on reflective practice, critical inquiry and clinical reasoning.

In 2009, the 'clinical procedures' for paramedics issued by the medical director of St John New Zealand, Dr Tony Smith, were renamed 'clinical guidelines'. These best-practice guidelines are more open-ended than the older-style procedures. Paramedics exercise more clinical judgment (for example, in determining drug dosage) and in providing treatments that are not described in the guidelines in cases where 'circumstances are exceptional' (St John New Zealand 2011–2013, p. 10). The updating of these guidelines involves a multidisciplinary committee reviewing available research to ensure that the guidelines are contemporary, that the understanding of pre-hospital care issues is advancing, and that sound clinical reasoning underpins the application of clinical guidelines. Most reasoning is based on experiences, evidence or data. The examination of the interrelationship of the elements of clinical problems enables debate about whether the status quo in current paramedic practice is clinically sound. The process of discussion and debate provides further clarification and generates questions that catalyse research.

International consensus statements provide evidence-based research that support changes to these clinical guidelines. In 1993, the International Liaison Committee on Resuscitation (ILCOR) formally adopted the mission statement: 'to provide a consensus mechanism by which the international science and knowledge relevant to emergency cardiac care can be identified and reviewed ... international guidelines will aim for a commonality supported by science' (Chamberlain, 2005, p. 158).

Undertaking resuscitative measures is the cornerstone of paramedic practice; clearly there is a need to understand this practice and, most importantly, whether these measures actually work. Changes to 'compression to ventilation' ratios are a good example. In some instances continuous chest compressions may improve outcomes (Nagao, Kikushima, Sakamoto, & Koseki, 2007). However, compressing the chest for long uninterrupted periods can be exhausting for paramedics (Deschilder, De Vos, & Stockman, 2007). Practice must be adapted accordingly. For example, a call for backup is not necessarily for advanced life support—it may simply be calling for more paramedics, more hands, to rotate and perform chest compressions.

In 1995, the Faculty of Pre-hospital Care of Royal College of Surgeons (Edinburgh) produced a consensus statement on the management of life-threatening chest injury. The college noted that there was little research on the best management for chest injuries and took the common sense approach to field needle chest decompression guidelines in tension pneumothorax based on in-hospital case reviews. In relation to the hierarchy of evidence, evidence provided by case studies is not considered the most robust

Guidelines
Information providing advice on how to interpret policy or procedure.

Hierarchy of evidence
A tool for evaluating research findings according to the degree of scientific rigour.

evidence, but it would clearly not be ethical to undertake double-blind trials just to prove equivocally that this consensus statement provided the best pre-hospital management plan, as some of the individuals in this design would get a placebo and would miss out on the life-saving intervention.

Consensus statements or research that is hospital-based may or may not translate to solving problems in the pre-hospital arena. It is important that research contributes to practice by solving problems, ensuring the advancement of clinical practice and improvement in patient health outcomes. Research into equipment design that is fit for the pre-hospital arena is one of the many relevant research topics for paramedics. The struggles of working with poorly designed equipment leads to frustration, and possibly adversely affects health outcomes. For example, pulse oximeters are ineffective in the cold and in shocked patients (Woodhouse, 1998).

Placebo
An apparently inert intervention used in research as a control to test the effectiveness of an active intervention.

CASE STUDY 23.2

SOTALOL VERSUS LIGNOCAINE

The RCT trial of sotalol versus lignocaine in out-of-hospital refractory cardiac arrest due to ventricular tachyarrhythmia in the New South Wales Ambulance Service in Sydney, Australia is a good example of paramedics being involved in the research process (Kovoor et al., 2005). The study was held over 43 months and stopped when the trial drugs expired. Unfortunately this was before the required sample size of 408 was achieved. The study of 151 cases was underpowered, but on analysis of the data the authors concluded that sotalol and lignocaine have similar efficacy and that the outcome for patients that have not responded after more than four shocks is poor; amiodarone is the drug of choice in refractory ventricular fibrillation although the use of it remains contentious. Multi-centre RCTs across Australasia will counter the challenge of sufficient numbers to ensure statistical significance and contribute to international consensus statements and guidelines.

RESEARCH LITERACY

Research literacy begins with learning to read research papers. It involves searching through databases for key articles, understanding the scientific method and scientific writing, gaining familiarity with common statistical analyses, and being able to critique the value of a study. Research comprehension skills are not easily acquired; this is why

Writing
The process of developing a written piece of work.

most paramedic degree programmes introduce research literacy, in a graduated way, from year one. When writing assignments, student paramedics are expected to reference not only the standard textbooks, but also key research findings. Being a healthy sceptic helps when reading research, along with an ability to argue a case for or against changes in paramedic practice, based on the evidence. Becoming research literate moves paramedics away from the technical-only towards a balanced mix of the technical and science-based practitioner.

RESEARCH ALIVE 23.1
LEARNING TO ASK QUESTIONS AND DEVELOPING RESEARCH OPPORTUNITIES

Hypothesis
A speculative explanation for a problem that can be tested by further research.

Research attempts to obtain the evidence to support or reject a **hypothesis**. In paramedic degree programmes, student paramedics are prepared for practice by being required to formulate a research question, do a literature review and produce a scientific poster. The questions range from proposed new treatments and new devices, finding effective professional approaches to cope with death and dying, the psychological health of paramedics who frequently work under duress, establishing the reasons for a high turnover among ambulance staff, and the philosophies underlying care delivery. These early rungs on the research ladder are extraordinary and powerful displays of enquiry.

Original research typically begins within postgraduate programmes, such as masters and doctoral degrees, but some of the most important and interesting questions have emerged from undergraduate students, such as:

- the accuracy in paramedic diagnosis of patients presenting with dyspnoea compared with emergency department diagnosis;
- gender inequity in acquisition of 12-lead ECGs from ambulance patients with non-traumatic chest pain;
- the best chest lead placement in females;
- autonomous thrombolysis; and
- exploring paramedic attitudes to advanced directives have been launched from the undergraduate programme.

Original research is worth pursuing as it establishes facts and evidence, pushing back ignorance, going out beyond the known horizon and exploring new territory. Sometimes the implications of research findings challenge accepted practices within ambulance services, and ultimately they may make a difference to the care of patients and their health outcomes.

EVIDENCE-BASED PARAMEDIC PRACTICE

Few people would disagree that all and any therapeutic intervention must be proven effective. Having an evidence-based approach to practice requires that evidence is assessed and evaluated. Paramedics must be familiar with the principles of evidence-based practice in order to make informed and insightful critiques of the quality and reliability of the evidence, and to be able to enhance and develop practice.

Reliability
The extent to which the same results are elicited when an investigation is repeated.

RESEARCH ALIVE 23.2
ANTIARRHYTHMIC DRUGS IN VF ARREST

For many years lignocaine was the antiarrhythmic drug used in VF (ventricular fibrillation) arrest. At least a generation of paramedics carefully memorised the lignocaine algorithm, an initial dose and a titrating infusion. However, there was no difference in long-term survival between receiving or not receiving antiarrhythmic drugs. Ong, Pellis, and Link (2011) in their systematic review, state:

> Despite the perceived necessity of antiarrhythmic drugs in cardiac arrest due to VT (ventricular tachycardia) or VF ... there is no conclusive evidence that antiarrhythmic agents improve survival. ... While some agents have shown an improved survival to hospital admission, none (including lignocaine) have shown an improved survival to discharge.(pp. 668–9)

If you asked experienced paramedics what they think of lignocaine, they would probably have been enthusiastically in favour of it because, in their experience, it worked. They could have explained the physiological basis of lignocaine's efficacy, including the slowing of spontaneous depolarisation. The research results were so at odds with years of front-line experience. So then, which is the better evidence that supports lignocaine's efficacy? Evidence-based practice strongly favours randomised trials over clinical experience. One anecdote concerning lignocaine noted that it was also the drug of choice for acute myocardial infarctions with frequent ventricular ectopic beats, and they would certainly disappear off the patient's ECG. When pointed out to a colleague that research on lignocaine provided evidence that there was no real benefit to the patient, he jokingly said:

> Let's keep giving the lignocaine anyway, because at least it benefits me! I feel a lot better when I see all those ventricular ectopic beats disappear!

[continued next page]

Of particular interest to paramedics is that lignocaine was replaced by amiodarone as the antiarrhythmic agent of choice after two RCTs were published around the turn of the millennium. The RCTs compared the two drugs, and amiodarone demonstrated better on-scene results. However, of note is that amiodarone has not yet been shown to improve discharge from hospital rates any more than lignocaine (Rea, Kane-Gill, & Rudis, 2006; Lee et al., 2006).

The first requirement for engaging with research is an enquiring mind, an attitude of curiosity, and the ability to question. Questions such as: 'We've always done it this way—but what's the evidence for that?' or 'What particular aspect of the way we do this is most important to the health outcome?' or 'In the face of this problem/difficulty, is there something new or different or better we could do?' For example, it is common for paramedics to believe that capillary refill time (CRT) should be less than two seconds (see Caroline, 1994). This is a way of assessing peripheral perfusion by seeing how quickly the nail bed of a patient returns to a normal colour after blanching. What was the evidence for this two-second rule? Apparently this timeframe for checking capillary refill was not originally based on any experimental evidence; rather, it was simply based on the personal experience of the original proponents, who arbitrarily decided that under 2 seconds was the normal value. Subsequent studies showed that CRT in normal people varies according to the person's sex (capillary refill takes longer in females), their age (capillary refill takes longer in the elderly), and the ambient temperature (capillary refill takes longer on a cold day). That paramedics would benefit from being familiar with the CRT research is aptly summarised by Lewin and Maconochie (2008).

SUMMARY

Climbing the rungs of the research ladder is both daunting and exciting. If Paramedics compare their own discipline to disciplines with long research histories, it may seem impossible but if the viewpoint taken is one of excitement not bound by traditional constraints, the opportunities to add new knowledge in pre-hospital care are bound only by F.E.A.R: False Expectations Appearing Real. It is worth reflecting on the fact that fear has rarely stopped a paramedic in a resuscitation setting. The stage is set for more research-active paramedics, a greater contribution to the body of knowledge, and consolidation of research-led practice as an essential cornerstone to clinically sound, reasoned paramedic practice.

REFLECTION POINTS

Taking a personal perspective, would you or those close to you like to be part of an unscheduled, unapproved, pre-hospital research project?

STUDY QUESTIONS

1 Which are the most useful antiarrhythmic drugs in VF cardiac arrest?
2 Should you ask a top-notch, highly experienced paramedic (an 'expert') for his/her opinion on the most useful antiarrhythmic drugs?
3 If in your initial search you only find rat studies, should you consider these as a valid basis for change in paramedic practice?
4 And finally, which sort of research will yield the most reliable evidence on antiarrhythmic drugs?

ADDITIONAL READING

Ball, L. (2005). Setting the scene for the paramedic in primary care: a review of the literature. *Emergency Medicine Journal, 22*(12), 896–900.

Bledsoe, B. E., Porter, R. S., Cherry, R. A., & Armacost, M. R. (2006). Paramedic care, principles & practice. *Prehospital Emergency Care, 10*(4), 522–523.

REFERENCES

Caroline, N. (1994). *Emergency care in the streets* (4th ed.) Sudbury, MA: Jones and Bartlett Publishers and American Academy of Orthopedic Surgeons.

Chamberlain, D. (2005). The International Liaison Committee on Resuscitation (ILCOR)—past and present: Compiled by the Founding Members of the International Liaison Committee on Resuscitation. *Resuscitation, 67*(2), 157–161.

Deschilder, K., De Vos, R., & Stockman, W. (2007). The effect on quality of chest compressions and exhaustion of a compression–ventilation ratio of 30:2 versus 15:2 during cardiopulmonary resuscitation—a randomised trial. *Resuscitation, 74*(1): 113–118.

Iscoe, S., Beasley, R., & Fisher, J.A. (2011). Supplementary oxygen for nonhypoxemic patients: O_2 much of a good thing? *Critical Care, 15*(3), 305.

Kovoor, O., Love, A., Hall, J., Kruit, R., Sadick, N., & Ho, D (2005). Randomized double-blind trial of sotalol versus lignocaine in out-of-hospital refractory cardiac arrest due to ventricular tachyarrhythmia. *Internal Medicine Journal, 35*(9), 518–525.

Lewin, J., & Maconochie, I. (2008). Capillary refill time in adults. *Emergency Medicine Journal, 25*, 325–326.

Lee, C., Pollak P.T., Wee, V., Al-Hazmi, A., Martin, J., & Zarnke, K.B. (2006). The use of amiodarone for in-hospital cardiac arrest at two tertiary care centres. *Canadian Journal of Cardiology, 22*, 199–202.

Nagao, K., Kikushima, K., Sakamoto, T., Koseki, K. (2007). Cardiopulmonary resuscitation by bystanders with chest compressions only (SOS-KANTO): an observational study. *The Lancet, 369*(9565), 920–926.

Ong M. E. H., Pellis, T., & Link, M. S. (2011). The use of antiarrhythmic drugs for adult cardiac arrest: A systemic review. *Resuscitation 82*, 665–670.

Rawles, J. M., & Kenmure, A. C. F. (1976). Controlled trial of oxygen in uncomplicated myocardial infarction. *British Medical Journal, 1*, 1121–1123.

Rea, R. S., Kane-Gill S. L., & Rudis, M. I. (2006). Comparing intravenous amiodarone or lignocaine, or both, outcomes for inpatients with pulseless ventricular arrhythmias. *Critical Care Medicine 34*, 1617–1623.

Ronning, O. M., & Guldvog, B. (1999). Should stroke victims routinely receive supplementary oxygen? A quasi-randomised controlled study. *Stroke, 30*, 2033–2037.

Smith, T. (2011). *Clinical practice guidelines 2011–2013*. Auckland: St John New Zealand.

Snowden, D. (2002). Complex acts of knowing: Paradox and descriptive self-awareness. *Journal of Knowledge Management, 6*(2), 100–111.

St John New Zealand.(2013). *Clinical practice guidelines, 2011–2013*. Auckland: Author.

Woodhouse, J. I. (1998). A field evaluation of pulse oximetry in two arduous environments, *Journal of the Royal Army Medical Corps, 144*(3), 159–60.

WEBSITES

American Heart Association—resources for health professionals:
http://www.heart.org/HEARTORG/HealthcareResearch/Healthcare-Research_UCM_001093_SubHomePage.jsp

Australasian Journal of Paramedicine:
http://ro.ecu.edu.au/jephc

CHAPTER 24

PODIATRY

KEITH ROME

CHAPTER OVERVIEW

This chapter covers the following topics:

- Quantitative podiatric research
- Qualitative podiatric research
- Outcome measures used in podiatry

KEY TERMS

Behaviour	Phenomenology
Clinical trial	Philosophy
Critical thinking	Randomised clinical trial
Ethnography	Reliability
Expertise	Treatment
Normative	Validity

Expertise
Expert skills and knowledge.

Critical thinking
The application of sceptical inquiry to examine knowledge claims and taken-for-granted assumptions.

Clinical trial
A formally structured approach to research which includes standards and processes for identifying the problem and investigating it.

Randomised clinical trial
A highly specialised and prescriptive approach to research often used within the health sector. It isolates the trial population into active and control groups and investigates the outcomes for each group.

Over the last decade there has been an exponential increase in the quantity and quality of podiatric medicine-related research. In the context of medicine, Sackett, Rosenberg, Gray, Haynes and Richardson (1996) define evidence-based practice as '… the conscientious, explicit, and judicious use of current best evidence in making decisions about the care of individual patients. The practice of evidence-based medicine involves integrating individual clinical expertise with the best available external clinical evidence from systematic research' (p. 71). Traditionally, podiatric practitioners have favoured previous experience, existing practice, professional training and peer opinion as guides for everyday decision-making regarding patients' care. Health-care podiatric research and evidence-based practice is also being used more and more in the development of clinical policies, both formal and personal, which are used to inform health-care decision-makers and control variation in clinical management decisions for similar clinical situations (Muir Gray, Haynes, Sackett, Cook, & Guyatt, 1997). It is therefore important that podiatrists become acquainted with and use evidence-based principles to ensure they are involved in the development of clinical policy that takes into account the circumstances and wishes of the patient and can be safely and effectively applied. Evidence-based practice can be seen as being applied to individual patients via the clinical decision-making process, which is informed by research and knowledge, is acted upon using critical thinking, and is reviewed and reflected upon in light of how each individual case responds (Redmond, Keenan, & Landorf, 2002).

QUANTITATIVE PODIATRIC RESEARCH

In the world of evidence-based medicine, Sackett et al. (1996) argue that research should be evaluated according to a hierarchy of evidence. A greater weight should be given to randomised controlled trials as the gold standard upon which clinicians should base their clinical decisions, placing less reliance on uncontrolled clinical trials. For example, in a systematic review the authors reported 28 studies relating to the use of foot orthoses in the rheumatoid foot (Clarke, Rome, Plant, O'Hare, & Gray, 2006). Of these, eight were randomised clinical trials; six were non-randomised case control or comparison studies; 10 further articles included audits, case studies and review articles; and two published reports from the Cochrane Controlled Trials Register. The authors concluded that there is limited and conflicting evidence upon which to base clinical practice and, if podiatric medical practice is to be based on rigorous evidence, then more high-quality randomised controlled trials are required to inform clinical practice.

CASE STUDY 24.1

LINKING QUANTITATIVE RESEARCH AND PRACTICE

A recent article published in Australia illustrates that the use of a randomised clinical trial research design can have an impact on clinical practice (Spink et al., 2011). The aim of the study was to determine the effectiveness of a multifaceted podiatry intervention in preventing falls in community-dwelling older people with disabling foot pain. The study design was a randomised controlled trial. The participants included 305 community-dwelling men and women with disabling foot pain and an increased risk of falling. One hundred and fifty-three were allocated to a multifaceted podiatry intervention and 152 to routine podiatry care, with 12 months' follow-up. The multifaceted podiatry intervention consisted of foot orthoses, advice on footwear, a subsidy for footwear (NZ$125—A$100—voucher), a home-based programme of foot and ankle exercises, a falls-prevention education booklet, and routine podiatry care for 12 months. The control group received routine podiatry care for 12 months. The main outcome measures were (1) the proportion of fallers and multiple fallers; (2) falling rate, and (3) injuries resulting from falls during follow-up.

The results demonstrated that 264 falls occurred during the study. Two hundred and ninety-six participants returned all 12 calendars: 147 (96%) in the intervention group and 149 (98%) in the control group.

Adherence was good, with 52% of the participants completing 75% or more of the requested three exercise sessions weekly, and 55% of those issued orthoses reporting wearing them most of the time. Participants in the intervention group ($n = 153$) experienced 36% fewer falls than participants in the control group. The proportion of fallers and multiple fallers did not differ significantly between the groups. Significant improvements in the intervention group compared with the control group were found for the domains of strength (ankle eversion), range of motion (ankle dorsiflexion and inversion/eversion), and balance (postural sway on the floor when barefoot and maximum balance range wearing shoes).

The authors concluded that a multifaceted podiatry intervention reduced the rate of falls in community-dwelling older people with disabling foot pain. The components of the intervention are inexpensive and relatively simple to implement, suggesting that the programme could be incorporated into routine podiatry practice or multidisciplinary falls prevention clinics.

KEITH ROME

QUALITATIVE PODIATRIC RESEARCH

Qualitative research attempts to verify or generate knowledge gleaned from gathering broad descriptive information in a natural setting. The techniques used to evaluate the information based on the philosophy of knowledge are wide and varied. The most common techniques include structured observation, documentary sources, interviews and survey methods (Redmond et al., 2002). Categorisation of qualitative research design is often based on the theoretical underpinning of a particular research question, such as examining the culture of a group of people (ethnography), investigating the 'lived' experience (phenomenology), and developing theories that are grounded in reality (grounded theory). There have been a number of articles pertaining to podiatry published within the qualitative domain, but they are relatively limited compared to those in the quantitative domain. For example, a qualitative design was employed in order to provide a rich and deep understanding of the impact of foot ulceration on health-related quality of life in patients and to understand patients with rheumatoid arthritis perceptions of their journey (Firth, Nelson, Briggs, & Gorecki, 2011).

Philosophy
The study of thought, meaning and existence.

Ethnography
The process of recording and describing human behaviour.

Phenomenology
The study of human experience and consciousness.

CASE STUDY 24.2

LINKING QUALITATIVE RESEARCH AND PRACTICE

A UK study illustrates rheumatoid arthritis patients' experiences of wearing therapeutic footwear (Williams & Graham, 2010). Specialist 'therapeutic' footwear is recommended for patients with diseases such as rheumatoid arthritis (RA) as a beneficial intervention for reducing foot pain, improving foot health, and increasing general mobility. However, many patients choose not to wear this footwear. Recommendations from previous studies have been implemented but have had little impact in improving this situation. The aim of this study was to explore RA patients' experiences of this footwear to ascertain the factors which influence their choice to wear it or not.

Ten females and three males with RA and experience of wearing specialist footwear were recruited from four National Health Service orthotic services. Semi-structured interviews were carried out in the participants' own homes. A hermeneutic phenomenological analysis of the transcripts was carried out to identify themes.

Thematic analysis revealed the participants' feelings about their footwear and their experiences of the practitioners involved in providing the footwear. In addition, further themes were revealed from the female participants: feelings about their feet, behaviour associated with the footwear, and their feelings about what would have improved their experience.

The authors concluded by stating that unlike any other intervention specialist therapeutic footwear replaces something that is normally worn and is part of an individual's body image. It has much more of a negative impact on the female patients' emotions and activities than previously acknowledged and this influences their behaviour with it. The patients' consultations with the referring and dispensing practitioners are pivotal moments within the patient–practitioner relationship that have the potential to influence whether patients choose to wear the footwear or not.

Behaviour
The response of a living thing (including people) to stimulation.

OUTCOME MEASURES USED IN PODIATRY

Outcome measurement involves using evaluative instruments to detect change within individuals or groups over time. Outcome measures often reported in the literature include range of motion, foot pain, plantar pressure, healing time, comfort and walking speed. Evidence-based practice relies on methods of measuring outcomes that can detect change over time. Self-reported outcome instruments have been used by clinicians and by researchers to assess the effect of treatment interventions directed at individuals with foot- and ankle-related pathological conditions and subsequent impairments (Otter et al., 2010; Landorf, Radford, & Hudson, 2010).

Treatment
The act of carrying out an intervention for the purpose of alleviating or curing a problem.

CASE STUDY 24.3

OUTCOME MEASURES IN GOUT AND FOOT PAIN

The aim of a New Zealand study was to evaluate the impact of acute gout on foot pain, impairment, and disability (Rome, Frecklington, McNair, Gow, & Dalbeth, 2012). This prospective observational study recruited 20 patients with acute gout flares. Patients were recruited from emergency departments, hospital wards and rheumatology outpatient clinics throughout Auckland,

[continued next page]

KEITH ROME

New Zealand. Patients were recruited at the time of the flare (the baseline visit) and then reassessed at a follow-up visit once the acute flare had resolved six to eight weeks after the initial assessment. General and foot-specific outcome measures were also recorded at each visit, including foot pain, impairment and disability.

The results found that the foot was affected by acute gout in 17 (85%) patients. Objective measures of joint inflammation, including swollen and tender joint counts and C-reactive protein levels, significantly improved at the follow-up visit compared with the baseline visit. At baseline, high levels of foot pain, impairment and disability were reported. All patient-reported outcome measures of general and foot-specific musculoskeletal function improved at the follow-up visit compared with the baseline visit. However, pain, impairment and disability scores did not entirely normalise after resolution of the acute gout flare.

The authors concluded that patients with acute gout flares experience severe foot pain, impairment and disability. These data provide further support for improved management of gout to prevent the consequences of poorly controlled disease.

If treatment outcomes are to be appropriately measured, clinicians and researchers need to select a suitable instrument and properly interpret the obtained scores. Grimmer-Somers, Lekkas, Nyland, Young and Kumar (2007) report that not only should outcomes measures used be valid, reliable and sensitive to detect change in the population of interest over time (responsiveness), but they should also be appropriate to the stakeholders involved and to all detectable subgroups of the subjects recruited. However, many of the foot-related, patient-reported outcome measures have limited evidence regarding their validity and responsiveness to change, limiting their use in clinical intervention and population studies (Riskowski, Hagedorn, & Hannan. 2011).

Validity
Fitness for purpose.

RESEARCH ALIVE 24.1
RESEARCH INFLUENCING PRACTICE

JUSTIFICATION OF USING RANDOMISED CLINICAL TRIALS
Clinicians often use foot orthoses to manage the symptoms of plantar fasciitis. Although there has been considerable research evaluating the effectiveness of orthoses for this condition, there is still a lack of scientific evidence that

is of suitable quality to fully inform clinical practice. Randomised controlled trials are recognised as the 'gold standard' when evaluating the effectiveness of treatments. Landorf, Keenan, and Herbert (2004) discuss why randomised controlled trials are so important, the features of a well-conducted randomised controlled trial, and some of the problems that arise when trial design is not sound. The authors then evaluate the available evidence for the use of foot orthoses, with particular focus on published randomised controlled trials. From this study it seems that foot orthoses do have a role in the management of plantar fasciitis and that prefabricated orthoses are a worthwhile initial management strategy. At this time, however, it is not possible to recommend either prefabricated or customised orthoses as being better, and it cannot be inferred that customised orthoses are more effective over time and therefore have a cost advantage. Additional good-quality randomised controlled trials are needed to answer these questions.

INTEGRATING PODIATRIC RESEARCH INTO THE CLINICAL SETTING
An article by Keenan and Redmond (2002) is aimed at introducing clinicians to current concepts in research, and outlining how they may be able to apply these concepts to their own clinical practice. Implementing research in clinical practice empowers practitioner and patient choice, and provides a mechanism for professional development as individuals and as a group. Ultimately, and without a doubt most importantly, incorporating good-quality research into clinical decision-making improves the care podiatrists provide for patients.

OUTCOME MEASURES NEED TO BE VALID AND RELIABLE
Accurately measuring, reporting and comparing outcomes are essential for improving health care delivery in podiatry. A review of the literature was undertaken to measure foot function (pressure and/or gait parameters), foot pain and foot-related disability in rheumatoid arthritis (RA), and to investigate the clinometric quality of these measures (van der Leeden et al., 2008). A systematic search was conducted in Medline, CINAHL, Embase and Sportdiscus. Standardised criteria, extended with levels of evidence, were applied to assess the quality of the clinometric studies and the properties (reliability, validity, and responsiveness) of the described instruments.

Reliability
The extent to which the same results are elicited when an investigation is repeated.

A variety of measurement instruments were identified. Only 16 instruments have been studied for their measurement properties in rheumatoid arthritis (RA) patients: seven for assessing foot function, three for measuring foot-related disability, and six for measuring both foot pain and foot-related disability. Thirteen instruments were rated for reliability, of which 10 were rated positively on different levels of evidence. The authors concluded by suggesting

[continued next page]

KEITH ROME

that the review offers a basis for choosing the most appropriate instruments for measuring foot function, foot pain and foot-related disability in RA patients, both for clinical practice and for research.

NORMATIVE VALUES ARE IMPORTANT FOR CLINICIANS IN CLINICAL PRACTICE

The Foot Posture Index (FPI) is a validated method for quantifying standing foot posture, and is being used in a variety of clinical settings. There have however, been no normative data available to date for comparison and reference. A UK study aimed to establish normative FPI reference values (Redmond, Crane, & Menz, 2008). The authors retrieved articles reporting FPI data that were identified by searching online databases. The data sets included information relating to age, gender, pathology (if relevant), FPI scores and body mass index (BMI) where available.

The results showed that a slightly pronated foot posture is the normal position at rest. A 'U' shaped relationship existed for age, with minors and older adults exhibiting significantly higher FPI scores than the general adult population. There was no difference between the FPI scores of males and females. No relationship was found between the FPI and BMI. Systematic differences from the adult normals were confirmed in patients with neurological and idiopathic pes cavus (high-arched feet), indicating some sensitivity of the instrument to detect a pathological foot-type population.

The authors concluded that a set of population norms for children, adults and older people have been derived from a large sample. Foot posture is related to age and the presence of pathology, but not influenced by gender or BMI. The normative values identified may assist in classifying foot type for the purpose of research and clinical decision-making.

Normative
Relating to the norms that form expectations about how people should behave, individually and as a society.

The use of good evidence to support a specific treatment is essential and it is important to understand and appreciate the differences between quantitative and qualitative approaches to podiatric research (Redmond et al., 2002). While practitioners may not need to understand the finer details of research design they have a professional responsibility to ensure they are up to date and able to judge the relevance and appropriateness of published evidence in the clinical setting.

SUMMARY

An evidence-based approach to podiatry is necessary so that clinicians and students can integrate sound knowledge within the clinical setting. The aims of the chapter are to provide students with examples from the literature and case studies utilising the different research approaches within podiatry. Outcome measures have been highlighted as pivotal. Many of the foot-related, patient-reported outcome measures have limited evidence regarding their validity and responsiveness to change, limiting their use in clinical intervention and population studies. There is a great need for valid and reliable instruments and surveys to measure foot health.

REFLECTION POINTS

- Do you think podiatric research is necessary to inform clinical practice?
- Qualitative research within podiatry is limited. What evidence refutes this comment?
- Why is it important to use outcomes measures in podiatry?
- In your first clinical session with patients, which valid and reliable outcome measures will you be using?

STUDY QUESTIONS

1 List the five levels of evidence and illustrate your answer with examples from the podiatric literature.
2 Name three research approaches in qualitative research and give examples of each approach within the podiatric literature.
3 What are the key principles of a good outcome measure?
4 Describe six valid and reliable outcome measures used in podiatric practice.
5 Why are normative values important in clinical practice?

ADDITIONAL READING

Campbell, J. (2007). *Guide to research for podiatrists*. Cumbria: M&K Update Ltd.

Mathesion, I. (2008). *A podiatrist's guide to using research*. Edinburgh: Elsevier/ Butterworth Heinemann.

REFERENCES

Clarke, H., Rome, K., Plant, M., O'Hare, K., & Gray J. (2006). Clinical and cost-effectiveness of foot orthoses for the management of rheumatoid arthritis: critical review. *Rheumatology, 45*, 139–145.

Firth, J., Nelson, E. A., Briggs, M., & Gorecki, C. (2011). A qualitative study to explore the impact of foot ulceration on health-related quality of life in patients with RA. *International Journal of Nursing Studies, 48*, 1401–1408.

Grimmer-Somers, K., Lekkas, P., Nyland, L., Young, A., & Kumar, S. (2007). Perspectives on research evidence and clinical practice: A survey of Australian physiotherapists. *Physiotherapy Research International, 12*, 147–161.

Keenan, A. M., & Redmond, A. C. (2002). Integrating research into the clinic: What evidence based practice means to the practising podiatrist. *Journal of the American Podiatric Medical Association, 92*, 115–122.

Landorf, K. B., Keenan, A. M., & Herbert, R. D. (2004). Effectiveness of different types of foot orthoses for the treatment of plantar fasciitis. *Journal of the American Podiatric Medical Association, 94*, 542–549.

Landorf, K. B., Radford, J. A., & Hudson, S. (2010). Minimal Important Difference (MID) of two commonly used outcome measures for foot problems. *Journal of Foot and Ankle Research, 14*(3), 7.

Muir Gray, J. A., Haynes, R. B., Sackett, D. L., Cook, D. J., & Guyatt, G. H. (1997). Transferring evidence from research into practice: developing evidence-based clinical policy. *ACP J Club, 126*, A14–6.

Otter, S. J., Lucas, K., Springett, K., Moore, A., Davies, K., & Cheek, L. et al. (2010). Foot pain in rheumatoid arthritis prevalence, risk factors and management: an epidemiological study. *Clinical Rheumatology, 29*, 255–71.

Redmond, A. C., Crane, Y. Z., Menz, H. B. (2008). Normative values for the Foot Posture Index. *Journal of Foot and Ankle Research, 31*(1), 6.

Redmond, A. C., Keenan, A. M., & Landorf, K. (2002). 'Horses for courses': the differences between quantitative and qualitative approaches to research. *Journal of the American Podiatric Medical Association, 92*, 159–169.

Riskowski, J. L., Hagedorn, T. J., & Hannan, M. T. (2011). Measures of foot function, foot health, and foot pain: American Academy of Orthopedic Surgeons Lower Limb Outcomes Assessment: Foot and Ankle Module (AAOS-FAM), Bristol Foot Score (BFS), Revised Foot Function Index (FFI-R), Foot Health Status Questionnaire (FHSQ), Manchester Foot Pain and Disability Index (MFPDI), Podiatric Health Questionnaire (PHQ), and Rowan Foot Pain Assessment (ROFPAQ). *Arthritis Care Research, 63*(S11), S229–S239.

Rome, K., Frecklington, M., McNair, P. J., Gow, P., & Dalbeth, N. (2012). Foot pain, impairment and disability in patients with acute gout flares; A prospective observational study. *Arthritis Care Research, 64*, 384–388.

Sackett, D. L., Rosenberg, W. M., Gray, J. A., Haynes, R. B., & Richardson W. S. (1996). Evidence based medicine: what it is and what it isn't. *British Medical Journal, 312,* 71–72.

Spink, M. J., Menz, H. B., Fotoohabadi, M. R., Wee, E., Landorf, K. B., Hill, K. D., et al. (2011). Effectiveness of a multifaceted podiatry intervention to prevent falls in community dwelling older people with disabling foot pain: randomised controlled trial. *British Medical Journal, 16,* 342.

van der Leeden, M., Steultjens, M. P., Terwee, C. B., Rosenbaum, D., Turner, D., Woodburn, J., et al. (2008). A systematic review of instruments measuring foot function, foot pain, and foot-related disability in patients with rheumatoid arthritis. *Arthritis & Rheumatism, 59,* 1257–1269.

Williams, A. E., & Graham, A. S. (2010). 'My feet: visible, but ignored …' A qualitative study of foot care for people with rheumatoid arthritis. *Clinical Rehabilitation, 26;* 952–959.

WEBSITES

Australasian Podiatric Rheumatology Specialist Interest Group:
  http://www.aprsig.co.nz

Foot and Ankle Research Review:
  http://www.researchreview.co.nz/nz/Clinical-Area/Other-Health/Foot-Ankle.aspx

Journal of American Podiatric Medical Association:
  http://www.japmaonline.org

Journal of Foot & Ankle Research:
  http://www.jfootankleres.com

Podiatry Arena:
  http://www.podiatry-arena.com

Podiatry Today:
  http://www.podiatrytoday.com

CHAPTER 25

PSYCHOLOGY

PANTEÁ FARVID, JASON LANDON AND CHRIS KRÄGELOH

CHAPTER OVERVIEW

This chapter covers the following topics:

- Psychology and research
- Key themes
- Learned behaviour
- The developmental
- How is psychological research carried out?
- Evaluating psychological research

KEY TERMS

Applied
Behaviour
Conditioning
Empirical
Mental
Mind
Unconscious

Psychology is a hugely diverse discipline. Research and practice in this area ranges from examining the biological to the social, the applied to the theoretical. The term 'psychology' itself refers to an interest in understanding the workings of the mind, human behaviour and establishing general principles around 'what makes people tick': the way people act, feel or behave in specific contexts. Some key areas of research, teaching and practice within psychology include clinical psychology, counselling psychology, health psychology, neuropsychology, behavioural psychology, evolutionary psychology, developmental psychology, cross-cultural psychology, indigenous psychology, feminist psychology, positive psychology and social psychology.

Applied
Put to practical use.

Mind
That which thinks, reasons and perceives.

Behaviour
The response of a living thing (including people) to stimulation.

PSYCHOLOGY AND RESEARCH

Psychological research extends beyond psychological disorders, distress and treatment. It is incredibly varied, spanning *basic* and *applied* areas, including various domains of practice, with many links to other disciplines (such as biology, neuroscience, mathematical sciences, sociology, gender studies and business). So what does psychological research *do*? Typically, psychological research seeks to understand and improve things. This can mean, for example, examining racism and sexism with the aim of combating prejudice, understanding the signs and reasons for depressive states and the best behavioural or therapeutic interventions for people displaying these, understanding the relationships between brain function and behaviour, examining the links between media exposure to violence and its effects on behaviour, and understanding how people construct (or put together and enact) their identities in different social contexts. In any of the varied research fields, the idea is to understand behaviour, to be able to contribute to theory and deal with (apply the theory to) the myriad issues people face in the contemporary social context.

RESEARCH ALIVE 25.1
TOPICS EXAMINED IN PSYCHOLOGY

The diversity of psychology as a discipline means that the topics examined, or areas researched, are also expansive. Some of the most common research areas include the following.

[continued next page]

Addiction and gambling	Language acquisition
Ageing	Learning and memory
Aggression	Mass media
Anxiety	Natural disasters
Autism	Neurological disorders
Brain Injury	Obesity
Bullying	Personality
Children	Prejudice and inequality
Culture and ethnicity	Psychological disorders
Death and dying	Psychological well-being
Dementia	Rehabilitation
Depression	Relationships
Disability	Sex and sexuality
Eating disorders	Sexual abuse and assault
Education	Shyness
Emotion and affect	Sleep
Environment	Sport and exercise
Ethics	Stress and coping
Fatigue	Suicide and self-harm
Gender roles	Therapy
Group behaviour	Trauma
Human rights	Violence
Identity	Women and men
Immigration and settlement	Workplace issues

Source: Adapted from American Psychological Association, http://www.apa.org, 2013

KEY THEMES
THE UNCONSCIOUS MIND

Unconscious
The part of the human mind that the individual is unaware of.

Empirical
Relating to a scientific approach to defining knowledge based on objective information and processes.

Mental
Relating to the mind.

The sorts of things that psychologists study, and how they go about that study, relate to the broad theoretical movements happening at any particular time within the discipline and wider fields of academia. The unconscious mind is a classic area of interest for psychological theory. Psychoanalysis, a set of theories established by Sigmund Freud (1856–1939) over 100 years ago, seeks to make sense of human behaviour through understanding the unconscious. Psychoanalysis is a difficult theory to test in an empirical way; however, the notion that some mental processes occur below the level of conscious awareness remains important in psychology.

LEARNED BEHAVIOUR

From very early on in the development of the field, psychologists have had an interest in behaviour analysis and modification. Part of this research includes understanding how people *learn* to behave. Ivan Pavlov's (1849–1936) well-known research on the salivation reflex in dogs documented how somewhat automated learning can take place in regular daily activities.

The type of conditioning described by Pavlov's experiments is an *involuntary* process (examples are salivation, the eye-blink response, sexual responses, galvanic skin response and emotional responses) and because of its reflexive nature, it is somewhat limited in the behaviours it can be used to explain. Behaviour that is under voluntary control is called operant behaviour, and operant behaviours are learned through the consequences that follow them. The behaviourist B. F. Skinner (1904–90) was very interested in how particular behaviours occur under specific environmental conditions, based on the reinforcement and punishment that follow them. Traditionally, research in the area of behaviour analysis has been conducted in tightly controlled experimental settings (and often using non-human subjects). Today, the strong experimental tradition remains, and links to the biological sciences are strengthening. For example, applied behaviour analysis (Cooper, Heron, & Heward, 2006) is used in a large range of settings from clinical and community applications, to business and industrial environments (see http://www. abainternational.org).

Conditioning
A process of using reinforcement to develop a behavioural response.

RESEARCH ALIVE 25.2
GAMBLING IN AOTEAROA NEW ZEALAND

In some form, gambling has been a feature of New Zealand society (and its economy) virtually since the first European contact; it is generally viewed as a legitimate recreational or entertainment activity. Gambling includes a diverse range of activities in a variety of settings, many of which have substantially greater hours of operation and greater availability throughout communities than alternative recreational activities. 'Pathological' gambling was recognised as a mental disorder with its inclusion in the DSM-III (American Psychiatric Association, 1980) and subsequent revisions. The term 'problem gambling' has been used in a variety of ways; in most situations it is used to indicate all patterns of gambling that disrupt personal, family, or vocational pursuits (Lesieur, 1998).

In Aotearoa New Zealand, the vast majority of people seeking help for gambling problems cite electronic gaming machines (EGMs) as their primary mode of harmful gambling. The core feature underlying the operation of these

[*continued next page*]

PANTEÁ FARVID, JASON LANDON AND CHRIS KRÄGELOH

machines is a simple variable-ratio schedule of reinforcement (Skinner, 1953; Ferster & Skinner, 1957). That is, the EGM provides a win unpredictably based on an average number of plays. The EGMs also include more sophisticated features such as several schedules, other win-related features, graphical displays, lights and music. If you play a machine, even for a short period of time, you will encounter a win feature of some sort—these frequent albeit small wins encourage gamblers to continue playing. As you can see, the importance of operant conditioning (small wins) and respondent conditioning (sounds, music and graphics) are a key part of why people gamble more than they intend, and some develop harmful patterns of gambling.

The Gambling and Addictions Research Centre at AUT University investigates a range of issues related to how the features of gambling products might lead them to be more harmful or safer and how exposure to various gambling products has influenced gambling problems at a population level. Currently, large research projects are investigating issues such as the incidence and prevalence of problem gambling in a nationally representative sample, the effectiveness of various phone-based and face-to-face interventions for gambling problems, the impact of game features on gambler behaviour, the effectiveness of various regulated EGM-based interventions on gambling harm, the impact of gambling on Pacific peoples, and the relationship between problem gambling and family violence (see http://www.niphmhr.aut.ac.nz/research-centres/gambling-and-addictions-research-centre).

Some key researchers have extended the notion of learning to social contexts and situations to understand how people learn to behave in a variety of ways. For example, Bandura, Ross and Ross (1961) carried out a series of experiments looking at how 'vicarious' learning may occur in children. He showed videos to preschool children depicting an adult either attacking (hitting, punching) a blow-up clown 'Bobo' Doll, or sitting next to it quietly. The children who had witnessed the aggressive behaviour were then more likely to display aggression towards the doll. This indicated to Bandura that merely witnessing certain behaviours (even in the absence of reinforcement or punishment) could elicit that behaviour in people. Named *social learning theory*, this model posits that people learn from one another through modelling, imitation and mere observation, with or without directly encountering reinforcement or punishment (Bandura, 1977). Social learning theory has been applied in a variety of ways in psychological research, such as examining links between violence in media and aggression, childhood development, educational performance and anxiety disorders.

THE DEVELOPMENTAL

A significant part of psychological research has been devoted to understanding how people develop across their life span. A major focus of this research has been on understating human 'attachment'. For example, Harry Harlow (1905–81) was able to demonstrate, through his experiments with infant rhesus monkeys, that 'contact comfort' from a mother or caregiver figure was more important than food and water. Infant monkeys were more drawn to a wire 'mother' that was covered in comforting 'cloth' than a wire 'mother' that was left bare but provided milk. Softness and closeness were thus identified as important parts of early development and attachment.

One of the most influential developmental psychologists was Jean Piaget (1896–1980) who proposed the theory of 'equilibration'. After many years of working with children, he noted that cognitive development happens in stages (from birth to adolescence) where children seek to gain a balance between the information they receive, the experiences they have *and* the cognitive abilities they have: an evolving form of equilibration (Piaget, 1954). In one of his famous experiments, the liquid conservation task, Piaget was able to demonstrate that until children reach the age of 'concrete operations' they will judge the *same* amount of liquid poured in differently shaped beakers as more or less depending on the height of the beaker. The quantity of the beaker is not recognised as being 'conserved' despite the superficial changes in the shape of the container.

RESEARCH ALIVE 25.3
QUALITY OF LIFE RESEARCH

The World Health Organization Quality of Life Group (WHOQOL) defines health-related QOL as 'individual's perception of their position in life in the context of the culture and value systems in which they live and in relation to their goals, expectations, standards and concerns. It is a broad ranging concept, incorporating in a complex way individuals' physical health, psychological state, level of independence, social relationships, personal beliefs and their relationships to salient features of the environment,' (WHOQOL Group, 1995, p. 1405). This multifaceted definition thus encompasses a wide range of aspects in people's lives.

Complete measurement of the health status of a country requires more than experts analysing morbidity and mortality statistics and other socio-economic indicators, and more than the collective opinions by health professionals about the health of their patients. After all, one may be happy with one's life in spite of illness or disease. Therefore, people should be asked directly about

[continued next page]

PANTEÁ FARVID, JASON LANDON AND CHRIS KRÄGELOH

their QOL. In health service evaluation, subjective assessments compliment the more objective biomedical measures, and thus broaden the focus of measuring health by introducing more humanistic elements. Measuring subjective perceptions can also help improve communication between health professionals and their patients. For example, today, medicines to be approved by the US Food and Drug Administration and the European Medicines Agency often require QOL impact analysis.

WHOQOL questionnaires measure the extent to which people feel satisfied with their health and QOL irrespective of their level of physical functioning. The WHOQOL assessment thus takes into account individuals' physical health, psychological state, their functional status to carry out tasks of everyday living, their social wellbeing, personal beliefs, and environmental factors. The core questionnaires are the WHOQOL-100 and the abbreviated WHOQOL-BREF, which have been developed with the collaboration of many field centres in different countries, and they thus possess very good cross-cultural applicability (WHOQOL Group, 1995, 1998). Researchers at AUT University have recently founded the New Zealand WHOQOL Group (Billington, Landon, Krägeloh, & Shepherd, 2010), which conducts research in the area of QOL and assists other researchers using these tools. The WHOQOL-BREF has also now been validated for use with the general New Zealand population (Krägeloh, Kersten, Billington, Hsu, Shepherd, Landon, & Feng, 2013), and a version with specific New Zealand items is now also available (Feng, Krägeloh, Billington, & Hsu, 2011).

THE SOCIAL

Along with an interest in individual learning and development, psychological research has been eager to examine how people behave in particular *social* situations, under various conditions, in the presence (or imagined presence) of others. Social psychological research has traditionally been interested in understanding how power operates within society, how and why social injustices are carried out, how people respond to authority figures, and the processes of conformity.

In a similar vein, Haney, Banks and Zimbardo (1973) conducted what became known as the famous 'Stanford Prison Experiment' to map how social roles influence or dictate human behaviour in specific situations. For this study, a number of university students were recruited and assigned to the role of either prisoner or guard in a 'mock prison'. Surprisingly, the participants not only took on these assigned roles, but took them on so well that the experiment had to be terminated much earlier than planned. The guards, with all their allocated power, had become increasingly aggressive and cruel to the prisoners, who then became withdrawn, anxious and depressed. Although the participants were aware they were part of an *experiment*, 'the *role* of guard and prisoner were so compelling and powerful … that this simple truth was overlooked' (Aronson, Wilson, & Akert, 2013, p. 240) and their identity lost. Similar real-life events have recently occurred in places like Abu Ghraib prison during the second Gulf War, where guards who had little training or supervision were engaging in acts of abuse and dehumanisation towards the prisoners (Zimbardo, 2007). It would seem the roles assigned in society, whatever they may be, have great impact on how people enact their identities or behave in specific contexts.

HOW IS PSYCHOLOGICAL RESEARCH CARRIED OUT?

Methods used to carry out research in psychology vary significantly. There are experimental qualitative and quantitative methods. Research may involve human participants, animal subjects or social and textual resources. Researchers may use various machines that measure or map brain functioning (such as an EEG machine or MRI scanning), administer surveys or questionnaires, observe participants, conduct interviews, run focus groups or analyse clinical case material. The methods of data collection deployed, and the modes of analyses used, depend on the research topic, what the researcher is interested in examining, and the epistemological positioning of any given project. It is important to stress that psychology is a research discipline and any application derived from psychology needs to be grounded in empirical evidence.

Most psychological research follows the 'scientific method' (as used in the natural sciences). This means there is an interest in measurable phenomena, but these phenomena can include non-observable constructs such as personality or quality of life. Through the systematic collection and analysis of data, and consequent development of sets of models or related theories, psychologists seek to understand and explain human behaviour. Objectivity is seen as an important part of the research process. Research from this approach usually follows the principle of 'hypothetico-deductivism'. Rather than 'confirming' a theory (A follows B) and putting claims to the 'test', psychological research works by looking for disconfirmation, or *falsification* rather than *confirmation*. Discovering which claims are *not true*, by a process of elimination of claims, moves researchers closer to the truth (Willig, 2008). Within this approach, well-controlled experiments (where the variables are controlled and manipulated by the researcher in laboratories or applied settings) are the ideal (but not only) approach, and direct measures of behaviour, brain function, physiology and self-report via surveys and questionnaires which include validated psychometric scales, are often used. This approach places heavy importance on the reliability (are the results consistent or repeatable?) and validity of the measures (are we really measuring what we think we are?) to ensure results are objective and replicable.

CASE STUDY 25.1

CRITICAL PSYCHOLOGY

Alongside the mainstream or traditional methodological approaches described above, there is a *critical* branch of psychology that draws on postmodern theories (e.g., Post-structuralism, Foucauldian theory) and critical social theories (e.g., Marxism, feminism), in order to examine our world (and us within it) to foster social or political change (e.g., Parker, 2007). Critical approaches tend to deal with issues of power and domination, stating that our society is structured unequally (thorough categories like class, gender, sexuality and ablebodiedness). It has criticised mainstream psychology for being too *individualistic* and experimental in its research endeavours and seeks to fully contextualise research socially, politically and historically.

What sets critical psychology apart is the *Epistemology* (theory of knowledge and theorising around what counts as 'legitimate knowledge'), *Methodology* (considering how research should best proceed), and *Method(s)* (techniques or ways of gathering data) that it deploys. This type of research tends to be in-depth, exploratory, qualitative, discursive, and seek to identify and problematise many forms of dominant or taken-for-granted 'truths' that maintain unequal power relations within society (which have adverse outcomes on people's health and wellbeing).

Much of the critical work in psychology comes from critical social psychology (Gough & McFadden, 2001), with its core origination being: a critique of the traditional scientific model for understating people (a preference for relativist/constructionist approaches), acknowledging the importance of language in shaping our realities, a focus on the analysis of power relations within society, a social change orientation, an emphasis on diversity within research, striving for ethically rigorous research and promoting researcher reflexivity (e.g., Farvid, 2010). Critical psychology seeks to do socially and politically important work and has examined topics like modern racism (Wetherell & Potter, 1992), modern sexism (Gill, 1993), rape and sexual coercion (Gavey, 2005), sexual ethics (Beres & Farvid, 2010), and the inegalitarian portrayals of male and female sexuality in magazines (Farvid & Braun, 2006). It has a solid following in Europe and Australasia and spans research in health, social, political and liberation psychology.

EVALUATING PSYCHOLOGICAL RESEARCH

Robust psychological research utilises appropriate research methods to answer its overall research questions. For example, exploring the relationships between two variables (such as the temperature in a room and the cognitive functioning of students in that room) might lead to devising an experiment within a quantitative framework to test this. Alternatively, investigating the personal narratives of people when it comes to their daily experiences (of sexual relationships or working life) might utilise interviews within a qualitative framework. The main thing to remember is that doing robust research means making methodological choices that are clearly justifiable and appropriate given the research topic, and that the research process is made transparent within any document reporting its findings.

SUMMARY

As a hugely diverse discipline, psychology spans a variety of research topics, interests and methodological approaches. This chapter has provided an outline of some of the classic theories and studies in the history of psychology and how they relate to research or psychological theorising today. Some current local research happening in Aotearoa New Zealand has been showcased to demonstrate how psychological theory is applied to research and practice in the contemporary context.

REFLECTION POINTS

- How do your interests line up with the sorts of things psychological researchers are interested in?
- What did you learn from reading about the classic studies in psychology?
- How relevant do you think the classic psychology studies are today?
- What is the relevance of some of the newer and local research?
- What sorts of methods can you use when doing psychological research?
- How would you go about evaluating research done in psychology?

STUDY QUESTIONS

1   What is psychology?
2   What is psychology interested in and why?
3   How does psychological research relate to health-care practice?
4   How does psychological research get carried out?
5   What makes for good psychological research?

ADDITIONAL READING

King, L. (2008). *The science of psychology*. New York: McGraw-Hill..

Rieger, E. (Ed.) (2011). *Abnormal psychology: Leading researcher perspectives* (2nd ed.). Sydney: McGraw-Hill.

Stainton Rogers, W. (2011). *Social psychology: Experimental and critical approaches*. Maidenhead: Open University Press.

Weiten, W. (c2011). *Psychology: Themes and variations: Briefer version* (8th ed.). Belmont, CA: Wadsworth/Cengage Learning.

REFERENCES

American Psychiatric Association. (1980). *Diagnostic and statistical manual of mental disorders*, (3rd ed.). Washington, DC: Author.

Aronson, E., Wilson, T. D., & Akert, R. M. (2013). *Social psychology*. New Jersey: Pearson.

Bandura, A. (1977). *Social learning theory*. Englewood Cliffs, NJ: Prentice Hall.

Bandura, A., Ross, D., & Ross, S. A. (1961). Transmission of aggression through the imitation of aggressive models. *Journal of Abnormal and Social Psychology, 63*, 575–582.

Beres, M. A., & Farvid, P. (2010). Sexual ethics and young women's accounts of heterosexual casual sex. *Sexualities, 13*(3), 377–393.

Billington, R., Landon, J., Krägeloh, C. U., & Shepherd, D. (2010). The New Zealand WHOQOL Group. *New Zealand Medical Journal, 123*, 65–70.

Cooper, J. O., Heron, T. E., & Heward, W. L. (2006). *Applied behavior analysis* (2nd ed.). Upper Saddle River, NJ: Prentice-Hall.

Farvid, P. (2010). The benefits of ambiguity: Methodological insights from researching 'heterosexual casual sex' *Feminism & Psychology 20*(2): 232–237.

Farvid, P., & V. Braun (2006). "Most of us guys are raring to go anytime, anyplace, anywhere": Male and female sexuality in *Cleo* and *Cosmo*. *Sex Roles, 55*(5–6), 295–310.

Feng, J., Krägeloh, C., Billington, R., & Hsu, P. (2011). Selection of national items for the New Zealand World Health Organization Quality of Life Questionnaire: Preliminary analyses [working paper]. In R. Scherman & C. Krägeloh (Eds.), *Walking the talk: The 2011 collection of oral presentations from the AUT School of Public Health and Psychosocial Studies* (pp. 87–95). Auckland: Auckland University of Technology.

Ferster, C. B, & Skinner, B. F. (1957). *Schedules of reinforcement*. New York, NY: Appleton-Century-Crofts.

Gavey, N. (2005). *Just Sex? The cultural scaffolding of rape*. London: Routledge.

Gill, R. (1993). Justifying injustice: broadcasters' accounts of inequality in radio. In E. Burman, & I. Parker (Eds.), *Discourse analytic research: Repertoires and readings of texts in action* (pp. 75–93). London: Routledge.

Gough, B., & McFadden, M. (2001). *Critical social psychology: An introduction*. Houndmills: Palgrave.

Haney, C., Banks, W. C., & Zimbardo, P. G. (1973). Interpersonal dynamics in a simulated prison. *International Journal of Criminology and Penology, 1,* 69–97.

Krägeloh, C. U., Kersten, P., Billington, D. R., Hsu, P. H.-C., Shepherd, D., Landon, J., et al. (in press). Validation of the WHOQOL-BREF quality of life questionnaire for general use in New Zealand: Confirmatory factor analysis and Rasch analysis. *Quality of Life Research, 22*(6), 1451–1457.

Lesieur, H. R. (1998). Costs and treatment of pathological gambling. *The Annals of the American Academy of Political and Social Science, 556,* 153–171.

Parker, I. (2007). *Revolution in psychology: Alienation to emancipation*. London: Pluto Press.

Piaget, J. (1954). *The construction of reality in the child*. New York: Basic Books.

Milgram, S. (1974). *Obedience to authority: An experimental view*. New York: Harper & Row.

Skinner, B. F. (1953). *Science and Human Behavior*. New York: Free Press.

Wetherell, M., & Potter, J. (1992). *Mapping the language of racism*. Hemel Hempsted: Harvester.

WHOQOL Group. (1995). The World Health Organization Quality of Life assessment (WHOQOL): Position paper from the World Health Organization. *Social Science and Medicine, 41*(10), 1403–1409.

WHOQOL Group (1998). Development of the World Health Organization WHOQOL-BREF quality of life assessment. *Psychological Medicine, 28*(3), 551–558.

Willig, C. (2008). *Introducing qualitative research in psychology: Adventures in theory and method*. Berkshire: Open University Press.

Zimbardo, P. (2007). *The Lucifer effect: Understanding how good people turn evil*. New York: Random House.

WEBSITES

New Zealand Psychological Society:
   http://www.psychology.org.nz

Psychologist's Board:
   http://www.psychologistsboard.org.nz

British Psychological Society:
   http://www.bps.org.uk

American Psychological Association:
   http://www.apa.org

CHAPTER 26

PHYSIOTHERAPY

DUNCAN REID

CHAPTER OVERVIEW

This chapter covers the following topics:

- Historical overview of the development of research in physiotherapy
- Common research methodologies in physiotherapy
- Linking science with practice
- Future directions for research in physiotherapy

KEY TERMS

Case control trial

Clinical trial

Control

Positivist

Secondary sources

Systematic reviews

HISTORICAL OVERVIEW OF THE DEVELOPMENT OF RESEARCH IN PHYSIOTHERAPY

> Those of us who are charged with the care of the sick in whatever capacity have a duty and a responsibility to study and investigate all possible methods of treatment for the benefit of our patients. (Gandevia, 1958, p. 3)

In order to understand the development and importance of research in physiotherapy it is useful to reflect on how the profession developed and the historical influences on research.

Physiotherapy was established officially as a profession in the United Kingdom by three nurses and a midwife who formed the Society of Trained Masseurs (STM) in 1894 (Nicholls & Cheek, 2006). The formalisation of the profession of massage was seen by the medical profession at this time as a move to improve the quality of the training and reduce the use of unregulated massage provision, as well as improve the opportunities for women from middle and upper classes to work in valued occupations (Nicholls & Cheek, 2006). Once established as a legitimate profession, physiotherapy would need support from the medical profession to survive (Nicholls & Cheek, 2006). The relevance of this from a research perspective is that, since the inception of the profession, physiotherapy chose to accept the medical model as its base for knowledge and, in doing so, aligned itself with medicine (Miles-Tapping, 1985). This was initially a helpful move because of the social status that medicine had within society and because the profession had not been in existence long enough to develop its own knowledge base. Therefore, as research began to develop, it did so along a biomedical model.

Positivist
An approach that emphasises natural phenomena, objectivity and empirical scientific approaches to knowledge.

The biomedical model philosophically comes from the positivist social viewpoint. Disease was seen as a deviance from the normal social behaviour and the medical profession was seen as the group to control this deviance (Miles-Tapping, 1985). Doctors developed the skills to diagnose the sick and then had the technical skills to cure and return the sick to the work force. This in turn meant that the medical profession performed an important social function and gave medical practitioners high status within society. By aligning itself with a profession that held this high social status, physiotherapy was accorded some of this status and gained some legitimacy. Being subordinate to the medical profession meant that in the early days of the profession, physiotherapists were seen somewhat like technicians performing treatments under the direction and referral of the doctor (Miles-Tapping, 1985). Therefore, treatments were prescribed based on the medical world view and based on research undertaken within its paradigm.

However, over time physiotherapy did develop its own knowledge, and three important world events brought physiotherapy to the fore from a rehabilitation perspective: the two world wars in the first half of the twentieth century and the worldwide polio epidemic in the 1940s and 1950s. These major events created a need for a large number of people to require rehabilitation services, especially breathing exercises for those with damaged lungs and those post-surgery (Higgs, Smith, Webb, Skinner, & Croker, 2009). The use of breathing exercises postoperatively became the standard care between the 1940s and 1970s (Innocenti, 1995). With a greater amount of care being provided by physiotherapists, the need to evaluate the effectiveness of that care became apparent and, as medical research began to grow, by the 1990s research began to emerge questioning the value of commonly applied physiotherapy interventions (Higgs et al., 2009). Crosby (2000) has commented that as a profession grows and develops it needs to validate its own body of knowledge. The first archived clinical trial in physiotherapy was published in 1955 and since then the research base of physiotherapy has grown exponentially, in particular the number of randomised controlled trials (RCTs). In a review of the Physiotherapy Evidence Database (PEDro) undertaken by Moseley, Herbert, Sherrington and Maher (2002) it was found that there were 2,708 records of which 2,376 were RCTs and 332 were systematic reviews. By 2013 there were 23,000 randomised trials, systematic reviews and clinical practice guidelines in physiotherapy available on the website (http://www.pedro.org.au).

Physiotherapy education in New Zealand has been in existence for 100 years, with the first school of physiotherapy starting in Aotearoa New Zealand in 1913. New Zealand's progress has mirrored countries like Great Britain and Australia both in professional development and in research (Higgs et al., 2009). Early articles published in the *New Zealand Journal of Physiotherapy* (NZJP) were written by doctors covering the management of conditions that physiotherapists commonly treated, such as back pain and other musculoskeletal conditions (Morris, 1938). The first RCT published by a New Zealand physiotherapist in NZJP was written by Glendining (1979). This was a study investigating the effectiveness of two different doses of the drug fenoterol, used in the management of severe asthma.

Clinical trial
A formally structured approach to research which includes standards and processes for identifying the problem and investigating it.

Systematic review
A specific process for analysing similar studies for the purpose of informing practice and practitioners.

COMMON RESEARCH METHODOLOGIES IN PHYSIOTHERAPY

Physiotherapists in Aotearoa New Zealand engage in all levels and types of research. These range from questionnaire type surveys (Reid, Larmer, Robb, Hing, & McNair, 2002), single case studies (Laslett, 2009) and validation of outcome measures (McNair et al., 2007), through to randomised control trials (Reeve et al., 2010; Reid & McNair, 2011; Taylor et al., 2012), systematic reviews (McNair, Simmonds, Boocock, & Larmer, 2009; Viswanathan & Kidd, 2012) and guideline development (Accident Compensation Corporation, 2002, 2003; Accident Compensation and the New Zealand Guidelines Group, 2003). The details of what makes up quantitative or qualitative research are covered in other chapters, but the next section aims to provide an overview of some of the main types of research undertaken by New Zealand physiotherapists under the broad methodological headings.

QUANTITATIVE RESEARCH

In keeping with Sackett's (1998) definitions, evidence-based medicine has a hierarchy of evidence, with RTCs seen as the gold standard upon which clinical decisions could or should be made. The historical perspective above indicates that physiotherapists have sought to demonstrate their effectiveness in clinical areas via this model. Three examples of RCTs across the main discipline areas of musculoskeletal cardiothoracic and neurological physiotherapy are presented below.

Osteoarthritis (OA) is a common condition encountered by physiotherapists. Physical therapies are mentioned in a number of guidelines as effective in the management of OA (Birrell et al., 2008; Zhang et al., 2008). Stretching of arthritic joints is one potentially useful intervention applied in practice. Reid and McNair (2011) designed an RCT that compared six weeks of hamstring stretching on knee extension range of motion in a group of 20 people with osteoarthritis (OA) of the knee and another group of 19 without. The groups were randomised to four subgroups: those with OA that stretched and a **control** group with OA who did not, and two groups without OA (one group who stretched and a control group who did not). The stretching intervention was a 60-second hamstring stretch, repeated three times a day, five days a week for six weeks. The control groups undertook normal daily activities and did not stretch. After the six-week time frame there was no difference in the results between those with OA and those without, but the groups that stretched demonstrated a significant increase in knee extension range of motion, whereas the control groups did not. These results are useful in demonstrating that having OA is not a barrier to improving knee range of motion with a simple stretching intervention.

Physiotherapy interventions such as breathing exercises and a range of motion exercises to the shoulders and trunk region are routinely provided after chest surgeries such as thoracotomy, with the aim of preventing and treating postoperative pulmonary and musculoskeletal complications (Reeve, Denehy, & Stiller, 2007). The ability to test the effectiveness of such physiotherapy procedures was examined by Reeve et al., (2010). The primary aim of this study was to investigate if a targeted postoperative respiratory physiotherapy intervention decreased the incidence of postoperative pulmonary complications and length of stay for patients undergoing elective pulmonary resection via open thoracotomy. Seventy-six patients participated in a prospective, single-blind, randomised trial. Those in the treatment group received daily respiratory physiotherapy interventions until discharge. The control group participants received standard medical and nursing care involving a clinical pathway. The presence of postoperative pulmonary

Control
A research cohort not treated in an active way to provide a point of comparison

complications was assessed on a daily basis during hospitalisation as was length of stay. The results indicated no significant difference in the key outcomes for either group, with minimal postoperative complication being observed across the whole cohort. However, those patients with chronic lung conditions preoperatively had more complications postoperatively. The study demonstrates (with some caution) that targeted postoperative physiotherapy is not required following pulmonary resection.

Falls in the elderly are common, with a third to half of people over 65 years old falling each year (Campbell, Robertson, Gardner, Norton, & Buchner, 1997). Exercises to strengthen the lower limbs and improve balance may help to reduce the rate of falls in these populations. Some studies have shown that tai chi as a form of exercise is helpful in falls prevention (Logghe, Verhagen, & Rademaker, 2010), but is it superior to other forms of general exercise? Taylor et al., (2012) investigated the effectiveness of tai chi and low-level exercise in reducing falls in older adults to determine whether mobility, balance, and lower limb strength could also be improved with the programme. This RCT was a 20-week, community-based study involving 684 participants allocated to one of three groups: tai chi once a week ($n = 233$); tai chi twice a week ($n = 220$); or a low-level exercise program control group ($n = 231$). The number of falls per month was recorded, as were measures of mobility, balance and lower limb strength. The results of the study indicated no differences in the three groups, with all groups showing a reduction in falls and improvements in balance and strength over time. This study demonstrated that exercise, regardless of type, is important in reducing falls in elderly populations.

SYSTEMATIC REVIEWS

A systematic review is a very structured process that allows researchers and practitioners to analyse clinical trials (usually randomised) using a set of predetermined criteria and tools to assess the methodological quality of the reviewed studies. The review endeavours to see if there is consistency and consensus in the outcomes to guide best practice. For example, what does the current evidence say about the use of exercise therapy to manage those patients with OA of the hip?

A systematic review to answer this question was undertaken by McNair et al. (2009). Over 4,000 relevant articles were identified; however, only six studies that met the review criteria specifically examined the efficacy of exercise in the management of OA of the hip. The results found that, at that time, the studies were of such poor methodological quality that no conclusion could be drawn as to the most effective exercise to help patients with this problem. This seemingly negative result is common in systematic review, but provides opportunities for research to be designed with improved methodological quality in future.

QUALITATIVE RESEARCH

The categorisation of qualitative research design is shown in other chapters of this book to have a theoretical underpinning of a particular research question, such as examining the culture of a group of people (ethnography), investigating the 'lived' experience (phenomenology), and developing theories that are grounded in reality (grounded theory).

One such theory or methodology is discourse analysis. One philosopher who is known in this area is Foucault. Powers (1996) defined a discourse as a group of ideas or a pattern of thinking that can be identified in textual or verbal communication and can also be located in wider social structure. Foucaultian discourse analysis views discourses as relations of power and knowledge encoded in the social processes of language and action.

Nicholls and Cheek (2006) used a Foucaultian discourse analysis approach to examine the emergence of new forms of physiotherapy practice, in particular therapeutic massage. The purpose of a discourse analysis approach is to reveal the notions of power, in this case within the development of massage in the physiotherapy profession. The historical information on the emergence of massage in the physiotherapy profession was gathered via texts from a range of primary and secondary sources but mostly from archived materials in relevant libraries in the Chartered Society of Physiotherapy held in the Wellcome Institute Library, London. The data gathered were then critically analysed in the context of other political, social and historical writings of the time. The paper provides a critical reflection and analysis of factors that contributed to the implementation of massage as a legitimate therapy developed under the power of medicine and to the development of the physiotherapy profession through the instigation of the Society of Trained Masseurs (STM). This was the beginning of what is now known as the Chartered Society of Physiotherapy, the forerunner of other such physiotherapy associations and societies across the world. The qualitative research approach is well placed to analyse this text- or interview-driven data, and provides views and thoughts that cannot be captured in the qualitative methodology.

Secondary sources
References to publications or research that are found within another publication or source.

RESEARCH ALIVE 26.1
MIXED METHODS

One method of combining the best aspects of quantitative and qualitative research is to use a mixed methods approach (see Chapter 5 for more details). This methodology is not yet commonly used in physiotherapy, but a recent study by Larmer, McNair, Smythe and Williams (2011) used this approach to gain a greater understanding of the differences in perceived functional capabilities following an ankle sprain between patients and treating therapists. Forty patients who had suffered an acute ankle sprain participated in the study. Following discharge from treatment the treating therapist and the patient completed the same questionnaire assessing the perceived functional ability of the patient. A small number of patients were then interviewed about their perceptions of their function following discharge. The study found that the therapists rated the level of function higher than the patient did. The ability to then explore this difference in perception with a set of qualitative questions revealed that some patients were still fearful of doing difficult tasks but others actually could do more than they expected. These findings indicate that clinicians need to be aware that patients may have lower or different self-expectation of their level of ability following ankle rehabilitation at discharge than the treating professional judgment indicates. Having both quantitative and qualitative data to support these findings adds a further level of richness to the results and implications for practice.

LINKING SCIENCE WITH PRACTICE

Stretching of muscles is a common activity before and after sport, part of injury management and also injury prevention. Nearly everyone involved in sport will have undertaken a stretching procedure of some kind. But have you considered what type of stretch you should do, when you should do it, how often and how many times, and whether stretching has an influence on other movements? Stretching exercises are one of the most common types of exercises prescribed on a daily basis so these questions will be of interest to practising clinicians and health professional students.

CASE STUDY 26.1

LOW BACK PAIN

Low back pain is common in rowing (Reid & McNair, 2000). The position of the back at certain parts of the rowing stroke may be influenced by the flexibility of the hamstrings as they attach to the pelvis. Reducing the amount of flexion in the spine is considered helpful to reduce back pain. Tight hamstrings may increase the amount of flexion in the spine during the rowing stroke; therefore, reducing this tightness may be helpful to reduce low back pain. In order to

[continued next page]

DUNCAN REID

investigate if stretching the hamstrings would influence the pelvic position, a randomised control trial was undertaken with 43 school-age rowers (Reid, 2002). Rowers were randomised by school to a stretching group who did hamstring stretches and a control group who did not. The stretching intervention was a 30-second stretch to the hamstring muscles repeated three times, once per day for five days of the week over a six-week time frame. The movement of the pelvis during the rowing stroke was measured using the electronic goniometer. The results of the study indicated that those who stretched the hamstrings increased their knee extension range of motion by 10 degrees. Those who did not stretch showed no change in range of motion. The position of the pelvis was not altered by the stretching intervention. This finding is consistent with other research in the area (Stutchfield & Coleman, 2006). The relevance to clinical practice is that stretching to the hamstrings may not be required to influence the position of the pelvis in an attempt to reduce low back pain in rowers. The research did also indicate that the optimal level of hamstring stretching required to increase knee extension range of motion was per the prescription and also consistent with other research (Bandy & Irion, 1994; Bandy, Irion, & Briggler, 1997, 1998; Reid & McNair, 2004).

FUTURE DIRECTIONS FOR RESEARCH IN PHYSIOTHERAPY

Some researchers believe that the medically driven RCT model is the preferred methodology to continue to demonstrate the efficacy of physiotherapy interventions (Koes, 1997). Crosby (2000) also felt that the future of physiotherapy research would continue to be dominated in the near future by the use of the clinical trials (in particular, RCTs) to evaluate physiotherapy practice and that more physiotherapy higher degree theses will include RCTs, case control trials (CCTs) and systematic reviews.

Case control trial
A study design that compares two groups of similar people, where the members of one group have a condition that members of the other group do not.

There are others who feel that using only this model is not going to answer the questions that will be placed in front of the profession in the future. Bithell (2000) commented that, because of the reductionist concept of research derived from medicine and the physical sciences, this methodology is less appropriate than others for examining the array of factors that influence the outcomes of physiotherapy. Clinicians trying to implement findings from large group studies may well find that they do not apply to their patients. Therefore the future directions of physiotherapy research will be driven by a number of factors, including the types of questions to be asked and the best methodologies to answer them. A mixture of quantitative and qualitative research via such methodologies as mixed methods will provide a rich perspective of how best to provide evidence to support improved clinical outcomes in physiotherapy. However, it is clear from this chapter that the physiotherapy profession has already delivered a significant amount of high-quality research; it will continue to do so in future years.

SUMMARY

Physiotherapy research has grown from under the umbrella of medicine to be a legitimate profession and significant generator of research that justifies and challenges everyday practice and current knowledge. Physiotherapy has embraced all the established research methodologies and begun to work in emerging methods. Future research will be driven by clinicians and researchers challenging and questioning what is currently known as best practice and looking for improved ways to ensure patients get the most out of their physiotherapy experience. This will include robust randomised controlled trials, a greater emphasis on the qualitative experiences of the patients and new methodologies such as mixed methods.

REFLECTION POINTS

- Why do you think there is variation in clinical practice or outcomes from physiotherapy treatments?
- Does this variation challenge your current knowledge or thinking?
- How would you use current physiotherapy evidence to guide your clinical practice decisions?

STUDY QUESTIONS

1 Why has the randomised control trial been so often used in physiotherapy research?
2 Which sort of methodology is suited to your practice-based questions?
3 Which methodologies do you think will be more widely used in the future?

ADDITIONAL READING

Higgs, J., Smith, M., Webb, G., Skinner, M., & Croker, A. (Eds.). (2009). *Contexts of physiotherapy practice*. London: Churchill Livingstone Elsevier.

REFERENCES

Accident Compensation Corporation. (2002). *Managing soft tissue ankle injuries: a summary of recent research*. Retrieved from http://www.acc.co.nz/PRD_EXT_ CSMP/groups/external_providers/documents/internet/wcmz002487.pdf

Accident Compensation Corporation. (2003). *New Zealand Acute Low Back Pain Guide.* Wellington: Author.

Accident Compensation and the New Zealand Guidelines Group. (2003). *The diagnosis and management of soft tissue knee injuries: internal derangements best practice evidence based guidelines.* Wellington: Author.

Bandy, W., & Irion, J. (1994). The effect of time on static stretch on the flexibility of the hamstring muscles. *Physical Therapy, 74*(9), 845–850.

Bandy, W., Irion, J., & Briggler, M. (1997). The effect of time and frequency of static stretching on flexibility of the hamstring muscles. *Physical Therapy, 77*(10), 1090–1096.

Bandy, W., Irion, J., & Briggler, M. (1998). The effect of static stretch and dynamic range of motion training on the flexibility of the hamstring muscles. *Journal of Orthopaedic and Sports Physical Therapy, 27*(4), 295–300.

Birrell, F., Burke, M., Conaghan, P., Cumming, J., Dieppe, P., Dickson, J., et al. (2008). *Osteoarthritis. The care and management of osteoarthritis in adults.* London: National Institute for Health and Clinical Excellence (NICE). Retrieved from http://www.nice.org.uk

Bithell, C. (2000). Evidence-based physiotherapy: Some thoughts on 'best evidence'. *Physiotherapy, 86*(2), 58–60.

Campbell, A., Robertson, M., Gardner, M., Norton, R. N., & Buchner, D. (1997). Falls prevention over 2 years: a randomized controlled trial in women 80 years and older. *Age and Aging, 28*, 513–518.

Crosby, J. (2000). Physiotherapy research: A retrospective look at the future. *Australian Journal of Physiotherapy, 46*, 159–164.

Gandevia, B. (1958). The principles of clinical research. *New Zealand Journal of Physiotherapy, 2*(3), 3–14.

Glendining, S. (1979). The use of fenoterol (Berotec) respirator solution 0.5% in patients with severe asthma. *New Zealand Journal of Physiotherapy, 7*(2), 26–27.

Higgs, J., Smith, M., Webb, G., Skinner, M., & Croker, A. (Eds.). (2009). *Contexts of Physiotherapy practice.* Melbourne: Elsevier Australia.

Innocenti, D. (1995). An overview of the development of breathing exercises into the speciality of physiotherapy for heart and lung conditions. *Physiotherapy, 81*, 681–693.

Koes, B. (1997). Now is the time for evidence based physiotherapy [Editorial]. *Physiotherapy Research International, 2*(2), 4–5.

Larmer, P., McNair, P., Smythe, L., & Williams, M. (2011). Ankle sprains: patient perceptions of function and performance of physical tasks. A mixed methods approach. *Disability and Rehabilitation, 33*(23–24), 2299–2304.

Laslett, M. (2009). Manual correction of an acute lumbar lateral shift: maintenance of correction and rehabilitation; a case report. *Journal of Manual and Manipulative Therapy, 17*(2), 78–85.

Logghe, I., Verhagen, A., & Rademaker, A. (2010). The effects of tai chi on fall prevention, fear of falling and balance in older people: A meta-analysis. *Preventative Medicine, 51*, 222–227.

McNair, P., Prapavessis, H., Collier, J., Bassett, S., Bryant, A., & Larmer, P. (2007). The lower limb tasks questionnaire: an assessment of validity, reliability, responsiveness, and minimal important differences. *Archives of Physical Medicine and Rehabilitation, 88*(August), 993–1001.

McNair, P., Simmonds, M., Boocock, M., & Larmer, P. (2009). Exercise therapy for the management of osteoarthritis of the hip joint: a systematic review. *Arthritis Research and Therapy, 11*(3), 1–19.

Miles-Tapping, C. (1985). Physiotherapy and medicine: Dominance and control? *Physiotherapy Canada, 37*(5), 289–293.

Morris, S. (1938). Manipulation in the treatment of injuries. *New Zealand Journal of Physiotherapy*, (September), 10–12.

Moseley, A., Herbert, R., Sherrington, C., & Maher, C. (2002). Evidence for physiotherapy practice: A survey of the Physiotherapy Evidence Database (PEDro). *Australian Journal of Physiotherapy, 48*, 43–49.

Nicholls, D., & Cheek, J. (2006). Physiotherapy and the shadow of prostitution: The Society of Trained Masseurs and the massage scandals of 1894. *Social Science and Medicine, 62*, 2336–2348.

Powers, P. (1996). Discourse analysis as a methodology for nursing enquiry. *Nursing Inquiry, 3*, 207–217.

Reeve, J., Denehy, L., & Stiller, K. (2007). The physiotherapy management of patients undergoing thoracic surgery: a survey of current practice in Australia and New Zealand. *Physiotherapy Research International, 12*, 59–71.

Reeve, J., Nicol, K., Stiller, K., McPherson, K., Birch, P., Gordon, I., et al. (2010). Does physiotherapy reduce the incidence of postoperative pulmonary complications following pulmonary resection via open thoracotomy? A preliminary randomised single-blind clinical trial. *European Journal of Cardio-thoracic Surgery, 37*, 1158–1167.

Reid, D. (2002). *The influence of hamstring extensibility on lumbar and pelvic angles in rowers*. Auckland: AUT University.

Reid, D., Larmer, P., Robb, G., Hing, W., & McNair, P. (2002). The use of a vignette to investigate the physiotherapy treatment of an acute episode of low back pain: report of a survey of New Zealand Physiotherapists. *NZ Journal of Physiotherapy, 30*(2), 26–32.

Reid, D., & McNair, P. (2000). Factors contributing to low back pain in rowers. *British Journal of Sports Medicine, 34*, 321–325.

Reid, D., & McNair, P. (2004). Passive force, angle and stiffness changes after stretching of hamstring muscles. *Medicine and Science in Sports and Exercise., 36*(11), 1944–1948.

Reid, D., & McNair, P. (2011). Effects of a six week lower limb stretching programme on range of motion, peak passive torque and stiffness in people with and without osteoarthritis of the knee. *New Zealand Journal of Physiotherapy, 39*(1), 2–9.

Sackett, D. (1998). Evidence based medicine. *Spine, 23*(10), 1085–1086.

Stutchfield, B., & Coleman, S. (2006). The relationships between hamstring flexibility, lumbar flexion, and low back pain in rowers. *European Journal of Sport Science, 6*(4), 255–260.

Taylor, D., Hale, L., Schluter, P., Waters, D., Binns, E., McCraken, H., et al. (2012). Effectiveness of tai chi as a community-based falls prevention intervention: A randomized controlled trial. *Journal of American Geriatric Society, 60*, 841–848.

Viswanathan, P., & Kidd, M. (2012). Effect of continuous passive movement following total knee arthroplasty on knee range of motion and function: a systematic review. *New Zealand Journal of Physiotherapy, 38*(1), 14–22.

Zhang, W., Moskowitz, R., Abramson, S., Altman, R., Arden, N., & Bierma-Zeinstra, S. (2008). OARSI recommendations for the management of hip and knee osteoarthritis, Part II: OARSI evidence based, expert consensus guidelines. *Osteoarthritis and Cartilage, 16*, 137–162.

WEBSITES

Physiotherapy evidence database:
http://www.pedro.org.au

Physiotherapy New Zealand:
http://www.physiotherapy.org.nz

Journal of Physiotherapy:
http://www.elsevier.com/journals/journal-of-physiotherapy/1836-9553

Physical Therapy in Sport:
http://www.journals.elsevier.com/physical-therapy-in-sport

Australian Physiotherapy Association:
http://www.physiotherapy.asn.au

Accident Compensation Corporation (New Zealand):
http://www.acc.co.nz

Physical Therapy:
http://ptjournal.apta.org

Journal of Orthopaedic & Sports Physical Therapy:
http://www.jospt.org

CHAPTER 27

MEDICAL LABORATORY SCIENCE

COLLEEN HIGGINS, WEE-LEONG CHANG AND HOLLY PERRY

CHAPTER OVERVIEW

This chapter covers the following topics:

- Evidence-based practice for medical laboratory scientists
- What is personalised medicine?
- Pharmacogenetics and pharmacogenomics
- Understanding genetic variation
- Drug responsiveness
- Associating genotypes or haplotypes with disease and treatment responses
- Drug discovery
- Randomised controlled trials and medical laboratory science

KEY TERMS

Disease susceptibility

Drug responsiveness

Genotype

Haplotype

Personalised medicine

Pharmacogenetics

Pharmacogenomics

Medical laboratory scientists do not treat patients directly. However, the results that they produce are used every day in patient diagnosis. In the research context, being one step removed from the patient can make the research path as a medical laboratory scientist a little less clear than it is for health practitioners involved in direct patient contact. However, as part of the role, medical laboratory scientists have the opportunity to be involved with teams of health professionals in research which informs evidence-based medicine.

EVIDENCE-BASED PRACTICE FOR MEDICAL LABORATORY SCIENTISTS

One of the questions to ask of medical laboratory scientists is: 'Is the current test the best test for the patient?' Medical laboratory scientists are experiencing a period of rapid change as improvements in automation, imaging, molecular tools and information technology explode in number. As reviewed by Carbonnelle et al. (2011), identification of microorganisms causing disease is undergoing a radical technology change: from sugar fermentation testing to a method that measures the mass of individual molecules making up the sample as the basis of identification. In blood banking, molecular tools are becoming increasingly important to recognise new blood group antigens and match those of donors and patients (Reid, 2007). The molecular revolution is also leading to the ability to apply personalised medicine, whereby a patient's drug regimen is selected by whether or not they possess the gene that allows them to respond to that drug in the optimal way. Understanding genetic variation and how it influences disease susceptibility and drug responsiveness is further leading to the development of more sophisticated medicines. Some of the research that leads to these changes is discussed in the Case Study and Research Alive sections of this chapter. This research is invariably quantitative, and heavily dependent upon statistical analysis of data.

Personalised medicine Prevention, diagnosis and treatment of disease based on an individual's genetic profile.

Disease susceptibility The tendency or likelihood of acquiring a disease.

Drug responsiveness How a person responds to medication.

WHAT IS PERSONALISED MEDICINE?

For more than two millennia, clinical medicine has never wavered from its aspiration of being personalised. With the completion of the Human Genome Project (Venter et al., 2001), there has been a vast increase in the amount of information regarding genetic susceptibility to complex diseases and genetic variability in drug responses. Holistic analysis of human DNA, known as genomics, has become an integral part of modern drug development, and a large number of pharmaceutical companies are using this information to identify novel drug targets, to identify patient subpopulations that are likely to benefit from the therapy under development, or for other screening purposes (Xie & Frueh, 2005).

COLLEEN HIGGINS, WEE-LEONG CHANG AND HOLLY PERRY

The future of personalised medicine promises to offer the right treatment for the right patient at the right time. It is clear that much needs to be determined to fully understand how genetic background can influence susceptibility to disease and people's responses to treatment. While many genetic variants have been identified, making clinically relevant associations and the development of fast, accurate, sensitive and cheap diagnostic tools are enormous undertakings. Further, assessing the importance of these associations within different populations cannot be underestimated; several studies are being undertaken to establish which genetic variations occur at different frequencies between racial groups (for example, Wang et al., 2012). Understanding the role of genetic variation also has the potential to inform new drugs that target specific genotypes or haplotypes. The biggest challenge will likely be determining how environmental factors are involved.

Determining the relationships between people's genetic background, their likelihood of developing disease, their chances of responding to the available treatment and their environment—such as their age, gender, body mass, what they eat, what other drugs they are taking, how much they exercise and whether they smoke—presents a great, but exciting, challenge. While it is difficult to determine exactly how much influence any single risk factor has, it is possible to estimate the percentage of occurrence of a disease or trait that is due to genetic factors (heritability) and the percentage of occurrence of a disease or trait that is due to non-genetic factors like lifestyle and environment.

For example, it is estimated that genetic factors make up about 88% of the risk of developing type 1 diabetes, while the remaining 12% of the risk is due to non-genetic factors (such as virus exposure) (Atkinson & Eisenbarth, 2001). Personalised medicine must incorporate the knowledge of how genetic and non-genetic factors interact to perturb cellular regulatory networks, affecting cellular phenotypes, to determine a rationale for targeted prevention and treatment of disease (Schadt, Friend, & Shaywitz, 2009).

PHARMACOGENETICS AND PHARMACOGENOMICS

Pharmacogenetics
The study of variation between individuals within a single gene that causes different responses to drug treatment.

Pharmacogenomics
The study of how all the genes within the genome function and interact to bring about a drug response.

Pharmacogenetics is the study of variation between individuals within a single gene that causes different responses to drug treatments. With the sequencing of the human genome and the development of '-omics' disciplines of research, such as genomics and metabolomics, the term pharmacogenomics has begun to be used to describe how all the genes within the genome function and interact to bring about a drug response. The aetiology of many diseases, including common diseases such as diabetes, heart disease and cancer, is known to involve many genes and environmental factors. Genetic variation can give rise to an altered risk of developing a disease, it may cause a disease or it may influence how a patient responds to drug treatment. For example, the current model for drug development and treatment is 'one size fits all'. Clinical trials establish the average reaction to a particular drug when used against a specific disease. The problem with this approach is that not everyone responds in the same way. The role a person's genetics plays is not well understood for the majority of diseases. In order for patients to receive the best clinical outcome, it is important to understand what genetic variation is associated with particular diseases, the individual's risk of developing disease based on their genetic background, and then how they would respond to the available treatment. The fields of pharmacogenetics and pharmacogenomics are helping us to determine each of these more accurately. This will inevitably lead to more accurate and sensitive diagnostic tools, providing greater efficiency for the health sector and better outcomes for the patient.

UNDERSTANDING GENETIC VARIATION

Each person has two copies of the 22 autosomes plus two sex chromosomes. Chromosomes are made up of two strands of deoxyribonucleic acid (DNA) wound around each other; these strands are, in turn, made up of four different nucleotides (A, C, G and T) joined together (Watson & Crick, 1953; Klug, Cummings, Spencer, & Palladino, 2012). In the human genome there are 3 billion nucleotides and, while the order (or sequence) of the nucleotides in each chromosome has been determined (International Human Genome Sequencing Consortium, 2001), understanding the full extent of genetic variation between individuals (up to 0.1 per cent between unrelated individuals), and the impact of this variation, are being elucidated.

About 10 million common DNA variants have been reported through sequencing the human genome (International Human Genome Sequencing Consortium, 2001) and variant analysis (International SNP Map Working Group, 2001; International HapMap 3 Consortium, 2010). The majority of these variants are alterations of single nucleotides, called single nucleotide polymorphisms (SNPs), while other types of variation such as copy number variants (CNVs) due to loss or duplication of chromosomal DNA (Figure 27.1) also occur. The specific pattern of genetic variation is unique to each individual; no two people will have exactly the same combination of SNPs and CNVs unless they are identical twins. Which particular SNP or CNV is present in a person's genome is called their genotype, while the combination of SNPs and/or CNVs at different sites is their haplotype.

While there is not yet a cure for sickle cell anaemia, knowing that an individual has the genetic background to develop this condition, and possibly the background for a particular pathology, allows a life-long health management plan to be put in place. Genotyping is one of the diagnostic tools for sickle cell available to the health-care team, in addition to haemoglobin electrophoresis and high performance liquid chromotography. The 'best test' or best array of tests may vary in different settings, depending on such factors as availability of funding. Hospitals may use algorithms, taking into account their organisational setting, to determine the range of tests to use in diagnosis.

Genotype
The genetic make-up of an organism or cell; also refers to the specific set of alleles inherited for one gene.

Haplotype
A set of alleles (one of the possible alternative forms of a gene) from genes that are closely linked on a chromosome and inherited together.

FIGURE 27.1   NORMAL CHROMOSOME PAIRS, SINGLE NUCLEOTIDE
POLYMORPHISMS AND COPY NUMBER VARIANTS, COMPARED

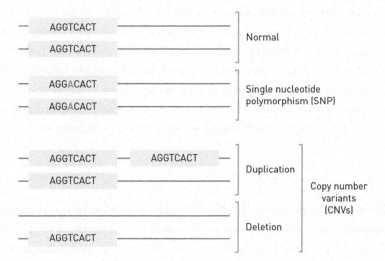

Each person has two copies of every chromosome (shown as grey lines), and each chromosome has the same or very similar DNA sequences, as shown for the normal chromosome pair. In some individuals, nucleotides might vary from the most common nucleotide in the population; these are called single nucleotide polymorphisms (SNPs). There may also be regions of a chromosome that have been duplicated, or deleted. These types of mutations are called copy number variants (CNVs).

CASE STUDY 27.1

DISEASE SUSCEPTIBILITY: SICKLE CELL ANAEMIA

The first disease-associated SNP described is that of sickle cell anaemia (Ingram, 1956). Red blood cells (RBCs) carry a protein called haemoglobin, which transports oxygen from the lungs to the rest of the body. This protein is made up of four subunits: two each of the alpha-globin and beta-globin. Patients with sickle cell anaemia make an atypical beta-globin protein, leading to the formation of haemoglobin S (HbS). A mutation in both copies of the beta-globin gene at nucleotide position 20 causes the 6th amino acid of the protein to change from a hydrophilic glutamate to a hydrophobic valine (Figure 27.2), creating a hydrophobic patch on the protein. Under low oxygen conditions as found in tissues, the hydrophobic patches of different HbS molecules join together forming a rod, which causes the distortion of the RBCs into the sickle shape. When the RBCs return to the oxygen–rich environment of the lungs, the HbS proteins fall apart and the RBCs return to their normal shape. This alternating rod formation and release causes RBCs to become less flexible, which has longer term affects for circulation, causing blockages and potentially secondary pathophysiological events such as stroke or heart attack.

FIGURE 27.2   THE NUCLEOTIDES SEQUENCES FOR NORMAL
HAEMOGLOBIN AND MUTATED HAEMOGLOBIN IN SICKLE
CELL ANAEMIA, COMPARED

Sequence for normal haemoglobin:
GTG CAC CTG ACT CCT GAG GAG AAG TCT   nucleotide
Val His Leu Thr Pro Glu Glu Lys Ser   amino acid

Sequence for mutated haemoglobin, HbS:
GTG CAC CTG ACT CCT GTG GAG AAG TCT   nucleotide
Val His Leu Thr Pro Val Glu Lys Ser   amino acid

The first 27 nucleotides of the healthy haemoglobin gene and the mutated HbS gene are shown, with the amino acid (protein) sequences they encode underneath. The 17th nucleotide is mutated from an adenine nucleotide to a thymine, creating the HbS version of the gene. This change causes the 6th amino acid of the protein to change from glutamate to valine.

Current laboratory diagnosis includes review of the peripheral blood smear, followed by haemoglobin electrophoresis and confirmatory diagnosis with high performance liquid chromotography. In patients where a rapid diagnosis is required, the sickle solubility test can be done (Wethers, 2000a).

While there are many disease features that are commonly experienced by sickle cell anaemia patients, there are many that can vary from patient to patient. In general, one gene affects a single trait, but many individual genes are known to affect many traits; that is, they are pleiotropic. Sickle cell anaemia is a pleiotropic trait; the HbS gene affects not just the haemoglobin molecule, but also multiple organs. Further, all patients have the same mutation but there are individual differences in the severity of the condition and how the condition progresses. Understanding the genetic basis for these differences is an important area of research. For example, Darbari et al. (2008) showed that an SNP at position -840 within the control region of the UDP-glucuronosyltransferase 2B7 (UGT2B7) gene (changing the nucleotide from a G to an A) affects how efficiently the liver can clear the analgesic morphine. This study, together with many others, suggests that pain management for sickle cell anaemia could be more personalised. Other studies are also highlighting roles for SNPs in the development of other pathologies of the disease (Fertrin & Costa, 2010).

DRUG RESPONSIVENESS

Drug responsiveness is probably controlled by many genes, and possibly by particular variants of those genes. The challenge now is to determine which SNP or CNV genotypes or haplotypes are associated with responsiveness to treatment (positive, negative or no response).With this information, doctors will be able to predict how a patient may respond to the available treatment regimens.

ASSOCIATING GENOTYPES OR HAPLOTYPES WITH DISEASE AND TREATMENT RESPONSES

Associations between SNPs or CNVs and disease risk and treatment responsiveness must be determined experimentally. Generally the genetic variation of a group of diseased individuals will be compared to that of a group of healthy individuals (controls) for a large number of SNPs or CNVs. If drug responsiveness is the focus, responders would be compared to non-responders. To date, genome-wide association studies using microarray analysis has been effective for carrying out such comparisons. Variants of clinical interest have been identified using microarrays carrying millions of SNPs (Hindorff, et al., n.d.) and massively parallel sequencing techniques such as Illumina˚ sequencing will be used increasingly to confirm disease associations between the genome region of interest in a large number of people. For CNVs, cytogenetic techniques such as fluorescent in situ hybridisation, comparative genomic hybridisation, array comparative genomic hybridisation and massively parallel sequencing have assisted discovery (see Redon et al., 2006; Korbel et al., 2007; Wellcome Trust Case Control Consortium, 2010).

CASE STUDY 27.2

HERCEPTIN

It has become increasingly apparent that breast cancer is a heterogeneous disease. Laboratory diagnosis of breast cancer in most hospitals has traditionally been performed using cell culture and the direct hormone receptor assay, which are expensive and time-consuming. However, some breast cancers have a lot more human epidermal growth factor receptor 2 (HER2) protein on their surface, causing cells to grow and divide abnormally. This was found to be due to a CNV where the number of HER2 encoding genes was increased three- to 22-fold (Seshadri, Matthews, Dobrovic, & Horsfall, 1989; Paterson et al., 1991). Patients with high levels of HER2 can be treated with drugs that specifically target the receptor protein, such as lapatinib (Tykerb®) and trastuzumab (Herceptin®) (Figure 27.3). However, about two-thirds of HER2-positive patients do not respond to this treatment, suggesting other factors are involved. Studies are looking at potential roles for other genetic variation (e.g. Minuti et al., 2012).

FIGURE 27.3   HOW HERCEPTIN WORKS

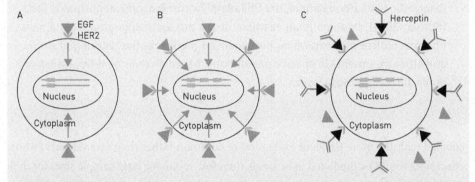

In healthy cells (A), the HER2 protein is expressed and binds epidermal growth factor (EGF), which in turn sends signals to genes in the nucleus to cause growth. In cells where the HER2 gene has been amplified (B), there is an overproduction of the HER2 protein, leading to more EGF being bound. The signals that cause growth are also amplified, leading to tumour development. Herceptin binds to HER2 in place of EGF (C), so that EGF can no longer affect the cells.

DRUG DISCOVERY

Understanding the impact of genetic variation will also lead to more intelligent drug design. The adoption of a personalised medicine strategy in drug discovery and development necessitates a paradigm shift from a linear process to an integrated and heuristic one. This new approach involves a series of research feedback loops where early stages of discovery, including selection and validation of drug targets, small-molecule screening and chemistry, and preclinical assessment of compounds will be linked with later stages of clinical development (Ginsburg & McCarthy, 2001). Molecular, pharmacological and patient clinical data will be captured at various phases and integrated in a 'knowledge management system' that will be used to facilitate rational drug design around molecular diseases (Ginsburg & McCarthy, 2001).

The major goal of pharmacogenetic research is development of genotype-based predictive tests of efficacy or toxicity. Despite some high-quality studies, in broad terms there are several features of the field as a whole that suggest that only a proportion of the positive associations reported are genuine. These include the small size of most studies

RESEARCH ALIVE 27.1
EXAMPLES OF PERSONALISED MEDICINE

One of the most innovative medications of recent years is imatinib (Kumar, 2011; Wethers, 2000b). Imatinib was the first of a new class of drugs that act by inhibiting a specific enzyme—in this case, a receptor called tyrosine kinase—that is characteristic of particular cancer cells. Because only certain cancers will respond to imatinib, it is prescribed only for patients identified by specific diagnostic tests (for example, the Philadelphia chromosome abnormality test) (Kumar, 2011). Imatinib is an example of the products emerging from a new pharmaceutical field known as personalised medicine: the tailoring of drugs and other treatments to specific populations, based on their genetic profiles or other differentiating factors.

coupled with the more frequent evaluation of common rather than rare variants (whose effect sizes would be predicted to be small, therefore requiring large sample sizes for their reliable detection); use of surrogate (usually continuous) outcome measures rather than more clinically relevant binary outcomes; and subgroup analyses with multiple hypothesis testing (Holmes et al., 2009). As more reliable information begins to emerge on genes influencing drug response from larger, better-designed whole genome and candidate gene studies, the focus will need to shift to the critical evaluation of the predictive performance of genetic tests in clinical practice, including studies of cost-effectiveness. To achieve a successful plan for personalised medicine, three elements of current research must be taken into account: (1) the prospects for innovation; (2) the right value proposition; and (3) the capabilities needed to deliver on that proposition (Wethers, 2000b). These will allow the combination of processes, technologies, knowledge, skills and organisation to develop over time to enhance the proficiency of personalised medicine.

RANDOMISED CONTROLLED TRIALS AND MEDICAL LABORATORY SCIENCE

Randomised controlled trials (RCTs) may be regarded as one gold standard for deciding whether or not to instigate new medicines or treatment regimens. Blood is governed by the *Medicines Act 1994* (NZ) and therefore it is reasonable to expect RCTs may be performed before transfusion is applied to particular medical conditions. However, unlike many medicines, blood is a human biological fluid and there are many known risks associated with blood transfusion. These include not only viral transmission risks (for example, hepatitis B) but also complications such as transfusion-related acute lung injury, transfusion-associated cardiac overload, alloimmunisation (the production of antibodies against red cell antigens) and sepsis from infected units, to name only a few. Therefore it is difficult to meet the strict conditions of an RCT when considering blood transfusion because it is unethical to randomly allocate individuals to an arm of the trial when, for instance, they may be more susceptible than usual to one or more of the complications of blood transfusion, or the study necessitates that transfusion to an individual in whom evidence-based criteria support the decision to transfuse (Vamvakas, 2012) is withheld. In transfusion research, it is more common to passively study individuals who have been transfused or not transfused, and compare the incidence of a variable of interest in these two groups. These observational cohort studies can be performed either prospectively or retrospectively (Vamvakas, 2001). Students are referred to two excellent books by Vamvakas (2001, 2012) for further discussion of these concepts.

SUMMARY

Medical laboratory scientists can and do practice from an evidence base. They are facing challenges due to rapid change in their practice, and it is important that they take the right direction when making choices about tests in the laboratory, informed by an evidence base. Although the promise of personalised medicine might seem far off, there is clear evidence that the traditional trial-and-error practice of medicine is eroding in favour of more precise marker-assisted diagnosis and treatment. For the patient, the benefits are clear: safer and more effective treatment of disease. For industry there appears an equally desirable outcome of this approach; increased efficiency, productivity and better product lines. The realisation of personalised medicine is not without challenges, yet many of these challenges are being addressed.

REFLECTION POINTS

- Why do you think research is necessary to inform medical laboratory science practice?
- Should a person's genome be sequenced at birth? Think about the ethical implications of this question and your answer.

STUDY QUESTIONS

1   Describe the terms 'pharmacogenetics' and 'pharmacogenomics'.
2   Compare and contrast genotyping and haplotyping, using examples from the literature.
3   Design a testing algorithm to associate a genotype with drug responsiveness.
4   Find further examples of haplotypes and/or genotypes associated with disease association risk, drug responsiveness, drug development and/or development of diagnostic tools.

ADDITIONAL READING

Klug, W. S., Cummings, M. R., Spencer, C. A., & Palladino, M. A. (2012). *Concepts of genetics* (10th ed.). San Francisco, CA: Pearson Education Inc.

REFERENCES

Atkinson, M. A., & Eisenbarth, G. S. (2001). Type 1 diabetes: new perspectives on disease pathogenesis and treatment. *The Lancet, 358*(9277), 221–229.

Carbonnelle, E., Mesquita, C., Bille, E., Day, N., Dauphin, B., Beretti. J., et al. (2011). MALDI-TOF mass spectrometry tools for bacterial identification in clinical microbiology laboratory. *Clinical Biochemistry, 44*, 104–109.

Darbari, D. S., van Schaik, R. H. N., Capparelli, E. V., Rana, S., McCarter, R., & van den Anker, J. (2008). UGT2B7 promoter variant -840G>A contributes to the variability in hepatic clearance of morphine in patients with sickle cell disease. *American Journal of Hematology, 83*, 200–202.

Fertrin, K. Y., & Costa, F. F. (2010). Genomic polymorphisms in sickle cell disease: implications for clinical diversity and treatment. *Expert Reviews in Hematology, 3*(4), 443–458.

Ginsburg, G. S., & McCarthy, J. J. (2001). Personalized medicine: revolutionizing drug discovery and patient care. *Trends in Biotechnology, 19*(12), 491–496.

Hindorff, L. A., MacArthur, J., Morales, J., Junkins, H. A., Hall, P. N., Klemm, A. K., et al. (n.d.). *A catalog of published genome-wide association studies*. Retrieved February 22, 2013, from http://www.genome.gov/gwastudies.

Holmes, M. V., Shah, T., Vickery, C., Smeeth, L., Hingorani, A. D., & Casas, J. P. (2009). Fulfilling the promise of personalized medicine? Systematic review and field synopsis of pharmacogenetic studies. *PloS ONE, 4*(12), e7960.

Ingram, V. M. (1956). A specific chemical difference between the globins of normal human and sickle-cell anaemia haemoglobin. *Nature, 178*(4537), 792–794.

International HapMap 3 Consortium. (2010). Integrating common and rare genetic variation in diverse human populations. *Nature, 467*, 52–58.

International Human Genome Sequencing Consortium. (2001). Initial sequencing and analysis of the human genome. *Nature, 409*, 860–921.

International Human Genome Sequencing Consortium. (2004) Finishing the euchromatic sequence of the human genome. *Nature, 431*, 931–945.

International SNP Map Working Group. (2001). A map of human genome sequence variation containing 1.42 million single nucleotide polymorphisms. *Nature, 409*, 928–933.

Klug, W. S., Cummings, M. R., Spencer, C. A., & Palladino, M. A. (2012) Concepts of genetics (pp. 238–314). San Francisco, CA: Pearson Education Inc.

Korbel, J. O., Urban, A. E., Affourtit, J. P., Godwin, B., Grubert, F., Simons, J. F., et al. (2007). Paired-end mapping reveals extensive structural variation in the human genome. *Science, 318*(5849), 420–426.

Kumar, D. (2011). The personalised medicine. A paradigm of evidence-based medicine [Review]. *Annali dell'Istituto Superiore di Sanita, 47*(1), 31–40.

Minuti, G., Cappuzzo, F., Duchnowska, R., Jassem, J., Fabi, A., O'Brien, T., et al. (2012). Increased MET and HGF gene copy numbers are associated with trastuzumab failure in HER2-positive metastatic breast cancer. *British Journal of Cancer, 107*(5), 793–799.

Paterson, M. C., Dietrich, K. D., Danyluk, J., Paterson, A. H. G., Lees, A. W., Jamil, N., et al. (1991). Correlation between c-erbB-2 amplification and risk of recurrent disease in node-negative breast cancer. *Cancer Research, 51*(2), 556–567.

Redon, R., Ishikawa, S., Fitch, K. R., Feuk, L., Perry, G. H., Andrews, T. D., et al. (2006). Global variation in copy number in the human genome. *Nature, 444*(7118), 444–454.

Reid, M.E. (2007). Overview of molecular methods in immunohematology. *Transfusion, 47*, 10S–16S.

Schadt, E. E., Friend, S. H., & Shaywitz, D. A. (2009). A network view of disease and compound screening. *Nature reviews. Drug discovery, 8*(4), 286–295.

Seshadri, R., Matthews, C., Dobrovic, A., & Horsfall, D. J. (1989). The significance of oncogene amplification in primary breast cancer. *International Journal of Cancer, 43*(2), 270–272.

Vamvakas, E. C. (2001). *Evidence based practice of transfusion medicine*. Bethesda, MA: AABB Press.

Vamvakas, E. C. (2012). *Decision making in transfusion medicine*. Bethesda, MA: AABB Press.

Venter, J. C., Adams, M. D., Myers, E. W., Li, P. W., Mural, R. J., Sutton, G. G., et al. (2001). The sequence of the human genome. *Science, 291*(5507), 1304–1351.

Wang, C., Wang, B., He, H., Li, X., Wei, D., Zhang, J., et al. (2012). Association between insulin receptor gene polymorphism and the metabolic syndrome in Han and Yi Chinese. *Asia Pacific Journal of Clinical Nutrition, 21*, 457–463.

Watson, J. D., & Crick, F. H. C. (1953). Molecular structure of nucleic acids. A structure for deoxyribose nucleic acid. *Nature, 171*(4356), 737–738.

Wellcome Trust Case Control Consortium. (2010). Genome-wide association study of CNVs in 16,000 cases of eight common diseases and 3,000 shared controls. *Nature, 464*(7289), 713–720.

Wethers, D. L. (2000a). Sickle cell disease in childhood: Part I. Laboratory diagnosis, pathophysiology and health maintenance. *American Family Physician, 62*(5), 1013–1020, 1027–1018.

Wethers, D. L. (2000b). Sickle cell disease in childhood: Part II. Diagnosis and treatment of major complications and recent advances in treatment [Review]. *American Family Physician, 62*(6), 1309–1314.

Xie, H.-G., & Frueh, F. W. (2005). Pharmacogenomics steps toward personalized medicine. *Personalized Medicine, 2*(4), 325–337.

WEBSITES

Genetics Home Reference:
ghr.nlm.nih.gov

Genetic variation databases:
http://www.humgen.nl/SNP_databases.html

International HapMap Project:
http://hapmap.ncbi.nlm.nih.gov

Molecular databases:
http://www.ncbi.nlm.nih.gov
http://genome.ucsc.edu

Online Mendelian Inheritance in Man:
http://omim.org

SNP database:
http://www.ncbi.nlm.nih.gov/books/NBK21088
http://www.ncbi.nlm.nih.gov/snp

The Human Genome Project:
http://www.ornl.gov/sci/techresources/Human_Genome/home.shtml
http://www.genome.gov/10001772

CHAPTER 28

HEALTH PROMOTION

HEATHER CAME AND JOANNE RAMSBOTHAM

CHAPTER OVERVIEW

This chapter covers the following topics:

- What is health promotion?
- Research and health promotion practice
- Planning and evaluation as the cornerstones of evidence

KEY TERMS

Contested	Tapu
Determinants	Tikanga
Equity	Tinana
Hauora	Te Tiriti o Waitangi
Hinengaro	Treaty of Waitangi
Kaupapa Māori	Wairua
Noa	

Determinants
Factors that lead to a
particular outcome.

Enjoyment of the highest available standard of health can be considered a fundamental human right. Health promotion is a broad-based discipline that encompasses a range of ways of working with communities to increase control over the determinants of health. This practice is underpinned by the principle that preventing disease and maintaining well-being is more effective than treating disease. The link between social determinants of health (e.g. socio-economic level, maternal education) and people's health outcomes is now well understood, as is the need to engage with people and communities in meaningful ways that recognise and respect both culture and the perspectives of individuals and groups within their own contexts.

Communities are groupings of people based on various similarities such as geography, age, sexuality, faith or ethnicity. No two communities are identical, so one of the core challenges of evidence-based health promotion is navigating the reality that what works for one community may not work for another. Research and evidence in the context of health promotion practice often have to be fine-tuned locally to accommodate the dynamics of particular cultural, political, social and environmental settings.

WHAT IS HEALTH PROMOTION?

Contested
Open to debate.

As a non-regulated profession, the boundaries of health promotion practice are contested and evolving. Raeburn and Rootman (1998) argue that the art and science of health promotion is the people-centred process of developing programmes with communities. Health promotion work requires imagination, creativity and 'street smarts' moderated by a commitment to rigour in both planning and evaluation. This work is often driven by a desire to 'make a difference' in the communities with whom health promotion practitioners work and live.

Equity
Equal rights for all
people in any situation.

In a global world, weighed down with health inequities and systemic discrimination, health promotion is grounded in values of social justice and a commitment to enhancing equity between groups of people. Empowerment is a key feature of health promotion practice wherein practitioners work with communities to increase control over the determinants of health (Laverack, 2004; Rissel, 1994). Advocacy, according to Carlisle (2000), is also a core competency for health promoters as they actively work to influence decision-makers to create policies and social and built environments that enhance well-being. Practice ethics (see Health Promotion Forum, 2011; Public Health Association, 2007) often lead practitioners to work with the most vulnerable, to ensure equitable access to what is described in the Ottawa Charter for Health Promotion (World Health Organization, 1986) as the prerequisites of health.

Health promotion transcends individual-based biomedical Western understandings of health and well-being. It is strongly influenced by indigenous understandings of the holistic nature of health and it embraces the World Health Organization's (1948) definition of health as a (collective) resource for everyday living. Within the context of Aotearoa, Durie's (1994) Te Whare Tapa Whā model, which includes the elements of taha wairua (spirituality) taha whānau (extended family), taha tinana (physical health), and taha hinengaro (mental/emotional health), is widely used. Health promoters are practitioners who contribute to the wider well-being of communities by engaging with them about their experiences and issues. This requires a range of expertise including that required to achieve objective (biomedical) health outcomes; it also involves wrestling with measuring concepts such as quality of life, social capital and community resilience (Cattan & Tilford, 2006).

Wairua
Spiritual well-being.

Tinana
Physical well-being.

Hinengaro
Mental well-being.

Within Aotearoa New Zealand health promotion practice is embedded in a practical understanding of the importance of Te Tiriti o Waitangi (the Treaty of Waitangi) as the founding document of New Zealand (Health Promotion Forum, 2011). Te Tiriti o Waitangi both reaffirms Māori sovereignty and critically establishes the terms of non-Māori settlement (Huygens, Murphy, & Healy, 2012). Aligned to the obligations of this covenant, the Health Promotion Forum (2000) advocates that practitioners apply Te Tiriti provisions of kāwantanga (governance), tino rangatiratanga (sovereignty) and ōritetanga (equity) within their practice to positively contribute to the achievement of Māori aspirations and the reduction in health inequities. Addressing indigenous health remains a global priority for health promotion (Gracey & King, 2009; King, Smith, & Gracey, 2009).

Te Tiriti o Waitangi and Treaty of Waitangi
The founding document of Aotearoa New Zealand signed between indigenous Māori and the British Crown in 1840.

Health promotion is therefore a complex, evolving and value-driven profession working with communities to increase the control over the determinants of health. Case Study 28.1 reflects how research evidence is used in health promotion practice.

CASE STUDY 28.1

TE TAI TOKERAU STRATEGIC PUBLIC HEALTH PLAN

The health promotion sector in Te Tai Tokerau (Northland) is similar to other rural provinces in Aotearoa New Zealand. There is a collection of Māori health providers, a local public health unit based at the District Health Board (DHB), Primary Healthcare Organisations and national Non-Governmental Organisations, all funded to deliver health promotion in the region. Health funders purchase a range of health promotion programmes aimed at addressing alcohol related harm, tobacco control, immunisation promotion, sexual and reproductive health, suicide prevention and core health protection services amongst others (Ministry of Health, n.d.).

[continued next page]

HEATHER CAME AND JOANNE RAMSBOTHAM

Te Tai Tokerau has a high Māori population and a strong interest in preserving the mana (esteem) of Te Tiriti o Waitangi and experiences high levels of deprivation (Ministry of Social Development, 2010; Te Rōpū Kai Hapai o Hauora o Te Tai Tokerau, 2008). In 2008 the Northland DHB and Te Tai Tokerau MAPO (Māori Co-Purchasing Organisation) Trust were commissioned to develop a strategic plan to strengthen the public health sector, and enable a more strategic approach to funding and service delivery.

The MAPO team approached this task from a kaupapa Māori paradigm and entered into a process of whanaungatanga (relationship building). A series of focus groups with open-ended questions were hosted by Māori providers supplemented by in-depth interviews with key Māori leaders from within and outside the health sector. Data analysis, framed around Durie's (1999) Te Pae Mahutonga, was informed by a review of published Māori health literature and document review of local evaluation and needs assessment reports. The team maintained dialogue with Māori public health leaders to ensure planning was aligned to Māori aspirations.

The DHB team, coming from a Western paradigm, undertook traditional epidemiological analysis of the patterns of morbidity and mortality across the populations of Northland, informed by central government data. A document review of existing public health contracts was undertaken to map gaps in service delivery. Strong emphasis was placed on developing an intersectoral approach to addressing health inequities within Northland.

The final plan, established after an intensive negotiation process of 25 iterations mediated through input from a representative advisory group, initiated a unique inclusive approach to public health research and planning. The Te Tai Tokerau approach is framed around Te Pae Mahutonga and incorporates kaupapa Māori understandings of hauora (health), traditional epidemiological analysis and reflects community aspirations in relation to health promotion priorities. This plan is an exemplar of the opportunities in utilising inclusive evidence to inform planning and practice.

Kaupapa Māori
Philosophy or agenda of the Māori community.

Hauora
Philosophy of health.

RESEARCH AND HEALTH PROMOTION PRACTICE

Kipuri (2009) argues that indigenous communities hold vast traditional knowledge, know-how and practices drawn from a wealth of experience transmitted orally from one generation to another. This collective knowledge forms the basis of traditional indigenous health systems worldwide. From a Western perspective, knowledge has usually been transmitted through the written word. Indigenous and Western forms of knowledge or evidence come from profoundly different ontological bases reflecting distinct understandings of the world.

Sir Mason Durie (1994) argues that traditional Māori public health was grounded in collective whānau lifestyles and intimate spiritual and practical connections with the natural environment. The application of tikanga was used to minimise disease and injury. Codes of behaviour governed by tapu, noa and rāhui (restrictions) were used to ensure survival, by protecting water supplies, food sources and the safety of whānau. This mātauranga (traditional knowledge) forms some of the evidence base for Māori health promotion practice (Durie, 2004).

Tikanga
Māori way of doing things; Māori protocol.

Tapu
A restricted or protected state, to be treated with the appropriate respect to ensure people are safe.

Noa
Normal (not sacred).

CASE STUDY 28.2

AUSTRALIAN INDIGENOUS PERSPECTIVES ON ACTIVE LIVING AND HEALTH

Concepts of health and wellness are often constructed and investigated in terms of particular cultural and scientific perspectives. It is important to ensure that any analyses of well-being are linked to the real and lived experiences of the communities being considered or served. Levels of physical activity have been linked to health outcomes and the risk of chronic disease. Increasing physical activity has also been demonstrated to improve the health of those with existing chronic disease. The burden of chronic disease in indigenous Australia is more than double that of non-indigenous Australians, and in remote rural locations such as the Northern Territory rates of chronic disease among indigenous people are even higher (Zhao, Conners, Wright, & Guthridge, 2008).

Thompson, Chenhall and Brimblecombe (2013) identified that there were few previous health promotion initiatives in remote communities targeting physical activity. They also found that cultural perspectives around this topic required exploration before health promotion activities that sought to improve chronic disease and health could be planned. They used a partnership approach with the community to investigate remote indigenous community members' perspectives on relationships between physical activity and health. Their conclusion was that in this remote setting, physical activity is about engagement with the natural environment and being 'on country' (traditional land). This is a different social concept to the Western-based understanding of physical activity as deliberate exertion as part of daily pursuits. Health promotion activities

[continued next page]

HEATHER CAME AND JOANNE RAMSBOTHAM

would need to recognise and be sensitive to these different perspectives to have any positive impact. This study highlights the value of partnership and community engagement in the health promotion research context.

There have been many waves of health promotion knowledge development. Since the 1950s, the International Union for Health Promotion and Education (IUHPE) has kept abreast of developments in the field and has acted as both a peak global agency and research clearinghouse for the sector (International Union of Health Promotion and Education, n.d). Over decades, the IUHPE has published reports and journals benchmarking the effectiveness of health promotion initiatives with a broad range of strategic partners including the World Health Organization.

These waves of practice have often been linked to scientific advances in epidemiological understandings of patterns of disease and/or injury. The major breakthrough of the 1950s was Sir Richard Doll (1950) establishing the link between smoking and cancer. Other health research later identified the link between diet/exercise and diabetes/obesity/heart disease, and between alcohol misuse and liver disease. These breakthroughs dominated fledgling health education initiatives, emphasising health professionals providing expert health advice and educational resources, throughout the 1960s. Throughout subsequent decades this work was further influenced by insights about (individual) human behaviour from the field of psychology and was enriched by learnings from social marketing, a field created as a means to facilitate social change.

RESEARCH ALIVE 28.1
BASELINE DATA FOR AOTEAROA NEW ZEALAND

Male Call (Worth, Saxton, Reid, & Segedin, 1997) was a substantial research project undertaken by the New Zealand AIDS Foundation (NZAF) in the late 1990s. This pioneering research was the first large-scale nationwide study exploring the socio-sexual characteristics of nearly 2000 men who have sex with men. The research was designed in dialogue with the wider gay community, driven by an urgent need to develop effective and efficient HIV prevention programmes. The research established a baseline set of data which continues to be used by the NZAF in the evaluation of its ongoing work in this area. The success of this evidence-based approach and the resulting culture and behaviour change via the health promotion interventions are reflected in the significant decline in HIV transmission rates in this community throughout the 2000s (Saxton et al., 2012).

CASE STUDY 28.3

REFUGEE CHILDREN IN AUSTRALIA AND IMMUNISATION STATUS

A large percentage of resettled refugee people in Australia are children under 18 years of age and their immunisation status is often unknown or, owing to a number of cultural and service barriers, they are inadequately immunised. This potentially puts them at greater risk of disease and preventable negative health outcomes than children immunised according to Australia's National Immunisation Program Schedule. Paxton, Rice, Davie, Carapetis and Skull (2011) studied data from a paediatric immigrant health clinic based at a Victorian hospital. They found that despite children having been in Australia for a median of eight months, only 33% had had an immunisation since their arrival. During this time children had multiple engagements with health care but opportunities were missed for catch up immunisation; only 15% of children had immunity to five major preventable diseases.

Studies such as this one provide a baseline understanding of a health issue in a particular group. Targeted health promotion activities, informed by health promotion values, can then be planned to address the health issue: in this case, appropriate options would include raising awareness of immunisation clinics in refugee communities and improving access through proactive provision of catch up immunisation.

In the 1990s, health researchers established that economic and social factors (such as income, poverty, education, employment and housing), and their distribution across a population, influence health status (Black, Davidson, & Whitehead, 1992). Some of these determinants of health (such as employment) are modifiable while others (such as ethnicity) are not. Building on this research, Wilkinson and Marmot (2003) isolated what they call a social gradient of health. Globally, when all other factors are controlled for, the lower the socio-economic position, the higher likelihood that health will be compromised. Tackling health inequities within (and between) countries (Pickett & Wilkinson, 2011) and addressing child poverty (Expert Advisory Group on Solutions to Child Poverty, 2012) remain core challenges facing the health promotion sector.

Governments are the main funders of health promotion programmes. Their commitment to public health and more specifically health promotion changes when different political parties come to power. Within Aotearoa New Zealand approximately three per cent of the overall health budget is committed to public health. This investment is often prioritised into minimising the risk factors for major preventable diseases such as heart disease, diabetes and some types of cancer in a quest to both drive down health-care costs and improve health status (Ministry of Health, 2013). The interventions often focus on lifestyle and behaviour changes—campaigns supporting people to quit smoking are a good example of this.

RESEARCH ALIVE 28.2
AUSTRALIAN NATIONAL HEALTH PRIORITIES

Many government funded health promotion activities are informed by the Australian National Health Priority Areas (NHPA) initiative, Australia's response to the World Health Organization's global strategy *Health for All by the Year 2000* and subsequent reports (Australian Institute of Health and Welfare, 2013). Extensive research over the last two decades has identified the following preventable diseases or conditions as requiring action, or high social and financial costs to Australian society will result:

- cancer;
- cardiovascular disease;
- injury prevention and control;
- mental health;
- diabetes mellitus;
- obesity;
- asthma;
- arthritis and musculoskeletal conditions;
- dementia.

The diseases and conditions targeted under the NHPA initiative were selected because it is forecast that with appropriate and focused health promotion intervention, significant gains in the health of Australia's population can be achieved (Australian Institute of Health and Welfare). Another closely related approach targeting the health of Australians is the Australian Government Department of Health National Chronic Disease Strategy, which provides an overarching framework that seeks to improve chronic disease prevention and care (Australian Institute of Health and Welfare).

The challenge for health promoters is to ensure lifestyle based interventions are grounded in health promotion values and address the wider socio-economic and cultural determinants of health. For instance efforts to promote the intake of fresh fruit and vegetables needs to recognise that many New Zealanders experience food insecurity (Carter, Lanumata, Kruse, & Gorton, 2010). Efforts to address uptake of smoking and misuse of alcohol need to recognise that the industries providing these substances continue to promote their products to young people (Bond, Daube, & Chikritzhs, 2010). Healthy public policy is potentially a powerful tool to neutralise the harmful effects of industry (Warwick-Booth, Dixey, & South, 2013).

CLINICAL REFLECTION 28.1: HEALTH PROMOTION IS EVERYONE'S BUSINESS

All health practitioner roles who have contact with people regarding any aspect of health can be said to be involved in health promotion. Where does the profession you are studying fit on the continuum below? What health promotion messages are you familiar with and where do they fit on the continuum?

TABLE 28.1   CONTINUUM OF HEALTH PROMOTION APPROACHES

Healthy public policy— settings and supportive environments	Community action for social and environmental change	Building capacity— programme planning and evaluation	Health education— skill development	Health information— social marketing	Screening, individual risk assessment, immunisation, and surveillance
Socio-environmental approach					
			Behavioural approach		
					Medical approach

Source: Adapted by Talbot and Verrinder (2010) from Labonte (1992), pp. 119–121.

RESEARCH ALIVE 28.3
THE AUSTRALIAN DEPARTMENT OF HEALTH AND AGING'S
GO FOR 2 & 5 PROGRAMME

The *2* and *5* in the title refer to the recommendation that we eat two serves of fruit and five serves of vegetables per day, an intake that many Australians do not achieve. This national health promotion programme was informed by

[continued next page]

extensive research into peoples' beliefs, habits and food choices, and targets causes of obesity (a condition which, as noted in Research Alive 28.2, is one of the Australian National Health Priority Areas). The programme takes a social marketing and behavioural perspective, with health promotion messages being delivered via television, internet and advertising in traditional print media, as well as in shopping centres and on shopping trolleys (Australian Department of Health & Aging, n.d.). Referring to Table 28.1 on page 379, you can see where this type of programme sits within the health promotion continuum.

PLANNING AND EVALUATION AS THE CORNERSTONES OF EVIDENCE

Planning and evaluation are core competencies identified for both health promotion and public health practitioners (Health Promotion Forum, 2011; Public Health Association, 2007). As a minimum requirement, it is expected all health promotion programmes have a formal plan of some kind and evaluation activities are undertaken to assess whether the objectives of that programme have been achieved (Waa, Holibar, & Spinola, 1998). Within a practice setting, evaluation efforts are usually proportional to the resources invested in the intervention and/or its possible impact. Although the terminology of evaluation varies across Aotearoa there are four main types widely used: formative, process, impact and outcome. The selection of those evaluation approaches is dependent on the design of the intervention.

Formative evaluation is often used at the beginning of an intervention to define a health issue and/or identify community concerns and needs. This is then developed further to establish what has been effective at either addressing similar problems or what approaches work with that particular (type of) community. Often this process involves gathering demographic and epidemiological data, reviewing relevant central and local government reports, local grey literature and relevant academic literature as available. In parallel, a process of whakawhanaungatanga (relationship-building) is undertaken and often a governance structure is established to embed community and/or strategic partners oversight of a programme (Moewaka-Barnes, 2000). Other examples of this type of research may be found in Dehar, Casswell, Duignan and Gourley (1993) and Henwood (2007).

Process evaluation involves systematically documenting what happens during the delivery of a programme. It involves collecting minutes, recording what is being done, how, when and how much it all costs. Process evaluation information is used as a routine monitoring procedure to refine the programme as it is being delivered, and enables duplication of the intervention. Examples of this approach may be found in Adams and Witten (2009), Schultz et al. (2007), and Brewin and Coggan (2002).

Impact evaluation examines the short-term and immediate impact of a programme. It primarily assesses to what extent a programme has achieved its planned objectives related to accomplishing change in knowledge, attitude, behaviour and/or environments (Rootman et al., 2001). Measurement of programme outcomes enables benchmarking to occur across disparate programmes and to isolate what works best to achieve what change with which type of communities. Building on the process evaluation, stakeholder perception and program reach can also be summarised within an impact evaluation and narrative gathered about the unintended outcomes of the intervention. Examples of this approach to research may be found in Bauman et al. (2003) and Edwards et al. (2008).

Outcome evaluation assesses the long term (five to 10 years) impacts of a health promotion intervention. Within such time frames, successful health promotion programmes should have made an attributable change in health status evidenced as mortality, morbidity and disability rates within a population. Qualitative outcome evaluation also attempts to capture how a programme has changed people's lives for the better. This approach can be found in Beautrais et al. (2007).

An intervention that is effective in one unique community may not transfer to another context. Some of the richness of health promotion practice is that there is always more than one way of doing things.

CLINICAL REFLECTION 28.2: WHAT HEALTH PROMOTION MESSAGES HAVE YOU BEEN EXPOSED TO?

How do we know if public health promotion activities make a difference and engage the wider community? Reflect on the health promotion messages you've been exposed to in the last week. Did they convey a relationship between behaviour and disease that would have been based on past research? Through what type of media was the message delivered? Was the message relevant to you or did it target another social group?

SUMMARY

Health promotion practice is dynamic, evolving and driven by values of social justice, collaboration, community engagement and, within Aotearoa New Zealand and Australia, a commitment to indigenous health and well-being. Over time health promotion practice has been informed by evidence from traditional indigenous understandings of health, epidemiological analysis, behaviour theory from psychology, and insights from critical social movements and global health promotion gatherings. At a flaxroots level, health promotion evidence is applied and generated on a daily basis by health promotion practitioners carrying out planning and formative, process, impact and outcome evaluation with communities.

HEATHER CAME AND JOANNE RAMSBOTHAM

REFLECTION POINTS

- What health promotion needs exist within your own community?
- How relevant do you think international health promotion research is to practice in Aotearoa New Zealand and Australia?

STUDY QUESTIONS

1   What are some of the fundamental values of health promotion practice?
2   Why is indigenous health important?
3   What are some of the major influences informing health promotion practice?
4   Why are planning and evaluation core competencies for health promotion?

ADDITIONAL READING

Department of Economic and Social Affairs. (Ed.). (2009). *State of the world's indigenous peoples (ST/ESA/328)*. New York, NY: United Nations, Secretariat of the Permanent Forum on Indigenous Issues. Retrieved from http://www.un.org/esa/socdev/unpfii/documents/SOWIP_web.pdf

Labonte, R. (1997). *Power, participation and partnership for health promotion*. South Carlton: Vic Health.

Laverack, G. (2004). *Health promotion practice. Power and empowerment*. London: Sage Publications.

McQueen, D., & Jones, C. (2007). *Global perspectives on health promotion effectiveness*. New York, NY: Springer International Union for Health Promotion and Education.

Pickett, K., & Wilkinson, R. (2011). *The spirit level: Why greater equality makes societies stronger*. New York, NY: Bloomsbury.

Raeburn, J., & Joubert, N. (1998). Mental health promotion: People, power and passion. *International Journal of Mental Health Promotion, 1*(1), 15–22.

Ratima, M. (2010). Māori health promotion—a comprehensive definition and strategic considerations. Auckland: Health Promotion Forum.

Robson, B., & Harris, R. (Eds.). (2007). *Hauora: Maori standards of health 4. A study of the years 2000–2005*. Wellington: Te Rōpū Rangahau Hauora a Eru Pōmare. Retrieved from http://www.hauora.maori.nz/hauora

Wise, M., & Signal, L. (2000). Health promotion development in Australia and New Zealand. *Health Promotion International, 15*(3), 237–248.

REFERENCES

Adams, J., & Witten, K. (2009). Community development as health promotion: Evaluating a complex locality-based project in New Zealand. *Community Development Journal, 44*(2), 140–157.

Australian Department of Health & Aging. (n.d.). *Go for 2 and 5 fruit and veg.* Retrieved from www.gofor2and5.com.au

Australian Institute of Health and Welfare. (2013). *National health priority areas.* Retrieved from www.aihw.gov.au/national-health-priority-areas

Bauman, A., McLean, G., Hurdle, D., Walker, S., Boyd, J., Van Aalst, I., et al. (2003). Evaluation of the national 'Push Play' campaign in New Zealand—creating population awareness of physical activity. *New Zealand Medical Journal, 116*(1179), 1–11.

Beautrais, A., Fergusson, D., Coggan, C., Collings, C., Doughty, C., Ellis, P., et al. (2007). Effective strategies for suicide prevention in New Zealand: A review of the evidence. *The New Zealand Medical Journal, 120*(1251), 2459,

Black, D., Davidson, N., & Whitehead, M. (1992). *Inequalities in health: The black report and the health divide.* New York, NY: Penguin.

Bond, L., Daube, M., & Chikritzhs, T. (2010). Selling addictions: Similarities in approaches between big tobacco and big booze. *Australasian Medical Journal, 1*(3), 325–332.

Brewin, M., & Coggan, C. (2002). Evaluation of a New Zealand indigenous community injury prevention project. *Injury Control and Safety Promotion, 9*(2), 83–88.

Carlisle, S. (2000). Health promotion, advocacy and health inequalities: a conceptual framework. *Health Promotion International, 15*(4), 369–376.

Carter, K., Lanumata, T., Kruse, K., & Gorton, D. (2010). What are the determinants of food insecurity in New Zealand and does this differ for males and females? *Australian and New Zealand Journal of Public Health, 34*(5), 602–608.

Cattan, M., & Tilford, S. (2006). *Mental health promotion: A lifespan approach.* Berkshire: McGraw-Hill.

Dehar, M., Casswell, S., Duignan, P., & Gourley, G. (1993). Formative evaluation of Heartbeat Awards in schools. *Evaluation Journal of Australasia, 5,* 30–42. A56.

Doll, R. (1950). Smoking and carcinoma of the lung. *British Medical Journal, 2*(4682), 739–748.

Durie, M. (1994). *Whaiora: Māori health development*. Auckland: Oxford University Press.

Durie, M. (2004). Understanding health and illness: Research at the interface between science and indigenous knowledge. *International Journal of Epidemiology, 33*(5), 1138–1143.

Edwards, R., Thomson, G., Wilson, N., Waa, A., Bullen, C., O'Dea, D., et al. (2008). After the smoke has cleared: Evaluation of the impact of a new national smoke-free law in New Zealand. *Tobacco Control, 17*(1), e2–e2.

Expert Advisory Group on Solutions to Child Poverty. (2012). Solutions to child poverty in New Zealand: Evidence for action. Wellington: Children's Commission.

Gracey, M., & King, M. (2009). Indigenous health part one: determinants and disease patterns. *The Lancet, 374*(9683), 65–75.

Health Promotion Forum. (2000). TUHA-NZ: Treaty understanding of Hauora in Aotearoa New Zealand. Retrieved from http://www.hauora.co.nz/resources/Tuhanzpdf.pdf

Health Promotion Forum. (2011). Ngā kaiakatanga hauora mō Aotearoa: Health promotion competencies for Aotearoa-New Zealand. Retrieved from http://www.hpforum.org.nz/assets/files/Resources/Final%20Sep%202011.pdf

Henwood, W. (2007). Māori knowledge: A key ingredient in nutrition and physical exercise health promotion programmes for Māori. *Social Policy Journal of New Zealand, 32*. Retrieved from http://www.msd.govt.nz/about-msd-and-our-work/publications-resources/journals-and-magazines/social-policy-journal/spj32/32-maori-knowledge-a-key-ingredient-in-nutrition-and-physical-exercise-health-promotion-programmes-pages181-190.html

Huygens, I., Murphy, T., & Healy, S. (2012). *Ngāpuhi speaks*. Whangarei: Network Waitangi Whangarei, Te Kawariki.

International Union of Health Promotion and Education. (n.d.). *The European bureau: A pioneer role*. Retrieved from http://www.iuhpe.org/uploaded/Regions/EURO/IUHPE.EURO_Background1968-1985_ENG.pdf

King, M., Smith, A., & Gracey, M. (2009). Indigenous health part two: The underlying causes of the health gap. *The Lancet, 374*(9683), 76–85.

Kipuri, N. (2009). Culture. In Department of Economic and Social Affairs (Ed.), *State of the world's indigenous peoples (ST/ESA/328)* (pp. 51–78). New York, NY: United Nations. Retrieved from http://www.un.org/esa/socdev/unpfii/documents/SOWIP_web.pdf

Labonte, R. (1992). Health inequities in Canada: Models, theory and planning. *Health Promotion International, 7*(2), 119–121

Laverack, G. (2004). *Health promotion practice. Power and empowerment*. London: Sage Publications.

Ministry of Health. (n.d.). *Public health service handbook: Service specifications*. Wellington: Author.

Ministry of Social Development. (2010). *The social report 2010*. Retrieved from http://socialreport.msd.govt.nz/documents/the-social-report-2010.pdf

Moewaka-Barnes, H. (2000). Kaupapa Maori: Explaining the ordinary. *Pacific Health Dialog, 7*(1), 13–16. Retrieved from http://www.kaupapamaori.com/assets//explaining_the_ordinary.pdf

Paxton, G., Rice, J., Davie, G., Carapetis, J., & Skull, J. (2011). East African immigrant children in Australia have poor immunisation coverage. *Journal of Paediatrics and Child Health, 47*, 888–892.

Pickett, K., & Wilkinson, R. (2011). *The spirit level: Why greater equality makes societies stronger*. New York, NY: Bloomsbury.

Public Health Association. (2007). *Generic competencies for public health in Aotearoa-New Zealand*. Retrieved May 20, 2010, from http://www.pha.org.nz/documents/GenericCompetenciesforPublicHealthMarch2007.pdf

Raeburn, J., & Rootman, I. (1998). *People-centred health promotion*. Chichester: John Wiley & Sons.

Rissel, C. (1994). Empowerment: The holy grail of health promotion? *Health Promotion International, 9*(1), 39–47.

Rootman, I., Goodstadt, M., Hyndman, B., McQueen, D., Potvin, L., Springett, J., et al. (2001). *Evaluation in health promotion: Principles and perspectives* [European Series, No. 92]. Denmark: World Health Organization.

Saxton, P., Dickson, N., Griffiths, R., Hughes, A. J., & Rowden, J. (2012). Actual and undiagnosed HIV prevalence in a community sample of men who have sex with men in Auckland, New Zealand. *BMC Public Health, 12*(1), 92.

Schultz, J., Utter, J., Mathews, L., Cama, T., Mavoa, H., & Swinburn, B. (2007). The Pacific OPIC project (Obesity Prevention in Communities): Action plan and interventions. *Health Promotion in the Pacific, 14*(2), 147–154.

Talbot, L. & Verrinder, G. (2010). *Promoting health: A primary health care approach* (4th ed.). Chatswood: Elsevier.

Te Rōpū Kai Hapai o Hauora o Te Tai Tokerau. (2008). *Te Tai Tokerau strategic Maori health plan 2008–2013*. Retrieved from http://www.northlanddhb.org.nz/images/stories/documents/ttt%20maori%20strategic%20plan%20final.pdf

Thompson, S., Chenhall, R., & Brimblecombe, J. (2013). Indigenous perspectives on active living in remote Australia: A qualitative exploration of the socio-cultural link between health, the environment and economics. *BMC Public Health, 13*(473), 1–11.

Waa, A., Holibar, F., & Spinola, C. (1998). *Programme evaluation: An introductory guide for health promotion*. Auckland: Alcohol and Public Health Research Unit and Whariki.

Warwick-Booth, L., Dixey, R., & South, J. (2013). Healthy public policy. In R. Dixey (Ed.), *Health promotion: Global principles and practice*. Oxfordshire, England: CABI.

Wilkinson, R., & Marmot, M. (2003). *Social determinants of health: The solid facts*. Retrieved from http://www.euro.who.int/__data/assets/pdf_file/0005/98438/e81384.pdf

World Health Organization. (1948). *Constitution*. Retrieved from http://www.who.int/governance/eb/who_constitution_en.pdf

World Health Organization. (1986). Ottawa Charter for Health Promotion *Proceedings of the 1st International Conference on Health Promotion*. Ottawa: World Health Organization.

Worth, H., Saxton, P., Reid, A., & Segedin, R. (1997). *Male call: Report one: Methodology and demographic characteristics*. Auckland: New Zealand AIDS Foundation.

Zhao, Y., Conners, C., Wright, J., & Guthridge, S. (2008). Estimating chronic disease prevalence among the remote Australian population of the Northern Territory using multiple data sources. *Australian and New Zealand Journal of Public Health, 32*, 307–313.

WEBSITES

Health Promotion Forum of New Zealand:
http://www.hpforum.org.nz

International Union of Health Promotion and Education:
http://www.iuhpe.org

The Treaty (of Waitangi) to you:
http://www.treaty2u.govt.nz/the-treaty-up-close/treaty-of-waitangi

CHAPTER 29

ORAL HEALTH

NAOMI HEAP, SUSAN SHAW AND SUSAN CARTWRIGHT

CHAPTER OVERVIEW

This chapter covers the following topics:

- The context of oral health
- Research into oral health
- The future of oral health research
- Research and oral health therapy

KEY TERMS

Cariogenic

Fluoride

Interprofessional learning

Oral therapists

Professional cultures

Professionalisation

Theory–practice gap

Professionalisation
The process of a
group of practitioners
becoming recognised
as a profession.

The professions of dental therapy and dental hygiene have developed within the wider context of dentistry. The current practice environment for these two professions emphasises supervision and guidance from registered dentists. The transfer of education for therapists and hygienists into the tertiary education sector (universities) marks a process of identity development and professionalisation that other professions such as nursing, midwifery, podiatry, occupational therapy and physiotherapy have already embarked upon. Such recognition and the emergence of professional identity enabled these other professions to assert their own research interests and agenda, and to distinguish themselves from one and other and also from medicine. The history of the education and practice of dental therapists and dental hygienists has been so closely entwined with that of dentistry that it can be difficult to identify the unique skills and contribution of these two professions to oral health. Dental research emphasises empirical approaches to a biomedical perspective of health and practice and, as a result, most of practice-related research available to hygienists and therapists comes from this perspective.

THE CONTEXT OF ORAL HEALTH

Oral health issues are considered within the public health agenda and have been identified as having an impact on well-being across the world (Petersen, 2003). Aotearoa New Zealand has a unique history in the provision of oral health care. Oral health was defined within the public health agenda at the beginning of the twentieth century and led to the establishment of dental nurse training and of the school dental service (Satur & Moffat, 2010), reflecting the view that schools are a good place to provide oral health care (Kwan, Petersen, Pine, & Borutta, 2005) The provision of oral health care has evolved through a complex history of legislation and regulation, which has limited the scope of practice in relation to age groups able to be treated as well as the professional supervision and responsibility of practitioners. While the role of the dental therapist has existed for a long time (previously, as school dental nurses), dental hygiene is a relatively new profession to Aotearoa New Zealand (Coates, Kardos, Moffat, & Kardos, 2009). Despite the political and social history of publically funded and accessible health care, the practice of dentistry has remained largely within the private sector in New Zealand. The practice of dental hygiene is closely linked to the provision of private sector care whereas dental therapy remains state funded for those under the age of 18 years.

An enviable goal would be to develop cohesive and integrated oral health care that is accessible to the wider community based upon best evidence. The current emphasis on interprofessional education and practice has led to the evolution of dual-qualified graduates leaving university with undergraduate degrees in oral health that enable them to register as therapists and hygienists. This poses challenges in terms of professional territories and access to funding for the provision of services, all of which require changes to existing models and professional cultures.

Professional cultures
The ways of thinking,
talking and interacting
that develop within
defined groups of
practitioners.

RESEARCH INTO ORAL HEALTH

Fluoride is closely associated with oral health and its use involves much debate (Block, 2009; Carstairs, 2010; Fischman, 1997; Spencer, 1998). The relationship between fluoride and oral health may be considered a piece of observational research carried out by a practitioner. While there had been interest in the minerals and other factors that may influence oral health in the diet and environment for many years, investigation into fluoride emerged in the twentieth century. Frederick McKay is considered to have been the instigator of research into the effects of fluoride on oral health (Pizzo, Piscopo, Pizzo, & Giuliana, 2007). The early adoption of fluoridation of civic water supplies in Aotearoa New Zealand has been attributed to research collaborations and other links between various disciplines and government agencies within the context of a strong public health agenda in the early twentieth century (Akers, 2008).

Fluoride
A mineral associated with prevention of tooth decay in humans.

CASE STUDY 29.1

MILK AND TEETH

Milk has long been associated with strong teeth. There is some evidence that the calcium in milk assists with remineralisation. The consumption of dietary calcium has been shown to have a positive impact on bone mineral content in children (Huncharek, Muscat, & Kupelnick, 2008). However, it does not follow that milk prevents dental caries. While milk is less cariogenic (causative of dental decay and caries) than honey and carbonated drinks, human milk is more cariogenic than bovine milk. Protracted exposure to artificial milk formula and human breast milk can have a negative impact on oral health (Bowen & Lawrence, 2005). Recent research linking milk with oral health has focused on using milk as a mechanism to deliver fluoride (fluoride-fortified milk) (Bánóczy, Petersen, & Rugg-Gunn, 2009; Merritt, Qi, & Shi, 2006) rather than for its own benefits.

It is possible that the emphasis on drinking milk through public health messages in Aotearoa New Zealand (as in Figure 29.1) is more closely linked to our identity as a dairy product-producing nation rather than to any specific research about the generic benefits of milk on teeth.

Cariogenic
Relating to a process or element that promotes tooth decay.

[continued next page]

FIGURE 29.1   A 1940S ADVERTISEMENT PROMOTING COW'S MILK

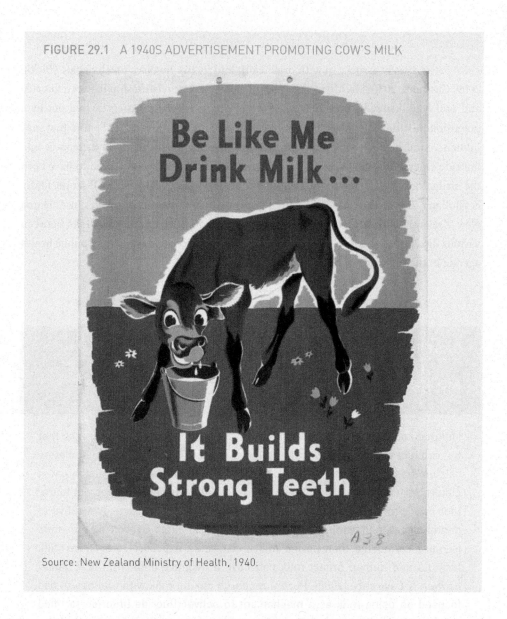

Source: New Zealand Ministry of Health, 1940.

THE FUTURE OF ORAL HEALTH RESEARCH

The existence of research about practice does not necessarily translate into changed practice. 'It is well documented that the translation of knowledge into clinical practice is a slow and haphazard process. This is no less true for dental healthcare than other types of healthcare' (Clarkson, Ramsay, Torgerson, & Vale, 2010, p. 57). As a result, various initiatives exist to attempt to address the theory–practice gap, such as practice-based research networks (Curro, et al., 2011) and an emphasis on evidence-based knowledge within the professions (Hendricson, et al., 2011; Kwok, Caton, Polson, & Hunter, 2012).

Theory–practice gap
The gap between what is known about practice and when or how it changes to reflect that knowledge.

These programmes engage practitioners in the research process, enabling them to contribute to the development of knowledge and understanding the links between research and practice, rather than being passive recipients of published information.

The links between oral health and general health are strong. Poor oral health is linked to bone and joint pathologies, diabetes and cardiovascular disease (Rautemaa, Lauhio, Cullinan, & Seymour, 2007). The negative impact of poor nutritional intakes caused by decreased function further exacerbates physical health conditions in all ages (McKenna et al., 2012; Kwan, et al., 2005). Psychological effects are also indicated where self-esteem and quality of life are affected by aesthetics and functionality (Huff, Kinion, Kendra, & Klecan, 2006). And conversely, disease processes, for example tooth loss and halitosis, have both physiological and psychological consequences (Davis, Fiske, Scott, & Radford, 2000). The changing demographics and, therefore, illness and disability experiences of the public are reflected in the oral health needs of the communities of which they are a part. New uses for existing medications, such as intermittent intravenous bisphosphonate infusions to treat osteoporosis in addition to their uses in palliative care (Reginster, Malaise, Neuprez, Jouret, & Close, 2007), require that oral health practitioners are informed and appreciate that any oral health-related side effects may become more prevalent. The general emphasis on the need for evidence is not confined to health professionals and is well understood by informed individuals and groups within society in general. This requires that practitioners are aware of how to access and analyse information and new knowledge relevant to their practice (Chiappelli, Newman, Sunga, Concepcion, & Edgerton, 2003; Iqbal & Glenny, 2002; Worthington, Glenny, Mauleffinch, Daly & Clarkson, 2010) and possibly how to counter poorly informed but easily accessed information and opinion widely available for public access, as found on the internet.

CASE STUDY 29.2

HISTORICAL MESSAGES LACKING EVIDENCE?

In 1940 the New Zealand Department of Health published this image of Keith, the cocker spaniel, 'chewing hard' to encourage strong white teeth. There is mixed opinion on whether canine dental health is positively affected by chewing bones and, in relation to human oral health, studies show that dental abrasion and fractures occur from the regular introduction of hard foreign objects to the oral cavity (Ashcroft & Joiner, 2010). This raises questions of the evidence behind the slogan 'Chew hard like Keith ... for strong white teeth.'

[continued next page]

NAOMI HEAP, SUSAN SHAW AND SUSAN CARTWRIGHT

FIGURE 29.2 CHEWING DOES NOT NECESSARILY IMPROVE TOOTH STRENGTH, DESPITE PROMOTIONS LIKE THIS ONE

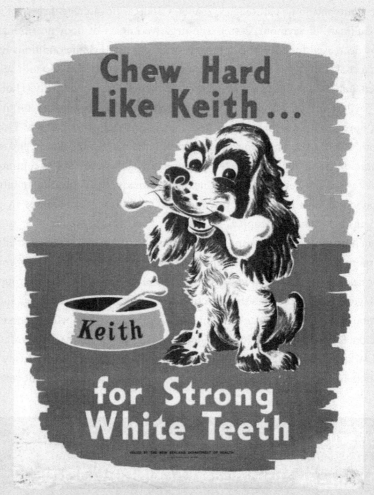

Source: New Zealand Department of Health 1940.

Therefore the rationale supporting this promotion should be considered in the context of the research of its day. During the 1930s Mellamby and Pattison (1932) published work on nutritional effects on dental health, which could have been a strong influence here. 'Experimental work on dogs and other animals has shown that for the normal development of the teeth the diet should include abundant vitamin D and calcium, and not be overweighted with cereals'

(Mellamby & Pattison, 1932, p. 507). In addition the chewing gum company Wrigley were at the time supporting independent research, indicating that chewing had positive effects on dental health. We can see how these two areas of study may have influenced the content of this oral health promotion, but it could be argued that the concept of 'chewing hard' is something of a leap from the groundbreaking work of the time, and although Keith the cocker spaniel may well have had improved dental health it is unlikely that many humans had stronger or whiter teeth as a result of this campaign.

RESEARCH AND ORAL HEALTH THERAPY

The movement of dental therapy and dental hygiene education into research-rich university environments has occurred within recent years in a number of nations including Canada (Cohham, 2004), Australia (Satur & Moffatt, 2010) and Aotearoa New Zealand (Coates, et al., 2009). There are now two universities in Aotearoa New Zealand graduating dual-qualified therapists and hygienists from three-year undergraduate degrees. There is a move to refer to this as oral health therapy, undertaken by oral therapists. Both curricula emphasise health promotion and the socio-political context of practitioners and service users, and closely link theory and practice throughout. One of the reasons for moving health professional education from industry-based or skills-based situations into universities was to increase the profile and development of the profession (Cohan, 2004). The evolution of a research profile and fields of expertise for other health professional groups such as nursing and midwifery can also be traced via the provision of education within tertiary education settings.

> **Oral therapists**
> Practitioners utilising the skills of dental therapy and dental hygiene.

Professions historically considered subordinate to medicine and dentistry have the potential to establish their own identities within the critical and interprofessional context of tertiary education. This constructs an environment where various scopes of practice are seen as making meaningful contributions to the provision of health care and disability support rather than as a hierarchical environment where 'others' are the 'helpers' of the dominant groups. This transition to establishing a research-based field of knowledge and expertise for dental therapists and hygienists is still in its infancy, but the experience of other 'allied' professions suggests this separate identity will be more clearly defined in time. Whether the education of oral health therapists resides alongside dental and medical education or other groups of health professionals is irrelevant if a true commitment to interprofessional learning and practice exists in concert with shared and meaningful access to resources and expertise.

> **Interprofessional learning**
> Learning that involves students engaging (learning with and about) their professional groups.

NAOMI HEAP, SUSAN SHAW AND SUSAN CARTWRIGHT

RESEARCH ALIVE 29.1
CARIES MANAGEMENT

Prevention of dental disease, particularly dental caries, has long been the focus for dental professionals. Materials exist that have contributed to the pursuit of this goal, most notably those that contain fluoride. There is international consensus that the most probable reason for the decrease in dental caries in industrialised countries (since 1970) has been the widespread exposure to fluoride, and, from a global perspective, the regular use of fluoride toothpaste (Bratthall, Hansell Peterssen, & Sundberg, 1996).

Why then does so much dental decay still exist? In the recent New Zealand Oral Health Survey (Ministry of Health, 2010) it was found that only one in four dentate adults aged 18–24 years was caries-free. How can some people be disease-free while others still develop carious lesions? This is a complex problem, but part of the solution could lie in how prevention of disease is practised.

Research from the University of Sydney has shown that, when prevention is practised according to a 10-step 'caries management system,' a decreased rate of dental caries results. Caries can be stopped, reversed and prevented (Curtis, Evans, Sbaraini & Schwarz, 2008). This system requires a change in mindset for many practitioners who have been educated to fill any defects they see on radiographs in case the defects should progress to become large cavities. Additionally, the 'models of caries management and reimbursement which have been heavily skewed toward "drilling and filling"' (Ismail et al., 2013, p. e12) need to change. Diagnostics need to improve, with the recognition that large proportions of radiolucencies on bitewing radiographs that extend to the dentino-enamel junction and beyond are not cavitated. Evans, Pakdaman, Dennison and Howe (2008) led research to develop a system for remineralisation of these lesions using fluoride varnish and improved oral hygiene techniques, among other things. They developed a system that informs the patient of their condition and guides practitioners to apply more thorough preventive regimens using more frequent recalls.

The system developed by Evans et al. (2008) is similar to other systems around the world, namely the International Caries Detection and Assessment System (ICDAS) from the United Kingdom and Caries Management by Risk Assessment (CAMBRA) from the United States. These systems and others were reviewed in a recently published article which highlights the importance of following a systematic approach when dealing with this prevalent chronic disease (Ismail et al., 2013).

An improved approach to the treatment of dental caries could help to increase numbers in the 'caries-free' category in years to come.

The chance to create new research agendas presents opportunities to draw on research from a range of fields of knowledge and human endeavour which may broaden perspectives and create synergies for practitioners, patients and funding and commissioning agencies. Links with architecture, planning, sociology, management, business, education and psychology could assist with exploring issues of building design and location, patient experience and the place of oral health care in society.

SUMMARY

The move of education to the tertiary sector has enabled the relatively young professional disciplines of dental therapy and dental hygiene to develop distinct identities. This in time will lead to the emergence of a research profile and agenda for these professions that will no doubt be distinct from, while complementary to, dentistry. This is an opportunity for practitioners and students of dental therapy and dental hygiene to consider the research questions and approaches that resonate with their practices and the wider environment. The historical emphasis on oral health promotion along with the current interest in interprofessional learning and practice are likely to play a part in these developments.

REFLECTION POINTS

- What do you think are the important historical events in oral health practice?
- Why is dental research on oral health practice important?
- What research questions do you think are important for the future of oral health practice?

STUDY QUESTIONS

1 What are the major potential research topics for oral health therapy?
2 Have health promotion messages related to oral health been based on sound research?
3 How can research influence practice in the oral health sector?

ADDITIONAL READING

Rugg-Gunn, A. J., Hackett, A. F., Appleton, D. R., Jenkins, G. N., & Eastoe, J. E. (1984). Relationship between dietary habits and caries increment assessed over two years in 405 English adolescent school children. *Archives of Oral Biology, 29*, 983–992.

Rugg-Gunn, A. J., Roberts, G. J., & Wright, W. G. (1985). Effect of human milk on plaque pH *in situ* and enamel dissolution *in vitro* compared with bovine milk, lactose and sucrose. *Caries Research, 19*, 327–334.

Satur, J., & Moffat, S. (2010). A history of oral health practice (dental therapy and dental hygiene) in Australia and New Zealand. In A. K. L. Tsang (Ed.), *Oral health therapy programs in Australia and New Zealand.* Queensland: Knowledge Books and Software.

REFERENCES

Akers, H. F. (2008). Collaboration, vision and reality: water fluoridation in New Zealand (1952–1968). *The New Zealand Dental Journal, 104*(4), 127–33.

Ashcroft, A. T., & Joiner, A. (2010). Tooth cleaning and tooth wear: a review. *Proceedings of the Institution of Mechanical Engineers, 224*(J6), 539–549.

Bánóczy, J., Petersen, P. E., Rugg-Gunn, A. J. (Eds.). (2009). *Milk fluoridation for the prevention of dental caries.* Geneva: World Health Organization.

Block, K. (2009). Deep structure and controversy: re-reading the fluoridation debate. *Health Sociology Review, 18,* 246–259.

Bowen, W. H., & Lawrence, R.A. (2005). Comparison of the cariogenicity of cola, honey, cow milk, human milk, and sucrose. *Pediatrics, 116*(4), 921–926.

Bratthall, D., Hansell Peterssen, G., & Sundberg, H. (1996). Reasons for the caries decline: what do the experts believe? *European Journal of Oral Science, 104,* 416–422.

Carstairs, C. (2010). Cities without cavities: democracy, risk and public health. *Journal of Canadian Studies, 44*(2), 146–170.

Chiappelli, F., Newman, P.M., Sunga, E., Concepcion, E., & Edgerton, M. (2003). Evidence-based practice in dentistry: benefit or hindrance. *Journal of Dental Research, 82*(6), 6–7.

Clarkson, J., Ramsay, C., Torgerson, C., & Vale, L., (2010). The translation research in a dental setting (TRiaDS) programme protocol. *Implementation Science, 5*(1), 57–67.

Coates, D. E., Kardos, T. B., Moffat, S. M., & Kardos, R. L. (2009). Dental therapists and dental hygienists educated for the New Zealand environment. *Journal of Dental Education, 73*(8), 1001–1008.

Cohhan, S. J. (2004). Evidence-based practice and the professionalization of dental hygiene. *International Journal of Dental Hygiene, 2,* 152–160.

Curro, F. A., Grill, A. C., Thompson, V. P., Craig, R. G., Vena, D., Keenan, A. V., et al., (2011). Advantages of the dental practice-based research network initiative and its role in dental education. *Journal of Dental Education, 75*(8), 1053–1060.

Curtis, B., Evans, R. W., Sbaraini, A., & Schwarz, E. (2008). The monitor practice programme: Is non-invasive management of dental caries in private practice effective? *Australian Dental Journal, 53*, 306–313.

Davis, D. M., Fiske, J., Scott, B., & Radford, D. R. (2000). The emotional effects of tooth loss: a preliminary quantitative study. *British Dental Journal, 188*(9), 503–506.

Evans, R. W., Pakdaman, A., Dennison, P. J., & Howe, E. L. C. (2008). The caries management system: an evidence based prevention strategy for dental practitioners. Application for adults. *Australian Dental Journal, 53*, 83–92.

Fischman, S. L. (1997). The history of oral hygiene products: how far have we come in 6000 years? *Periodontology 2000, 15*(1), 7–14.

Hendricson, W. D., Rugh, J. D., Hatch, J. P., Stark, D. L., Deahl, T., & Wallmann, E. R. (2011). Validation of an instrument to assess evidence-based practice knowledge: attitudes, access and confidence in the dental environment. *Journal of Dental Education, 75*(2), 131–144.

Huff, M., Kinion, E., Kendra, M. A., & Klecan, T. (2006). Self-esteem: a hidden concern in oral health. *Journal of Community Health Nursing, 23*(4), 245–255.

Huncharek, M., Muscat, J., & Kupelnick, B. (2008). Impact of dairy products and dietary calcium on bone-mineral content in children: results of a meta-analysis. *Bone, 43*, 312–321.

Iqbal, A., & Glenny, A-M. (2002). General dental practitioners' knowledge of attitudes towards evidence-based practice. *British Dental Journal, 13*(10), 587–591.

Ismail, A. L., Tellez, M., Pitts, N., Ekstrand, K. R., Ricketts, D., Longbottom, C., et al. (2013). Caries management pathways preserve dental tissues and promote oral health. *Community Dentistry and Oral Epidemiology, 41*, e12–e40.

Kwan, S. Y. L., Petersen, P. E., Pine, C. M., & Borutta, A. (2005). Health-promoting schools: an opportunity for oral health promotion. *Bulletin of the World Health Organization, 83*(9), 677–685.

Kwok, V., Caton, J. G., Polson, A. M., & Hunter, P. G. (2012). Application of evidence-based dentistry: from research to clinical periodontal practice. *Periodontology 2000, 59*(1), 61–74.

McKenna, G., Allen, P. F., Flynn, A., O'Mahony, D., DaMata, C., Cronin, M., et al. (2012). Impact of tooth replacement strategies on the nutritional status of partially-dentate elders. *Gerodontology, 29*(2), e883–e890.

Mellamby, M., & Pattison, L. (1932). Remarks on the influence of a cereal-free diet rich in vitamin D and calcium on dental caries in children. *British Medical Journal, 1*, 507.

Merritt, J., Qi, F., & Shi, W. (2006). Milk helps build strong teeth and promotes oral health. *Journal of the California Dental Association, 34*(5), 361–366.

Ministry of Health. (2010). *Our oral health: Key findings of the 2009 New Zealand oral health survey.* Wellington: Ministry of Health.

Petersen, P. E. (2003). The world oral health report 2003; continuous improvement of oral health in the 21st century—the approach of the WHO global oral health programme. *Community Dentistry and Oral Epidemiology, 31*(Supplement 1), 3–24.

Pizzo, G., Piscopo, M. R., Pizzo, I., & Giuliana, G. (2007). Community water fluoridation and caries prevention: a critical review. *Clinical Oral Investigations, 11*, 189–193.

Rautemaa, R., Lauhio, A., Cullinan, M. P., & Seymour, G. J. (2007). Oral infections and systemic disease—an emerging epidemic in medicine. *Clinical Microbiology and infection, 13*(11), 1041–1047.

Reginster, J-Y., Malaise, O., Neuprez, A., Jouret, V-E., & Close, P. (2007). Intermittent bisphosphonate therapy in postmenopausal osteoporosis progress to date. *Drugs and Ageing, 24*(5), 351.

Satur, J., & Moffat, S. (2010). A history of oral health practice (dental therapy and dental hygiene) in Australia and New Zealand. In A. K. L. Tsang (Ed.), *Oral health therapy programs in Australia and New Zealand.* Queensland: Knowledge Books and Software.

Spencer, A. J. (1998). New or biased, evidence on water fluoridation? *Australian and New Zealand Journal of Public Health, 22*(1), 149–154.

Worthington, H. V., Glenny, A. M., Mauleffinch, L. F., Daly, F., & Clarkson, J. (2010). Using Cochrane reviews for oral diseases. *Oral Diseases, 16*(7), 592–598,

WEBSITES

Borrow Foundation:
http://www.borrowfoundation.org

New Zealand Dental & Oral Health Therapists:
http://www.nzoral.org

CHAPTER 30

COUNSELLING

CAROLINE DAY AND ROBIN SUTCLIFFE

CHAPTER OVERVIEW

This chapter covers the following topics:

- Historical overview of the development of research in counselling
- Common research methodologies in counselling research
- Linking science with practice
- Future directions for research in counselling

KEY TERMS

Applied
Internet
Methodology
Model
Rigour
Scientist–practitioner

Research in counselling in Aotearoa New Zealand could be said to be in its infancy, partly due to the way that counselling as a profession has evolved. The education of counsellors has only recently moved into the university sector and therefore into an environment in which research is resourced and encouraged.

HISTORICAL OVERVIEW OF THE DEVELOPMENT OF RESEARCH IN COUNSELLING

Counselling describes different practices that occur in many varied contexts such as social work and within schools, community agencies and private practice (Miller, 2001). It can also be seen as having been woven from several developmental strands. The first of these is the church-based charity work that is credited with leading to the development of social work (Healy, 2008). The second was the marriage guidance movement, an initially voluntary organisation that in New Zealand was implemented in 1949 and that aimed to reduce delinquency in communities by reducing the number of 'broken homes' (Penny, Epston, & Agee, 2008). Marriage guidance has been through several incarnations and is currently called Relationships Aotearoa, one of the biggest employers of counsellors in Aotearoa New Zealand (Relationships Aotearoa, n.d.). The third strand is vocational guidance and counselling which began in North America in the early 1900s and was introduced into schools in New Zealand in the 1960s. In 1974 the New Zealand Guidance and Counselling Association was established; it was renamed the New Zealand Association of Counsellors in 1990.

It can be difficult to define counselling and how to research it (Anderson, 1991). Bunce (1992) stated that there had been ongoing questioning of the value of using traditional 'quantitative, empirical, models of experimental methodology' (p. 4) to research counselling.

Models of education, practice and research have been based on perspectives from North America and the United Kingdom (Bunce, 1992). According to Beutler (1990) prior to the 1960s practitioners were concerned with researching the process as it applied to their everyday practice whereas researchers were concerned with providing evidence of the outcomes of counselling. Researchers were seen by practitioners to be using inappropriate methodologies to investigate topics that were not necessarily relevant to them and to present the findings in ways that were difficult to translate into practice (Bunce, 1992). There were corresponding views held by researchers that practitioners were perhaps unwilling to either educate themselves in the understanding and application of different methodologies or to actively engage in formal evaluation of their work.

Methodology
Particular principles, rules and processes for undertaking research.

Model
A framework for describing concepts.

Applied
Put to practical use.

This divide was less evident in Aotearoa New Zealand as most who were engaged in research were educators and/or practitioners (Bunce, 1992).

Counselling practice from the 1960s was influenced by Carl Rogers's person-centred theory (Mearns & Thorne, 2007) as well as the shifting societal awareness of the importance of individual freedom and self-determination (Aubrey, 1977). According to Hill (1982, cited in Anderson, 1991) Rogers was open to his work being scrutinised, an attitude which was in contrast to that of many psychoanalytic psychotherapists and counsellors at the time. By the mid-sixties the divide between counselling practice and counselling research had begun to break down and the 'empiricalisation of process research became noticeable with the development of instruments to measure the constructs of person-centred therapy' (Beutler, 1990, p. 263).

As the education of counsellors evolved in New Zealand there was developing recognition of the need to acknowledge the New Zealand context, and away from the 'prevailing monoculturalism of Western psychological theory and counselling practice' (Crocket, Flanagan, Winslade, & Kotze, 2011a, p. 6). As a New Zealand approach to counselling began to evolve from the late 1980s, questions were asked about the applicability of overseas models to Aotearoa New Zealand. There was growing interest from New Zealand counselling practitioners towards models that were collaborative and co-constructed (White & Epston, 1990) as well as towards those with a social justice or ecological stance that took account of the social context of clients (Waldegrave, Tamasese, Tuhaka, & Campbell, 2003).

According to Bunce (1992), at this time much of the research was 'based on a scientist–practitioner model of practice' (p. 2), but not all practitioners agreed with this model. This model was based on the concept of practitioners who were actively involved in reading and applying research findings to their practice. However, as many practitioners had not been educated within the university sector or with an emphasis on research-based practices, they did not identify with this model of practice. There was growing interest in Aotearoa New Zealand for a researcher–practitioner model, involving 'collaboration between researchers and practitioners and from practitioners initiating research relating to their own or others' practice' (Bunce, 1992, p. 4). An example of this was David Epston's model using video recordings of client sessions that the practitioner and client would view together and 'observe, gather data, develop hypotheses, undertake experiments, and construct new explanations' (Bunce, 1992, p. 4).

Scientist–practitioner
A professional who engages with science as they practice.

From the 1990s there has been a growing appreciation of qualitative methods. Prior to this there was poor understanding of these methodologies, and the research was viewed as lacking in rigour (Bunce, 1992). Action research was also being used quite extensively because it was an approach that positioned practitioners as researchers and experts.

Rigour
The degree to which research process and findings stand up to challenge.

COMMON RESEARCH METHODOLOGIES IN COUNSELLING RESEARCH

Counsellors in Aotearoa New Zealand and overseas have tended to regard the work they are engaged in with clients as evidence-based and, furthermore, that they are 'knowledgeable about current counselling research and its implications for clinical practice' (Manthei, 2006, p. 59). This is despite the relative—until recently—paucity of published research in counselling. Of the research available, there has been a predominance of quantitative research, particularly that research which is focused on the counsellor's experience (Berrios & Lucca, 2006). According to Manthei (2006), there is a need for further study of the client's experience of counselling and, further, that this research needs to use qualitative methodologies in order to capture more fully the clients' understandings of 'their inner experience of the process of counselling' (p. 60).

QUANTITATIVE RESEARCH AND COUNSELLING

Quantitative methodologies have predominated in the counselling field until recently, and still have a certain dominance (McLeod, 2010). Counselling researchers commonly used the survey method as a means for gathering and analysing data reasonably simply, and indeed the survey method is one that is still widely encountered in counselling research. There are many researchers in Aotearoa New Zealand studying counselling who avail themselves of this method (Raffensperger & Miller, 2005; Paton, 2005; Everts & Withers, 2006; Crocket, 2011).

CASE STUDY 30.1

COUNSELLING EFFECTIVENESS

A survey conducted by Young, Wiggens-Frame and Cashwell (2007) on members of the American Counselling Association asked participants to rate their abilities and effectiveness as counsellors against a set of religious and spiritual competencies, along with rating whether those competencies were achievable in counselling practice. The results indicated that 53% of the 500 participants agreed that practising within established competencies was achievable and that they felt confident to be able to do so. Additionally, the survey found that half of the participants felt a need for further training, along with experiencing less confidence in their counselling abilities.

The researchers suggest that this study provides a sense of how counsellors view practising within a set of theoretical competencies, along with identifying the importance of ongoing development and training for practising counsellors.

Manthei (2011) studied the success of a community counselling centre by distributing a questionnaire to former counselling clients. One of the aims of the research was to compare the results with results from earlier studies of the agency. The questionnaire comprised three parts: part one asked clients if they had attended counselling in the past and, if so, how many counsellors they had; part two asked what the clients had tried in terms of problem-solving and seeking help; and part three asked clients how well they were managing over various times—before counselling, during counselling and after counselling. The results indicated that the clients experienced satisfactory outcomes in terms of what the agency had set out to achieve—to offer affordable and accessible support to people walking in from its community. These results were also consistent with the findings from the previous studies. Despite constraints such as a small sample size, more women clients than men and more older people, the study concluded that overall the agency offered 'a successful, self-sustaining service' (Manthei, p. 85), along with identifying areas for development and discussion within the agency. This too was consistent with earlier findings. Manthei suggests that data-gathering over many years from one agency can assist with long-term planning and also help with resourcing, developing policies and implementing a more cost-effective, efficient service to the community.

QUALITATIVE RESEARCH AND COUNSELLING

McLeod (2010) made a call for narrative case studies to feature in qualitative counselling research more widely than they currently do. He stated there is 'considerable evidence' that qualitative methods have an important role to play in practice: 'perhaps a greater role than any other form of research and enquiry' (p. 205). Such methods are better able to capture the lived experience of participants, perhaps more than any other (Bedford & Landry, 2010). These authors also suggest that narrative inquiry is particularly appropriate, with its focus on 'the construction of life stories in the development of individual identity' (Bedford & Landry, p. 152). Additionally, narrative inquiry acknowledges the researcher's experience within the study area and this is made visible in the research itself. Narrative inquiry has become increasingly popular (Sliedrecht & Kotze, 2008; Gossman, 2011; Marsden, 2011).

RESEARCH ALIVE 30.1
NARRATIVE INQUIRY

Sliedrecht and Kotze (2008) utilised narrative inquiry when they focused their research on the former patients of a spinal unit and their experiences of counselling. As the researchers state, by allowing for the experience of the patients to be central to the study, space was opened for 'illness and disability narratives to be storied' (Sliedrecht & Kotze, p. 72). This study examined illness narratives: loss, grief and hope; acceptance of losses; and holding hope, among other narratives. The study's conclusion was written from the perspective of what the researchers had noticed and learnt, and included the importance of noticing 'the possible filtering out of stories of struggle and difficulty' (Sliedrecht & Kotze, p. 84) that patients can engage in. One of the researchers reported discovering the importance of 'talking with patients about the destination they are reaching for' and 'being open to hear multiple and at times competing stories of disability' (Sliedrecht & Kotze, p. 84).

MIXED METHODS AND COUNSELLING

Mixing both qualitative and quantitative methods is also a relatively recent addition to counselling research. It has its proponents, including Kottler and Shephard (2004), who describe a replication or match between mixed methods research and the ways in which practitioners engage in the work with clients. They suggest there is a tendency to emphasise the counselling relationship in qualitative research whereas the focus in quantitative research is on the counsellor's perception of the work. Combining both qualitative and quantitative methods would therefore attend to both the counselling relationship and the experience of the counsellor, thereby allowing for a more accurate representation of counselling in research.

With the emphasis in qualitative research on the relationship and the focus in quantitative research on the counsellor's perception of the work, there is an inherent framework for both to be represented in research.

Hertlein and Lambert-Shute (2007) undertook a quantitative study on students enrolled in counselling training. They distributed a survey via the internet and asked what factors had been influential in leading them to decide which particular training programme to enrol in, by ranking factors such as clinical aspects of the training; whether the training was a personal match; and research opportunities, among others. This survey was followed up with a qualitative set of discussion questions with the intention of elucidating the findings from the survey, including whether or not their

Internet
The electronic means (and protocols) to connect computer users to information from a vast array of sources.

chosen programme of study was meeting expectations. The findings suggest that ongoing evaluation of training programmes is important as well as refining the marketing of counselling training programmes, given the factors that influence in students' choices.

LINKING SCIENCE WITH PRACTICE

Links between research and practice in the counselling field are relatively recent. Despite an expectation in the late 1980s and early 1990s that practitioners would avail themselves of published work in order to stay abreast of developments in the field, many instead preferred to research their own practices, even though this style of research was regarded by 'academic writers at that time as an inferior substitute of little validity' (Evans, 2008, p. 56). This led to studies that suggested there was a commonly held view among practitioners of a gap between research and practice. Since the mid-1990s, however, there has been a greater interest in the counselling field of the relevance of research and how this affects and influences practice. This was in part influenced by qualitative methodologies which, by then, had 'developed in strength and sophistication' (Evans, p. 57), along with action research emerging as a method.

Evans (2008) summarised the importance of research specifically in terms of the beneficial effects on practice as well as the benefits of both using and conducting research in counselling. This included noting the importance of the *Health Practitioners Competence Assurance Act 2003* (Ministry of Health, 2003) in producing an expectation that 'practice is based on research that has been rigorously produced through scientifically appropriate design and methodology' (Evans, p. 60). There are, therefore, increasing demands on practitioners to develop a practice based on research, and to utilise research to inform practice development.

McLeod (1999) stated that the idea of a 'scientist–practitioner' began in North America in the 1950s, and ultimately led to clinical psychology becoming a profession. He stated that the description 'scientist–practitioner' is most evident in this area of the helping professions, and also underpins practitioners using a cognitive-behavioural approach to counselling and therapy. He discussed the constraints of linking science with practice, pointing out that those principles that underpin 'mainstream scientific enquiry' (including rigour, objectivity and rationality) are difficult, perhaps even at times undesirable, principles to adopt in counselling research, which lends itself to partiality both because of the nature of the work and the 'inescapable moral visions of counselling' (McLeod, p. 18). Such notions are also described by Christopher (1996).

Karam and Sprenkle (2010) also discuss the constraints of the scientist–practitioner model: that although this may be realistic for doctoral students, it may not be such a good fit for Master's students whose primary ambition is to practise, rather than research. The authors coined the term 'research informed perspective' (Karam & Sprenkle, p. 307) in order to describe the differences between a 'scientist–practitioner framework' and a 'research-training model'. They suggest that it is important to 'infuse research into programs [sic] that desire to remain clinical in focus, but also research informed' (Karam & Sprenkle, p. 307). They offer 10 steps which they hope will help orient students and teachers towards 'research informed clinical practice' (Karam & Sprenkle, p. 314).

FUTURE DIRECTIONS FOR RESEARCH IN COUNSELLING

There is now an expectation that, along with other professional groups, research into counselling will be conducted within tertiary institutions (Crocket, Flanagan, Winslade, & Kotze, 2011b) and most educational programmes now include some research. Despite this, the task to engage practitioners to participate in, and apply, research to their practice— to become scientist–practitioners—continues. As Sheperis, Young and Daniels (2010) say: 'proponents of the scientist–practitioner model encourage counselors-in-training to approach all cases as formal research projects and to use empirical evidence in everyday practice' (p. 2). They suggest that future counsellors be trained to view their role in a new way. Whereas in the past training has focused on the development of clinical skills, they suggest the focus should now be on the development of skills that are integrated with research.

In 2002, the *New Zealand Journal of Counselling* republished an article from the British Association for Counselling and Psychotherapy (Goss & Rose, 2002) that promoted evidence-based practice. It suggested that practitioners should contribute to the evidence base by researching their own practice both quantitatively and qualitatively. According to Goss and Rose, randomised controlled trials offer the possibility of providing valuable evidence of effectiveness; they are, however, expensive to conduct and create difficulties when few counselling practitioners use single, pure theories or interventions. Another approach has been to use 'practice-based evidence', which seeks to research the reality of everyday counselling practice (Goss & Rose, 2002).

As the practice of counselling continues to develop a distinctly New Zealand approach, one that seeks to incorporate the principles of biculturalism and multiculturalism, and that more accurately reflects the local context, there is growing need to develop research methods that are culturally appropriate (Agee, Culbertson, Mariu, 2005; Bishop, 1996). As Agee, Culbertson and Mariu state, 'exciting developments are also evident in theorising Māori research methodologies, including the rising influence of post-colonialism' (p. 5).

SUMMARY

Research into counselling in Aotearoa New Zealand has been slow to have an impact outside of academia and the education of counsellors. This is a result of a combination of traditional ways of learning counselling and the nature of the activity itself. Until recently, quantitative methods were the most used and tended to focus on the practitioners' experiences but, as understanding of qualitative methodologies has developed, these are being employed more often. As counselling training is becoming more established in tertiary institutions, research and practice are becoming more integrated. New Zealand approaches to practice and research, which take account of the bicultural and multicultural context, are evolving.

REFLECTION POINTS

- What might assist you to continue to read and apply research in your future practice?
- How would you use current counselling evidence to guide your practice decisions?

STUDY QUESTIONS

1 What might be some of the limitations in using quantitative methods in counselling research?
2 Which sort of methodology is suited to your practice-based questions?
3 Which methodologies do you think will be more widely used in the future?

ADDITIONAL READING

Crocket, K., Flanagan, P., Winslade, J., & Kotze, E. (2011). Considering counsellor education in Aotearoa New Zealand Part 1: Looking back in order to look forward. *New Zealand Journal of Counselling. Special Issue*, 2–21.

Karam, E. A. & Sprenkle, D. H. (2010). The research-informed clinician: a guide to training the next generation MFT. *Journal of Marital and Family Therapy, 36*(3), 307–319.

Manthei, R. J. (2004). Encouraging counsellors to become active researchers and users of research. *New Zealand Journal of Counselling, 25*(1), 70–81.

McLeod, J. (1999). *Practitioner research in counselling*. London: Sage Publications.

Sheperis, C. J., Young, J. S., & Daniels, M. H. (2010). *Counseling research: quantitative, qualitative and mixed methods*. Upper Saddle River, NJ: Pearson Education.

REFERENCES

Agee, M., Culbertson, P., & Mariu, L. (2005). A bibliography of literature related to Maori mental health. *New Zealand Journal of Counselling, 26*(2), 1–36.

Anderson, R. (1991). Counselling: A practice in search of an explanation. *New Zealand Journal of Counselling, 13*, 2–12.

Aubrey, R. F. (1977). Historical development of guidance and counselling and implications for the future. *Personnel and Guidance Journal, 55*(6), 288–295.

Bedford, A. W., & Landry, S. T. (2010). Narrative research: interpreting lived experience. In Sheperis, C. J., Young, J. S., & Daniels, M. H. (Eds.). *Counseling research: Quantitative, qualitative, and single subject design.* Upper Saddle River, NJ: Prentice Hall.

Berrios, R., & Lucca, N. (2006). Qualitative methodology in counselling research: recent contributions and challenges for a new century. *Journal of Counseling & Development, 84*, 174–186.

Beutler, I. E. (1990). Introduction to the special series on advances in psychotherapy process research. *Journal of Consulting and Clinical Psychology, 58*(3), 263–264.

Bishop, R. *Collaborative research stories: Whakawhanaungatanga.* Palmerston North: The Dunmore Press.

Bunce, J. (1992). Counselling research and practice: The New Zealand experience. *New Zealand Journal of Counselling, 14*(2), 2–9.

Christopher, J. C. (1996). Counseling's inescapable moral visions. *Journal of Counseling and Development, 75*, 17–25.

Crocket, K. (2011). Teaching professional ethics in counsellor education in Aotearoa New Zealand. A small survey study. *New Zealand Journal of Counselling. Special Issue,* 40–58.

Crocket, K., Flanagan, P., Winslade, J., & Kotze, E. (2011a). Considering counsellor education in Aotearoa New Zealand Part 1: Looking back in order to look forward *New Zealand Journal of Counselling. Special Issue,* 2–21.

Crocket, K., Flanagan, P., Winslade, J., & Kotze, E. (2011b). Considering counsellor education in Aotearoa New Zealand Part 2: How might we practise? *New Zealand Journal of Counselling. Special Issue,* 133–143.

Evans, Y. (2008). Counsellors and research. Exploring the benefits of researching other counsellors' experiences. *New Zealand Journal of Counselling, 28*(1), 56–71.

Everts, H., & Withers, R. (2006). A practitioner survey of interactive drawing therapy as used in New Zealand. *New Zealand Journal of Counselling, 26*(4), 15–30.

Goss, S., & Rose, S. (2002). Evidence based practice: A guide for counselors and psychotherapists. *New Zealand Journal of Counselling, 23*(2), 67–76.

Gossman, M. (2011). Trainee counsellor's perceptions of their experiences of recording for supervision. *New Zealand Journal of Counselling. Special Issue*, 59–75.

Healy, L. (2008). Exploring the history of social work as a human rights profession. *International Social Work, 51*(6), 735–748.

Hertlein, K. M., & Lambert-Shute, J. (2007). Factors influencing student selection of marriage and family therapy graduate training programs. *Journal of Marital and Family Therapy, 33*, 18–34.

Karam, E. A., & Sprenkle, D. H. (2010). The research-informed clinician: A guide to training the next generation MFT. *Journal of Marital and Family Therapy, 36*(3), 307–319.

Kottler, J. A., & Shephard, D. S. (2004). *Introduction to counseling: Voices from the field*. Belmont, CA: Thompson Higher Education.

Manthei, R. (2006). What can clients tell us about seeking counselling and their experience of it? *New Zealand Journal of Counselling, 26*(4), 59–75.

Manthei, R. (2011). The work of a Christchurch community counselling centre: How successful has it been with its clients? *New Zealand Journal of Counselling. Special Issue, 26*(2), 70–87.

Marsden, V. (2011). Enriching future therapeutic conversations with lesbian clients. *New Zealand Journal of Counselling, 31*(1), 53–69.

Mearns, D., & Thorne, B. (2007). *Person-centred counselling in action*. Los Angeles, CA: Sage Publications.

McLeod, J. (1999). *Practitioner research in counselling*. London: Sage Publications.

McLeod, J. (2010). *Case study research in counseling and psychotherapy*. London: Sage Publications.

Miller, J. H. (2001). *Professional faces: Professionalisation as strategy in New Zealand counselling, 1974–1998*. Unpublished doctoral dissertation, University of Canterbury, Christchurch, New Zealand.

Ministry of Health. (2003). *Health Practitioners Competence Assurance Act 2003*. Wellington: Authors.

Paton, I. E. M. (2005). How to have your cake and eat it too: counselling in private practice. *New Zealand Journal of Counselling, 26*(2), 55–69.

Penny, R., Epston, D., & Agee, M. (2008). A history of marriage guidance in New Zealand: A personal reflection. *New Zealand Journal of Counselling, 28*(2), 1–9.

Raffensperger, M., & Miller, J. (2005). Counselling services for adults with an intellectual disability: implications for counselling. *New Zealand Journal of Counselling, 26*(2), 37–54.

Relationships Aotearoa. (n.d.). Retrieved from http://www.relationshipsaotearoa.org.nz

Sheperis, C. J., Young, J. S., & Daniels, M. H. (2010). *Counseling research: quantitative, qualitative and mixed methods.* Upper Saddle River, NJ: Pearson Education.

Sliedrecht, S. & Kotze, E. (2008). Hope and loss. Multiple realities when bodies are injured. *New Zealand Journal of Counselling, 28*(1), 72–86.

Waldegrave, C., Tamasese, K., Tuhaka, F., & Campbell, W. (2003). *Just therapy—a journey: A collection of papers from the Just Therapy team New Zealand.* Adelaide: Dulwich Centre Publications.

White, M., & Epston, D. (1990) *Narrative means to therapeutic ends.* New York, NY: Norton.

Young, J. S., Wiggens-Frame, M., & Cashwell, C. S. (2007). Spirituality and counsellor competence: A national survey of American Counseling Association members. *Journal of Counseling and Development, 85,* 47–52.

WEBSITES

New Zealand Association of Counsellors:
http://www.nzac.org.nz

Relationships Aotearoa:
http://www.relationshipsaotearoa.org.nz

CHAPTER 31

MIDWIFERY

JUDITH McARA-COUPER AND MARION HUNTER

CHAPTER OVERVIEW

This chapter covers the following topics:

- Evidence and research in midwifery
- Exploring midwifery research and scholarship
- Evidence-based midwifery practice

KEY TERMS

Contested
Evidence-based practice
Hermeneutic
Interviews
Knowing
Partnership

From the beginning of time, evidence has informed childbirth and midwifery practice. Empirical evidence collected through observation and even experimentation was passed from one woman to another.

EVIDENCE AND RESEARCH IN MIDWIFERY

Women in ancient times recognised that mortality is reduced when they received emotional and physical support in labour. This led to women seeking out others, often their kinswomen, to be present at the birth of their children (Trevathan, 1987; Rosenburg & Trevathan, 2001), and over time the role of the midwife emerged. This ancient knowing of women is seen in twenty-first century research, which reports that continuous support of women in childbirth is associated with less pharmacological analgesia, less intervention and greater satisfaction with midwifery (Hodnett, Gates, Hofmeyr, Sakala, & Weston, 2011).

Over the centuries, 'knowledge and evidence' has been a contested space with certain groups gaining authority to determine what counts as evidence and best practice. Much of the early knowledge and evidence that informed childbirth and midwifery was empirical knowledge. Empiricists gathered raw data from the sense experience, which they viewed as the starting point of knowledge. Rationalists (in contrast to empiricists) claimed that the ultimate starting point for all knowledge is not the senses, but reason. This latter view maintains that without prior categories and principles supplied by reason people cannot organise and interpret their sense experience in any meaningful way. This way of thinking is greatly influenced by the Greek philosophers Socrates, Plato and Aristotle. These philosophers and their contemporaries believed in a linear perspective of the world and that the power to reason and the ability to think logically distinguished humans over and above other species. They also believed that a life guided by reason was a superior life.

Changes in the seventeenth century meant that childbirth, the way women gave birth, and the evidence that informed this process were reconceptualised. The midwifery body of knowledge based on empirical evidence grew from an understanding of birth as primarily being natural and normal, and something to be attended or waited on—not hurried along or interfered with (Arney, 1982). The reconceptualisation of birth, informed by the changes in the seventeenth century, increasingly meant that birth became a 'thing' to be 'managed' and 'handled' and no longer a process to be waited on or attended to (Katz-Rothman, 1989; Wagner, 1994). This understanding of birth still informs many birthing practices throughout the Western world. Midwifery is both an art and a science, and it is important that midwives embrace the scientific methods and also those ways of knowing that are often ignored by the mainstream, such as embodied knowing and intuitive knowledge (Davis, 1995). Midwives need to draw on all sources of knowledge and develop the ability to critique all evidence so that women are provided with the best care based on the best knowledge and evidence available.

Knowing
Understanding, through being informed and aware.

Contested
Open to debate.

EXPLORING MIDWIFERY RESEARCH AND SCHOLARSHIP

Midwifery in many countries has a history of existing under sustained political attack and even coming close to extinction as a model of care. In Aotearoa New Zealand the committed and powerful political action of women and midwives in the 1980s and 1990s led to the model of midwifery care in place in New Zealand today. Much of the argument against midwives and midwifery as a profession was made in the name of science as those who had a monopoly on scientific knowledge sought to undermine the midwifery body of knowledge (Farley, 2005). Research and evidence, along with science, raise issues of power, values and the world views that are promulgated by particular approaches to knowledge. Research involves people who are socially and culturally situated and who determine what questions should be researched, what resources should be allocated to particular research and what designs and approaches should be given authority and validity (Farley, 2005). Therefore, it is of the utmost importance that midwives become researchers and developers of their own body of knowledge and think critically about research and science to ensure that midwifery evidence informs midwifery practice.

Midwifery journals and publications have a relatively short history. The *Midwifery Digest* (Midirs) was established in 1986, and the well-known midwifery journals such as *Birth* (1973), *Midwifery* (1980s), *British Journal of Midwifery* (1993) were all first published in the latter quarter of the last century, with the *New Zealand College of Midwives Journal*'s first publication being in the first decade of this century. The existence of midwife researchers and academics is also relatively recent even in countries that have a long history of midwifery. In 1992, Lesley Page became the first Professor of Midwifery in the United Kingdom, followed by Mary Renfrew and Mavis Kirkham. In Scotland in 1997, Tricia Murphy Black was the first midwifery professor and in Wales in 2005 it was Billie Hunter who became the first Professor of Midwifery in Ireland, followed in 2006 by Marlene Sinclair (Sinclair, 2006).

In Aotearoa New Zealand, as in other countries, the rise of midwifery scholarship and research came second to the political action that was required to re-establish midwifery as a profession (Smythe, 2007). However, while political action brought about change, scholarship and research were needed to give credibility, structure and authority to the changes (Smythe, 2007). This is no more clearly seen than in the development of the unique partnership model of midwifery that was established in New Zealand. Guilliland and Pairman (1995) first documented the model in their monograph entitled 'The midwifery partnership: A model for practice.' Also in 1995 Valerie Fleming graduated with New Zealand's first doctorate in Midwifery and its title was 'Partnership, power and politics: Feminist perceptions of midwifery practice'. This was the first research in New Zealand on a midwifery topic and it shows how research and evidence can work

Partnership
Genuine and respectful relationship between people.

alongside political change to give credibility and authority to an emerging midwifery model of practice (Gilkison, 1995).

Joan Donley, the esteemed elder and leader of midwifery during all the political change of the 1990s, was a great believer that midwives needed the evidence to support midwifery autonomy and practice (Smythe, 2007). Midwives need to gain research skills so that they can decide what will be researched, and will have control over analysis of data and dissemination of findings as only in this way can 'practice wisdom be offered as evidence' (White, cited in Smythe 2007, p. 23). The scholars and researchers in Aotearoa New Zealand on whose shoulders the rest of us stand are Joan Donley, Valerie Fleming, Karen Guilliland, Sally Pairman, Liz Smythe, Gillian White, Marilyn Foureur and Cheryl Benn. These women, and others who have followed them, have led the way in the phenomenal rise in midwifery research and scholarship in the past 30 years. Smythe (2007) states that 'it is scholarship that builds a strong foundation for women focused, politically attuned, on midwifery practice' (p. 25).

EVIDENCE-BASED MIDWIFERY PRACTICE

A new era in maternity care was launched after four interrelated publications convinced readers about the significant benefits of evidence-based care. The publications were four small books: *The Oxford Database of Perinatal Trials*, *Effective Care in Pregnancy and Childbirth*, *A Guide to Effective Care in Pregnancy and Childbirth*, and *Effective Care of the Newborn Infant* (Fox, 2011). The authors recall using these books and sensing that a change was imminent where evidence would inform practice as opposed to practice prescribed according to the preference of the head obstetrician or general practitioner within each obstetric or maternity unit. These publications were a prelude to the Cochrane Collaboration in 1993 and brought readable evidence to the notice of doctors, midwives and consumers.

Evidence-based practice
Practice that is informed by the careful consideration and evaluation of relevant information, and client/patient and practitioner experience and preference.

The introduction of evidence-based practice (EBP), described as care shown to be effective in target populations, was not without opposition. Doctors criticised EBP for taking away the decision-making tailored to each individual patient (Fox, 2011; Walsh, 2007). Walsh affirmed that the Cochrane database enabled systematic reviews to change clinical care, and this database set maternity care ahead of other health disciplines at that time. Walsh laments that some midwives continue to express doubts about EBP in a similar manner to historic criticism by doctors. Midwives need to keep up with changes in EBP by being open to new learning, by putting aside their personal beliefs and not relying on historical ways of clinical care in all situations (Armstrong, 2010; Page, 1997; Powell-Kennedy, Doig, Hackley, Leslie, & Tillman 2012). A change in attitude and habits alongside access to research is necessary for EBP to be linked with practice (Page, 1997; Waters, Rychetnik, Crisp, & Barrett, 2009).

Walsh (2007) cautioned midwives against reliance upon extensive years of experience as some midwives practise ineffective procedures repetitively over 20 years, such as frequent episiotomy and/or artificial rupture of membranes. A commitment to EBP is essential for credibility in clinical practice and for professional wisdom to develop (Fahy, 2008; Halldorsdottir & Karlsdottir, 2011).

Evidence should be based on studies of large numbers to eliminate bias. Systematic reviews are ranked at the highest level of evidence (McGowan, 2012) and random controlled trials are ranked as close second in the research hierarchy (see Chapter 4). McGowan describes systematic reviews as a summary of evidence that overrides the necessity to read each individual study in the world of rapidly changing information related to care during pregnancy, intrapartum, postpartum and the neonate.

Qualitative research (see Chapter 3) tends to have had less credibility; however, this is changing with acknowledgment of studies informing midwifery care. Cowan, Smythe and Hunter (2011) published findings from a hermeneutic study uncovering women's experience of severe pre-eclampsia in New Zealand. The disease is confusing in its presentation and thus is often missed, according to Cowan's in-depth interviews with women who shared their experience. The study revealed that while symptoms might appear 'ordinary' or similar to common antenatal complaints, the midwife needs to rule out the possibility of pre-eclampsia to prevent the catastrophic event of undiagnosed early onset pre-eclampsia. Qualitative studies have informed additional areas of practice such as women's experience of breastfeeding (Dykes, 2011), perineal trauma (East, Sherburn, Nagle, Said & Forster, 2012); parental attachment; and satisfaction of maternity care (Ministry of Health, 2012).

Hermeneutic
A set of principles or a method of interpretation.

Interviews
Conversations held for the purpose of gathering information.

CASE STUDY 31.1

CONTINUOUS SUPPORT FOR WOMEN DURING CHILDBIRTH: COCHRANE COLLABORATION INTERVENTION REVIEW

Hodnett and colleagues (2013) conducted a review of the Cochrane Pregnancy and Childbirth Groups' Trials register to assess the effects of continuous, one-to-one support of women during labour and delivery compared with usual care. Continuous supportive care may involve emotional support, comfort measures, provision of information and advocacy. This was provided by health staff

[continued next page]

(midwife or nurse) or a person of the woman's choice, such as a doula, partner or friend. The review also sought to determine what other factors influence the provision of continuous support and labour, and the resulting birth outcomes. For example, were outcomes different if continuous support was provided by a person who was part of the birthing woman's social network? This was a large review that analysed data from 22 trials in 16 different countries and over 15,000 women. Results demonstrated that when compared to women without continuous support, those who had continuous support 'were more likely to give birth spontaneously (i.e. gave birth without caesarean, forceps or vacuum). In addition, [these] women were less likely to have intra-partum analgesia, were more likely to be satisfied, had slightly shorter labours and their infants were less likely to have low five-minute Apgar scores' (Hodnett et al., np). Support from a person outside the woman's social network whose role it is to provide continuous labour support, who is experienced, and who has relevant training (that is, a doula) appears to have the most benefit. The authors surmised that continuous support should be made available to all women as it has clinically meaningful benefits and causes no known harm, not impacting on complication rates or breast feeding initiation. There is a longstanding midwifery tradition across cultures of women being continuously supported by other women during labour and delivery; it is satisfying that this time-honoured practice is relevant to the modern midwifery context and is supported by evidence.

RESEARCH ALIVE 31.1
EVIDENCE-BASED LEARNING

Midwives need to move beyond learning only after 'seeing' an event in a clinical situation and learn from EBP by reading and engaging (Waters et al., 2009). A midwife shared with students her astonishment when a young pregnant woman, with no risk factors whatsoever, screened positive for gestational diabetes. The young woman had requested all screening procedures during her pregnancy; hence undertook diabetes screening with informed choice. She was subsequently diagnosed with gestational diabetes mellitus (GDM) and treated to stabilise her blood sugar levels and reduce the risk of foetal macrosomia. After seeing this young woman diagnosed with GDM, the midwife stated that she henceforth recommended that every client undertake GDM screening as diabetes is frequently a hidden disease. This case illustrates the reinforcement of 'seeing' an event; however, the evidence for routine screening of all women for GDM had been published for many years prior to this event. Midwives are obligated to provide current evidence and enable women to then make an informed choice. Diagnosis of GDM is known to reduce incidence of pregnancy and neonatal complications without increasing the caesarean rate (Crowther et al., 2005) and women had improved psychological outcomes (Simmons et al., 2006; Simmons, Rowan, Reid, & Campbell, 2008).

CASE STUDY 31.2

BREAST FEEDING DURATION: SYSTEMATIC REVIEW

It has long been recognised by agencies such as the World Health Organization that exclusive breast feeding for the first six months of life is beneficial for infants and mothers. However, when best to introduce solid foods with continued breastfeeding, in particular the resulting impacts on childrens' growth, development and health, has been debated. To investigate this topic, Kramer and Kakuma (2012) conducted a systematic review of 23 studies from both developed and undeveloped countries. Review results suggest that exclusive breast feeding for six months compared with earlier mixed feeding (solid food introduction at three to four months with continued breast feeding) reduces rates of gastrointestinal infection, a leading cause of infant morbidity and mortality in undeveloped countries. It also positively impacts mothers' health by promoting post partum weight loss and delaying subsequent pregnancy. Results also identified that the duration of exclusive breast feeding made no difference to infants' risks of allergic disease, obesity and iron deficiency, nor did it impact on growth rates, cognitive ability or behaviour.

Midwives are well placed to advise child bearing women about the optimal duration of breast feeding, to clarify related infant outcomes, and, at discharge, to refer women to ongoing community breastfeeding support.

Effective education is paramount to implementing evidence-based practice. Waters et al. (2009) suggested that there is a point in time when individual differences regarding the meaning of evidence need to be put aside and the profession agrees on a national strategy of education, while leaders work towards a positive culture that enables change. An example

JUDITH McARA-COUPER AND MARION HUNTER

of the sense of disconnection between practice and evidence can be found in an Australian qualitative study (Fenwick et al., 2012) of 16 new graduate midwives who reported that they 'found it difficult to comprehend why they were educated to question and use their initiative and yet in practice were required to obey orders and conform' (p. 2060). Armstrong (2010) in similar manner, acknowledged the dilemma for midwifery students who were taught EBP at university, yet practised according to the direction of their midwife practice mentor, sometimes in order to pass or get 'signed off'. There is often a conflict between historical routine care and EBP in clinical settings where midwifery mentors favour traditional practice and coerce students into similar beliefs. It is disheartening that hierarchical structures prevail and impede the application of EBP by student midwives and new graduate midwives.

RESEARCH ALIVE 31.2
COMPARING THE MANAGEMENT OF LABOUR

One large study assessing active versus physiological management of the third stage of labour in the United Kingdom was criticised as a number of midwives in the study did not know how to do physiological management, yet were conducting this 'newly learnt' method during data collection (Prendiville, Harding, Elbourne, & Stirrat, 1988). The fact that midwives were not experienced with use of physiological management of the third stage raises doubts about the study findings. On occasions, publications might reveal findings that are contrary to those from a previous study. In such cases, the reader or midwife needs to apply research skills, discernment and elimination of their own bias, and compare the context of each study with the context of the midwife's own practice setting.

In situations where 'evidence' is not available, the usual practice is to refer to local guidelines such as New Zealand College of Midwives (NZCOM) consensus statements and Royal Australian New Zealand College of Obstetricians and Gynaecologists (RANZCOG) guidelines. The National Institute for Health and Clinical Excellence (NICE) guidelines are renowned for rigour regarding maternity care (Halldorsdottir & Karlsdottir, 2011). Guidelines need to be updated frequently (usually at least every two or three years) and should recommend judicious use as opposed to routine use of interventions (such as artificial rupture of membranes, oxytocin augmentation and opioid analgesia).

Guidelines are particularly useful in the management of less common situations such as iron infusion, medication, and monitoring for pre-eclampsia or cardiac disorders and other complicated conditions. It is difficult to recall management for all aspects of maternity care; guidelines assist midwives with more common issues such as prolonged rupture of membranes, induction of labour, hypoglycaemia of the newborn and jaundice of the newborn.

RESEARCH ALIVE 31.3
WHAT DIFFERENCE HAS EVIDENCE MADE
TO MIDWIFERY PRACTICE?

TOPIC	EBP FINDINGS	AUTHORS AND YEAR
Discontinuing routine episiotomy for primigravidae	Perineal tears are more comfortable than episiotomy.	Sleep et al. (1984) Bick (2011)
Birthplace and outcomes for low risk women	Women without risk factors have less interventions when they commence labour in primary maternity units.	Davis et al. (2011) Hunter et al. (2011) Stapleton, Osborne, & Illuzzi (2013)
Continuity of care and analgesia	Continuous support in labour enables women to use less analgesia.	Hodnett et al. (2011)
Expertise in expectant management of third stage of labour	Expert midwives shared their experience of expectantly managing the third stage.	Begley, Guilliland, Reilly, & Keegan, (2012)
Exploring the protection, promotion and support of breastfeeding over 25 years	Removal of detrimental practices has improved breastfeeding rates.	Dykes, (2011)
Differentiating postpartum depression from other disorders	Beck distinguishes depression, panic disorder and post-traumatic stress disorder.	Beck, Gable, Sakala, & Declercq (2011)

SUMMARY

Midwives are expected to keep up to date with new research, treatments and interventions so that they are able to give women and their partners accurate information to inform their choices. Midwives are faced with the continual challenge of promoting physiological birth while being aware that detection of problems is in the interest of the woman and baby's well-being. Utilisation of EBP should foster confidence in physiological birth and timely interventions when deviations or complications are apparent.

REFLECTION POINTS

- Discuss how 'knowledge and evidence' has been a contested space with certain groups gaining authority in order to determine what counts as evidence and 'best practice'.
- What enables a group to gain authority and determine what counts as evidence?

JUDITH McARA-COUPER AND MARION HUNTER

- State what you think are the main factors in the 'midwifery body of knowledge'.
- What were the origins of evidence-based practice?
- Can you think of any barriers that might stop a midwife from practising in an evidence-based way?

STUDY QUESTIONS

1 How has the 'knowing' of women informed the body of knowledge around childbirth and childbirth practices?

2 How did the changes in the seventeenth century lead to a 'reconceptualisation of childbirth'?

3 How do the changes from the seventeenth century still influence the midwifery body of knowledge in the twenty-first century?

4 What link does research and scholarship have with the political action that led to the changes in the law around midwifery in the 1990s?

5 Why is it important that midwives do research about midwifery?

6 Discuss how evidence-based practice has contributed to changes within midwifery clinical practice.

7 How can qualitative research inform the findings of quantitative research?

8 What do midwives do when there is no research available related to a particular question or topic, and what documents can midwives refer to for guidance in practice?

9 Why should evidence-based practice 'foster confidence in physiological birth' and timely interventions when deviations or complications are apparent?

ADDITIONAL READING

Borbasi, S., & Jackson, D. (2011). *Navigating the maze of research: enhancing nursing and midwifery practice*. Chatswood: Elsevier.

Parry, D. C. (2008). 'We wanted a birth experience, not a medical experience': Exploring Canadian women's use of midwifery. *Health Care for Women International, 29*(8–9), 784–806.

REFERENCES

Armstrong, N. (2010). Clinical mentors' influence on student midwives' clinical practice. *British Journal of Midwifery, 18*(2), 114–123.

Arney, W. (1982). *Power and the profession of obstetrics*. Chicago: University of Chicago Press.

Beck, C., Gable, R., Sakala, C., & Declercq, E. (2011). Posttraumatic stress disorder in new mothers: Results from a two-stage U.S. national survey. *Birth, 38*, 216–227.

Begley, C., Guilliland, K., Reilly, M., & Keegan, C. (2012). Irish and New Zealand midwives' expertise in expectant management of the third stage of labour: The MEET study. *Midwifery, 28*, 733–739.

Bick, D. (2011). Evidence based midwifery practice: Take care to 'mind the gap'. *Midwifery, 27*, 569–570.

Cowan, J., Smythe, E., & Hunter, M., (2011). Women's lived experience of severe early onset preeclampsia: a hermeneutic analysis. In G. Thomson, F. Dykes, & S. Downe (Eds.), *Qualitative research in midwifery and childbirth: phenomenological approaches.* London: Routledge.

Crowther, C., Hiller, J., Moss, J., McPhee, A., Jeffries, W., & Robinson, J. (2005). Effect of treatment of gestational diabetes mellitus on pregnancy outcomes. *New England Journal of Medicine, 352*, 2477–2486.

Davis, D. (1995). Ways of knowing in midwifery. *Australian College of Midwives Incorporated Journal, 8*(3), 30–32.

Davis, D., Baddock, S., Pairman, S., Hunter, M., Benn, C., Wilson, D., et al. (2011). Planned place of birth in New Zealand: does it affect mode of birth and intervention rates in low-risk women? *Birth, 38*, 111–119.

Dykes, F. (2011). Twenty five years of breast feeding research in Midwifery. *Midwifery, 27*, 8–14.

East, C., Sherburn, M., Nagle, C., Said, J., & Forster, D. (2012). Perineal pain following childbirth: Prevalence, effects on postnatal recovery and analgesia usage. *Midwifery, 28.* 93–97.

Fahy, K. (2008). Evidence-based midwifery and power/knowledge. *Women and Birth, 21*, 1–2.

Farley, C. (2005). Midwifery research history. A Delphi survery of midwifery scholars. *American College of Nurse Midwives, 50*(2), 122–128.

Fenwick, J., Hammond, A., Raymond, J., Smith, R., Gray, J., Foureur, M., et al. (2012). Surviving not thriving: A qualitative study of newly qualified midwives experience of their transition to practice. *Journal of Clinical Nursing, 21*, 2054–2063.

Fox, D. M. (2011). Systematic reviews and health policy: The influence of a project on perinatal care since 1988. *The Milbank Quarterly, 89*(3), 425–449. Retrieved from http://www.jameslindlibrary.org

Gilkison, A. (1995). New Zealand's first doctorate in midwifery! *New Zealand College of Midwives Journal,* April, 12, 11.

Guilliland, K., & Pairman, S. (1995). *The midwifery partnership: a model for practice. Monograph series 95/1.* Wellington: Victoria University of Wellington, Department of Nursing and Midwifery.

Halldorsdottir, S., & Karlsdottir, S. I. (2011). The primacy of the good midwife in midwifery services: an evolving theory of professionalism in midwifery. *Scandinavian Journal of Caring Sciences, 25*, 806–817.

Hodnett, E. D., Gates, S., Hofmeyr, G. J., Sakala, C., & Weston, J. (2011). Continuous support for women during childbirth (review). *The Cochrane Library, 2.*

Hodnett, E. D., Gates, S., Hofmeyr, G. J., Sakala, C., & Weston, J. (2013). Continuous support for women during childbirth (review—updated). *Cochrane Database of Systematic Reviews, 7*, Art. No. CD003766.

Hunter, M., Pairman, S., Benn, C., Baddock, S., Davis, D., Dixon, L., et al. (2011). Do low risk women actually birth in their planned place of birth and does ethnicity influence women's choice of birthplace? *New Zealand College of Midwives Journal, 44*, 5–11.

Katz-Rothman, B. (1989). *Recreating motherhood. Ideology and technology in a patriarchal society.* New York, NY: W.W. Norton & Company.

Kramer, M. & Kakuma, R. (2012). Optimal duration of exclusive breast feeding. *Cochrane Database of Systematic Reviews, 8*, Art. No. CD003517.

McGowan, L. (2012). Systematic reviews: the good, the not so good and the good again. *British Journal of Midwifery, 20*(8), 588–592.

Ministry of Health (2012). *Maternity consumer surveys 2011.* Wellington: Ministry of Health.

Page, L. (1997). Evidence-based practice in midwifery: A virtual revolution. *Journal of Clinical Effectiveness, 2*(1), 10–13. Retrieved from http://ezproxy.aut.ac.nz/login?url=http://search.proquest.com/docview/208439772?accountid=8440

Powell-Kennedy, H., Doig, E., Hackley, B., Leslie, M., & Tillman, S. (2012). The midwifery two-step: A study of evidence based practice. *Journal of Midwifery & Women's Health, 57*, 454–460.

Prendiville, W., Harding, J., Elbourne, D., & Stirrat, G. (1988). The Bristol third stage trial: active versus physiological management of third stage of labour. *British Medical Journal, 297*(6659), 1295–1300.

Rosenberg, K. R., & Trevathan, W. R. (2001). The evolution of human birth. *Scientific American, 285*(5), 72–77.

Simmons, D., Rowan, J., Reid, R., & Campbell, N. (2008). Screening, diagnosis and services for women with gestational diabetes mellitus (GDM) in New Zealand: A technical report from the National GDM Technical Working Party. *New Zealand Medical Journal.* Retrieved from http://journal.nzma.org.nz/journal/121-1270/2950

Simmons, D., Wolmarans, L., Cutchie, W., Johnson, E., Haslam, A., Roodt, C., et al. (2006). Gestational diabetes mellitus: Time for consensus on screening and diagnosis. *The New Zealand Medical Journal, 119.* Retrieved from http://journal.nzma.org.nz/journal/119-1228/1807

Sinclair, M. (2006). History in the making: a personal chair in midwifery research for Northern Ireland [Editorial]. *Evidence Based Midwifery, 4*(3), 75.

Sleep, J., Grant, A., Garcia, J., Elbourne, D., Spencer, J., & Chalmers, I. (1984) West Berkshire perineal management trial. *British Medical Journal, 289,* 587–590.

Smythe, L. (2007). A hermeneutical analysis of the rise of scholarship in midwifery. *New Zealand College of Midwives Journal, 37,* 20–26.

Stapleton, S. R., Osborne, C., & Illuzi, J. (2013). Outcomes of care in birth centers: Demonstration of a durable model. *Journal of Midwifery & Women's Health, 58*(1), 3–14.

Trevathan, W. R. (1987). *Human birth: An evolutionary perspective.* New York, NY: Aldine de Gruyter.

Wagner, M. (1994). *Pursuing the birth machine.* Camperdown: ACE Graphics.

Walsh, D. (2007). *Evidence based care for labour and birth: a guide for midwives.* Oxon: Routledge.

Waters, D., Rychetnik, L., Crisp, J., & Barrett A. (2009). Views on evidence from nursing and midwifery opinion leaders. *Nurse Education Today, 29,* 829–834.

WEBSITES

Home Birth Aotearoa:
http://www.homebirth.org.nz

Joan Donley Midwifery Research Collaboration:
http://www.midwife.org.nz/research

Centre for Midwifery and Women's Health Research:
http://www.aut.ac.nz/study-at-aut/study-areas/health-sciences/research/centre-for-midwifery-and-womens-health-research

CHAPTER 32

INTERPROFESSIONAL LEARNING

ANTOINETTE McCALLIN AND BRENDA FLOOD

CHAPTER OVERVIEW

This chapter covers the following topics

- The changing context of interprofessional learning
- Key definitions
- Interprofessional learning research

KEY TERMS

Collaborative practice

Hypothesis

Interprofessional

Interprofessional collaboration

Interprofessional education

Interprofessional learning

Relationships

Interprofessional learning is defined as a formal or informal process whereby different professionals interact and learn from each other (Freeth, Hammick, Reeves, Koppel, & Barr, 2005). The evidence about interprofessional learning has developed gradually, as its importance in interprofessional working has been better understood. The reasons for the development are linked to the professional practice context, which has changed substantially in recent years. As the context changes, the type of knowledge that is needed for professional practitioners alters, and research evidence that is valued changes as well. Such change occurred in the area of interprofessional learning which, in the 1960s, was merged under the broad interprofessional umbrella that included interprofessional education and collaboration. Initially, understandings of interprofessional learning were vague in that learning together apparently occurred when different health professionals were involved in shared learning situations, even though students had no interaction at all (Miller, Freeman, & Ross, 2001). Research evidence about interprofessional learning was minimal.

THE CHANGING CONTEXT OF INTERPROFESSIONAL LEARNING

Initially health professionals and educators were not very interested in interprofessional learning. They wanted evidence about collaborative practice that was promoted as a new model of care in primary health care (World Health Organization, 1978). Changes from institutional to community care had raised all sorts of questions about models of care, but evidence about the strengths or weaknesses of the models was lacking. Collaborative practice was especially problematic, as health professionals had not learned how to collaborate. The World Health Organization (WHO) (1988) for instance questioned the effectiveness of multidisciplinary teamwork that dominated care. This resulted in a call for health professionals to learn how to work together in teams. The emphasis was on learning together and developing research evidence about teamwork. The change in direction was challenging for health professionals who were educated separately from each other and usually learned collaboration once they were qualified practitioners (McCallin, 2005). Nonetheless, the WHO (1988) report drew attention to the lack of evidence about interprofessional working and learning, and the need for research evidence to support decision-making (Casto & Julia, 1994; Leathard, 1994; Soothill, Mackay, & Webb, 1995). Research evidence about teams and teamwork followed (McCallin, 1999; Ovretveit, 1996).

Various interprofessional learning initiatives in pre-registration health professional education programmes followed (Cote, Lauzon, & Kyd-Strickland, 2008). Initiatives were driven by legislation, policy development, and health service modernisation

Interprofessional learning
Learning that involves students engaging (learning with and about) their professional groups.

Interprofessional
Relating to the interaction between two or more professionals.

Interprofessional education
Education in which students from various professions learn about, from and with each other.

Collaborative practice
Practice involving many health workers from different professional backgrounds working together with patients, families, carers and communities to deliver the highest quality of care.

(Bell et al., 2009; Hean, Macleod Clark, Adams, & Humphris, 2006; Philippon, Pimlott, King, Day, & Cox, 2005). Professional bodies in particular wanted evidence about the success of interprofessional learning and its effectiveness in developing collaborative skills for students.

The evidence was eventually evaluated in another WHO (2010) report that synthesises the research evidence about interprofessional education and collaborative practice, both of which need to be supported by interprofessional learning. The report emphasises the need for a new model of care to improve health outcomes for populations and manage the worldwide shortage of 4.3 million health workers. According to the WHO (2010), 'The health workforce [needs to be] more flexible, and better prepared to maximise limited resources' (p. 13). It summarises the baseline research evidence about knowledge in the interprofessional field. As such, it is useful in a changing context, as it draws attention to the need to prepare health professional students to think differently, so that they understand others' perspectives, and can solve patient problems in new ways (Barr, 2009). The overall goal of interprofessional learning is to ensure that undergraduate students learn collaborative skills that will improve the efficiency and sustainability of the health system (Ministry of Business, Innovation and Employment, 2009). Therefore, evidence about interprofessional learning is important to ensure that student learning opportunities are carefully facilitated and approaches to learning are supported with rigorous and reliable evidence.

In this chapter the scene has been set by outlining the changing context for the development of interprofessional learning. Next, key definitions are clarified, and a justification for interprofessional learning is provided. Then a selection of the interprofessional learning research is outlined, the evidence from the systematic reviews in the area is summarised, and future directions for research are identified.

KEY DEFINITIONS

Developing evidence about interprofessional learning has been challenging, because of the debate about how the concept is defined. In fact, several definitions had an influence on developing evidence in the interprofessional field (Reeves et al., 2011). This caused all sorts of confusion. Despite the problems, it is now clear that interprofessional learning is an active process, requiring interaction and engagement (Freeth et al., 2005). Learning proceeds more smoothly if participants are co-located, value others, learn about each other, trust and respect one another, and learn to have confidence in a colleague's knowledge base (Bainbridge & Woods, 2012). Not surprisingly, all of these factors influence learning potential. Clearly the learner cannot be passive in the process. At the same time interprofessional learning may occur spontaneously or it may be the result of more structured interprofessional education activities (Howkins & Bray, 2008).

In interprofessional education 'two or more professions learn with, from and about each other to improve collaboration and the quality of care' (Freeth et al., 2005, p. xv). The justification for emphasising this way of learning is outlined in Research Alive 32.1.

RESEARCH ALIVE 32.1
ENABLING INTERPROFESSIONAL LEARNING

The interprofessional way of working is promising, as it offers a potential solution to some of the challenges occurring in health care today. If students can understand why it is important for them to learn with professionals from other disciplines they may be better prepared to manage:

- the increasing complexity of problems affecting individuals, families, and communities and be more adaptable to developing new approaches to care that support an ageing population and people with chronic conditions (Barr & Low, 2012; Lewy, 2012; Thistlethwaite, 2012; WHO, 2010);
- interprofessional **relationships** and integrate the different specialisations (Barr & Low, 2012);
- rising health care costs and suggest innovative solutions to health and human resource issues (Barr & Low, 2012; Lewy, 2012; WHO, 2010);
- inter-agency fragmentation (Barr & Low, 2012; Lewy, 2012);
- quality and safety issues (Barr & Low, 2012; Lewy, 2012; Reeves et al., 2009);
- consumer expectations (McKeown, Malihi-Shoja, & Downe, 2010).

> **Relationships**
> The similarities and connections between people or variables in any given situation.

However, if interprofessional learning is to be promoted, students need clear guidelines for learning. The Canadian Interprofessional Health Collaborative (CIHC) (2010) developed a National Interprofessional Competency Framework which identifies the attitudes, knowledge, skills, and behaviour required for collaborative practice. While there are several international competency frameworks and the definitions and measurement associated with them are in question (Reeves, 2012), a framework is useful to provide direction for the development of research evidence. The competency areas outlined by the Canadian Interprofessional Health Collaborative (2010) include:

- interprofessional communication;
- patient/client/family/community-centred care;
- role clarification;
- team functioning;
- collaborative leadership; and
- interprofessional conflict resolution (p. 9).

Student and practitioner demonstration of interprofessional competencies is central to interprofessional learning, as they identify the collaborative skills already mentioned. The aim of the competencies is to promote interprofessional collaboration, which is 'the process of developing and maintaining effective interprofessional working relationships with learners, practitioners, patients, clients, families and communities to enable optimal health outcomes' (Thistlethwaite, 2012, p. 60). The fact that there are several competency frameworks suggests that research evidence would be useful to clarify exactly what is important for interprofessional collaboration. Despite differences, the emphasis in interprofessional learning is on developing knowledge about other professionals, understanding different approaches to client care, interprofessional communication, teamwork, and shared goal-setting.

The ultimate goal is to provide the best outcomes for clients. Figure 32.1 represents the sequence and outcome of interprofessional education, learning and collaborative practice. It illustrates that the development and delivery of effective interprofessional education supports interprofessional learning, which in turn promotes interprofessional collaboration. The ultimate goal is to improve the best possible health outcomes for clients.

Interprofessional collaboration
The process of practitioners from different professions working together in a meaningful way.

FIGURE 32.1   THE SEQUENCE AND OUTCOME OF INTERPROFESSIONAL EDUCATION, LEARNING AND COLLABORATIVE PRACTICE

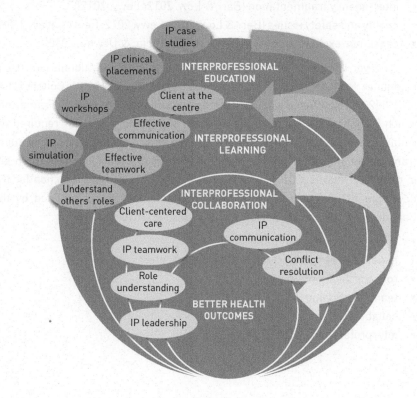

Learning together can be challenging and may depend on the attitudes students bring with them when they enter a programme (see Case Study 32.1).

CASE STUDY 32.1

INTERPROFESSIONAL ATTITUDES

Have you considered your attitudes towards other professional groups? Attitudes are based on assumptions, stereotypes and the previous experience of health professionals, or they may come from the way a profession is portrayed in the media. What does the research evidence say about interprofessional attitudes?

Perhaps not surprisingly, the attitudes of different professional groups affect a student's ability to learn with other health professionals. The evidence in one study (Coster et al., 2008) is quantitative and was collected four times during a student's course of study. Sixteen hundred and eighty three undergraduate health students were surveyed to measure their interprofessional attitudes. The students came from nine different professional groups (Coster et al., 2008). The measurement tools—the Readiness for Interprofessional Learning Scale, the Professional Identity Scale and the Contact Index—all have well-documented reliability and validity, suggesting that this evidence is trustworthy. The researchers found that undergraduate students had positive attitudes towards learning with other health professionals upon entry into a programme. However, attitudes about interprofessional learning declined significantly over the course of their studies. Students who began with negative attitudes did not change their mindset towards others at all. The researchers concluded that interprofessional education has little effect on changing interprofessional attitudes. Although the researchers were not clear about the reasons for the decline in attitudes, they concluded that there was some connection between readiness to learn with others and interference with professional identity.

Clearly, student attitudes have a significant influence on the interprofessional communication and teamwork that are the baseline collaborative skills. The research evidence suggests that interprofessional collaboration is more likely when undergraduate students are socialised to work interprofessionally with colleagues from different disciplines. Case Study 32.2 illustrates the importance of learning how to work with different health professionals in practice.

ANTOINETTE McCALLIN AND BRENDA FLOOD

CASE STUDY 32.2

INTERPROFESSIONAL TRAINING WARDS

Have you engaged in any interprofessional learning activities as an undergraduate student? What do you think you would gain from learning with other health professional students? While there is evidence about both the problems and benefits of undergraduate interprofessional learning experiences, a positive example is outlined below.

'Learning together to be able to work together' was the motto developed by a number of university hospitals in Sweden that went on to establish interprofessional training wards in the 1990s (Hylin, 2010). The interprofessional training wards provide interprofessional learning opportunities for health students and are located within a hospital or other care institution. Students work as part of an interprofessional team with real patients in the provision of high-quality patient care, independently but with supervision. They are able to develop their own professional role and in the process learn about the roles of others, as they develop knowledge and skills in effective communication, and promote patient-centred care (Hylin, 2010).

This research is based on four studies, which used a mix of quantitative and qualitative evidence. Evidence was collected from questionnaires and observations, and the researcher reported that students had a clearer understanding of their professional role and learning about the roles of other health professionals during the placement. Interestingly, the students found that team-building activities prior to the clinical learning experience improved teamwork and collaboration in the student teams (Hylin, 2010).

When students are learning, it can be challenging to know how to communicate professionally with those who come from other professions. What are some of the things you can do to make this easier?

How might you prepare yourself for this interprofessional communication?

Students need interprofessional learning opportunities so that they can engage in learning experiences that will prepare them for collaborative practice (Freeth, et al. 2005). But what evidence is there to support this **hypothesis**? What interprofessional content should be included? When should it be scheduled; pre- or post-registration? How might interprofessional learning be organised? Who should be involved? Interprofessional learning sounds reasonable, but becomes more complex when context and professional traditions are considered (Thistlethwaite, 2012).

Hypothesis
A speculative explanation for a problem that can be tested by further research.

INTERPROFESSIONAL LEARNING RESEARCH

Many approaches have been used to generate evidence about interprofessional learning. Most of the evidence is quantitative, although a few qualitative studies are now available. One excellent example of a valid and reliable (McFadyen, Webster, Strachan, Figgins, Brown, & McKechnie, 2005; McFadyen, Webster, & Maclaren, 2006) tool for quantitative measurement is the Readiness for Interprofessional Learning Scale (Parsell & Bligh, 1999). There is emerging evidence that well-planned and -executed interprofessional education with students, learning in groups with different disciplines, promotes the adoption of positive attitudes towards each other (Anderson, Thorpe, & Hammick, 2011). While there have been many developments in interprofessional learning, Thistlethwaite (2012) suggests there is little empirical evidence that interprofessional education is effective in changing attitudes towards different health professionals in practice. This was seen in the case study above. Overall, the quantitative evidence suggests that some students do not engage in interprofessional learning at all. While it may be offered in an educational setting, there are many questions about its sustainability in practice. In contrast, Pollard, Miers and Rickaby (2012) employed a qualitative design to generate evidence on extensive undergraduate interprofessional learning initiatives and their effectiveness in preparing practitioners to work interprofessionally after qualification. This evidence offers an alternative perspective of interprofessional learning. Results are quite limited though, as there were only 29 participants in the study. Although Pollard et al. conclude that interprofessional learning encourages changes in attitudes and perceptions towards other professions, Braithwaite et al. (2012) have evidence that organisational structures compromise interprofessional working and, despite the call for collaboration in practice, doctors in particular have not at all changed their attitudes towards working more closely with other health professionals.

Even though there is evidence emphasising the positive benefits of promoting interprofessional learning, the challenges also need to be considered. Newell-Jones (2008) reviews the evidence and identifies major issues that are now well recognised in the interprofessional field. Not surprisingly, the definitional confusion has caused problems because there have been different professional motives and expectations. Second, there is evidence that context, power and authority issues have a significant effect on interprofessional learning. In particular, professional identity, policy and accreditation changes highlight power and status differences, all of which influence evidence development. Third, there is evidence that cost-cutting is driving the need for interprofessional learning. Fourth, it seems that interprofessional learning is complex and this causes competing professional agendas. Finally, effective facilitation of interprofessional learning is critical and facilitators need to be experienced in managing interprofessional diversity and conflict.

Another gap in the evidence about interprofessional learning relates to the fact that there is no research showing that interprofessional learning improves collaboration and health outcomes for patients (Hammick, Freeth, Koppel, Reeves, & Barr, 2007; Pollard, Miers, Gilchrist, & Sayers, 2006). Salvatori, Berry and Eva (2007) have evidence that interprofessional learning promotes role understanding, communication and teamwork—this is a beginning. Suter and Deutschlander (2010) synthesise knowledge about interprofessional collaboration and report that students experiencing interprofessional clinical placements are more likely to seek interprofessional working situations once they are registered. Various research studies are evaluated in that report, although the conclusions are questionable if the methodology is examined closely. Not surprisingly, leaders and practitioners in the field have looked to the systematic reviews to judge the quality of the evidence.

An attempt to conduct a systematic review of interprofessional learning failed (Barr, 1998), as none of the studies available met the inclusion criteria (Cooper, Carlisle, Gibbs, & Watkins, 2001). Another systematic review (Barr, Koppel, Reeves, Hammick, & Freeth, 2005) reported that interprofessional education fostered interprofessional interaction and collaboration, both of which are fundamental to interprofessional learning. A later best evidence, systematic review (Hammick et al., 2007) found, however, that 'evidence to support the proposition that learning together will help practitioners and agencies work better together remains limited and thinly spread' (p. 735). This systematic review provides useful baseline empirical evidence in the area, as it goes beyond the anecdotal discussions that were typical at the time. Nevertheless, another updated systematic review (Reeves et al., 2010) concluded that, while some progress had been made in developing the interprofessional knowledge base, further rigorous evidence was required to see if interprofessional initiatives improved client outcomes and collaborative practice. The results of these reviews are important when considering the future of interprofessional learning.

SUMMARY

While interprofessional learning appears to be a promising concept to be incorporated into health professional education, the evidence supporting its inclusion is limited. Much has been written in the interprofessional field and many initiatives have been published. Yet evaluation of methodology in particular has rarely occurred. This raises questions about the quality of the knowledge informing interprofessional learning and practice. Similarly, interprofessional changes are seldom appraised and measurement tools to assist in this process are few and far between. Consequently, it is argued that there is extensive interprofessional literature that needs to be viewed with caution, as evidence in the field requires substantial development.

REFLECTION POINTS

- What other factors might influence your attitudes towards learning with students from other professions?
- Why do issues about your developing professional identity influence learning with other health professional students?
- What sort of learning activities might help students to develop a willingness to learn to work with other health professional students?
- If you consider the evidence presented overall in this chapter, what are your impressions about the emphasis on interprofessional learning?
- What are the advantages and disadvantages of interprofessional learning?
- What are some of the barriers and how might these be managed?
- How might you use current interprofessional learning evidence in your practice?

STUDY QUESTIONS

1 What has been the most common research methodology used in interprofessional learning research?
2 Which methodology might be better suited to answer practice-based research questions?

ADDITIONAL READING

Freeth, D., Goodsman, D., & Copperman, J. (2009). *Being interprofessional*. Cambridge: Polity Press.

Humphris, D., & Hean, S. (2004). Educating the future workforce: Building the evidence about interprofessional learning. *Journal of Health Services Research and Policy, 9,* 24–27.

McFadyen A. K., Webster V. S., & Maclaren W.M. (2006). The test-retest reliability of a revised version of the Readiness for Interprofessional Learning Scale (RIPLS). *Journal of Interprofessional Care, 20*(6), 633–639.

Meads, G., Ashcroft, J., Barr, H., Scott, R., & Wild, A. (2005). *The case for interprofessional collaboration in health and social care*. Oxford: Blackwell Publishing Ltd.

Pollard, K. C., Thomas, J., & Miers, M. (2010). *Understanding interprofessional working in health and social care: Theory and practice*: Palgrave Macmillan Limited.

Reeves, S., Lewin, S., Espin, S., & Zwarenstein, M. (2010). *Interprofessional teamwork for health and social care*. Oxford: Blackwell Publishing Ltd.

Reeves, S., Zwarenstein, M., Goldman, J., Barr, H., Freeth, D., Koppel, I., & Hammick, M. (2010). The effectiveness of interprofessional education: Key findings from a new systematic review. *Journal of Interprofessional Care, 24*, 230–241.

REFERENCES

Anderson, E. S., Thorpe, L. N., & Hammick, M. (2011). Interprofessional staff development: Changing attitudes and winning hearts and minds. *Journal of Interprofessional Care, 25*, 11–17.

Bainbridge, L., & Woods, V. I. (2012). The power of propositions: Learning with, from and about others in the context of interprofessional education. *Journal of Interprofessional Care, 26*, 452–458.

Barr, H. (1998). Cochrane review of outcomes from interprofessional practice. *Education in Health Change in Training and Practice, 11*, 402–403.

Barr, H. (2009). Interprofessional education as an emerging concept. In P. Bluteau, & A. Jackson (Eds.), *Interprofessional education: Making it happen*. London: Palgrave Macmillan.

Barr, H., Koppel, I., Reeves, S., Hammick, M., & Freeth, D. (2005). *Effective interprofessional education: Assumption, argument and evidence*. London: Blackwell Science.

Barr, H., & Low, H. (2012). *Interprofessional education in pre-registration courses: A CAIPE guide for commissioners and regulators of education*. Farnham: Centre for the Advancement of Interprofessional Education.

Bell, C., Dunston, R., Fitzgerald, T., Hawke, G., Lee, A., Lee, A., et al. (2009). *Interprofessional health education in Australia: The way forward*. Sydney: Australian Learning and Teaching Council. Retrieved December 19, 2012, from http://www.altc.edu.au/resources?text=Interprofessional+Health+Education+in+Australia%3+The+Way+Forward

Braithwaite, J., Westbrook, M., Nugus, P., Greenfield, D., Travaglia, J., Runciman, W., et al. (2012). Continuing differences between health professions' attitudes: The saga of accomplishing systems-wide interprofessionalism. *International Journal of Quality and Health Care, 25*(1), 8–15.

Casto, R. M., & Julia, M. C. (1994). *Interprofessional care and collaborative practice: Commission on interprofessional education and practice*. Pacific Grove, CA: Brooks/Cole.

Canadian Interprofessional Health Collaborative (CIHC). (2010). *A national interprofessional competency framework*. Retrieved from http://www.cich.ca/files/CIHC_IPCompetencies_Feb1210.pdf

Cooper, H., Carlisle, C., Gibbs, T., & Watkins, C. (2001). Developing the evidence base for interdisciplinary learning: A systematic review. *Journal of Advanced Nursing, 35*, 228–237.

Coster, S., Norman, I., Murrells, T., Kitchen, S., Meerabeau, E., Sooboodoo, E., et al. (2008). Interprofessional attitudes amongst undergraduate students in the health professions: A longitudinal questionnaire survey. *International Journal of Nursing Studies, 45*, 1667–1681.

Cote G., Lauzon C., & Kyd-Strickland, B. (2008). Environmental scan of interprofessional collaborative practice initiatives. *Journal of Interprofessional Care, 22*, 449–460.

Freeth, D., Hammick, M., Reeves, S., Koppel, I., & Barr, H. (2005). *Effective interprofessional education: Development, delivery and evaluation*. Oxford: Blackwell Science.

Hammick, M., Freeth, D., Koppel, I., Reeves, S., & Barr, H. (2007). A best evidence systematic review of interprofessional education. *Medical Teacher, 29*, 735–751.

Hean, S., Macleod Clark, J., Adams, K., & Humphris, D. (2006). Will opposites attract? Similarities and differences in students' perceptions of the stereotype profiles of other health and social care professional groups. *Journal of Interprofessional Care, 20*(2), 162–181.

Howkins, E., & Bray, J. (2008). *Preparing for interprofessional teaching: Theory and practice*. Oxford: Radcliffe.

Hylin, U. (2010). *Interprofessional education: Aspects on learning together on an interprofessional training ward*. Unpublished doctoral dissertation, Krolinska Institute, Stockholm, Sweden.

Leathard, A. (Ed.). (1994). *Going interprofessional: Working together for health and welfare*. London: Routledge.

Lewy, L. (2012). The complexities of interprofessional learning/working: Has the agenda lost its way? *Health Education Journal, 69*, 4–12.

McCallin, A. M. (1999). *Pluralistic dialoguing: A grounded theory of interdisciplinary teamwork*. Unpublished doctoral dissertation, Massey University, Palmerston North, New Zealand.

McCallin, A. M. (2005). Interprofessional practice: Learning how to collaborate. *Contemporary Nurse, 20*, 28–37.

McFadyen A. K., Webster V.S., Strachan, K., Figgins, E., Brown, H. & McKechnie, J. (2005). The Readiness for Interprofessional Learning Scale: A possible more stable sub-scale model for the original version of the RIPLS. *Journal of Interprofessional Care 19*(6), 595–603.

McKeown, M., Malihi-Shoja, L., & Downe, S. (2010). *Service user and carer involvement in health and social care education.* Oxford: Wiley-Blackwell.

Miller, C., Freeman, M., & Ross, N. (2001). *Interprofessional practice in health and social care.* London: Arnold.

Ministry of Business, Innovation and Employment. (2009). *Health delivery research landscape: An overview of New Zealand research capability and health delivery.* [Report to the Minister of Science and Technology] Wellington: Author.

Newell-Jones, K. (2008). Embedding interprofessional learning in postgraduate programmes of learning and teaching. In E. Howkins, & J. Bray (Eds.), *Preparing for interprofessional teaching: Theory and practice* (pp. 27–40). Oxford: Radcliffe.

Ovretveit, J. (1996). Five ways to describe a multidisciplinary team. *Journal of Interprofessional Care, 10*(2), 163–171.

Parsell G. & Bligh J. (1999). The development of a questionnaire to assess readiness of health care students for interprofessional learning (RIPLS). *Medical Education, 33*, 95–100.

Philippon, D. J., Pimlott, J. F. L., King, S., Day, R.A., & Cox, C. (2005). Preparing health science students to be effective health care team members: The interprofessional initiative at the University of Alberta. *Journal of Interprofessional Care, 19*, 195–206.

Pollard, K. C., Miers, M. E., Gilchrist, M., & Sayers, A. (2006). Comparison of interprofessional perceptions and working relationships among health and social care students: The results of a 3-year intervention. *Health and Social Care in the Community, 14*, 541–552.

Pollard, K. C., Miers, M. E., & Rickaby, C. (2012). 'Oh why didn't I take more notice?' Professionals' views and perceptions of pre-qualifying preparation for interprofessional working in practice. *Journal of Interprofessional Care, 26*, 355–361.

Reeves, S. (2012). The rise and fall of interprofessional competence. *Journal of Interprofessional Care, 26*, 253–255.

Reeves, S., Goldman, J., Gilbert, J., Tepper, J., Silver, I., Suter, E., & Zwarenstein, M. (2011). A scoping review to improve conceptual clarity of interprofessional interventions. *Journal of Interprofessional Care, 25*, 167–174.

Reeves, S., Zwarenstein, M., Goldman, J., Barr, H., Freeth, D., Hammick, M., & Koppel, I. (2009). Interprofessional education: Effects on professional practice and health care outcomes (review). *The Cochrane Library* 4.

Salvatori, P.S., Berry, S.C., & Eva, K.W. (2007). Implementation and evaluation of an interprofessional education initiative for students in the health professions. *Learning in Health and Social Care, 6,* 72–82.

Soothill, K., Mackay, L., & Webb, C. (Eds.). (1995). *Interprofessional relations in health care.* London: Edward Arnold.

Suter, E., & Deutschlander, S. (2010). Can interprofessional collaboration provide human health resources solutions? A knowledge synthesis. Retrieved July 12, 2011, from http://www.wcihc.ca

Thistlethwaite, J. (2012). Interprofessional education: A review of context, learning and the research agenda. *Medical Education, 46,* 58–70.

World Health Organization (1978). *Working interrelationships in the provision of community health care (medicine, nursing and medicosocial work): Report of a working group.* Florence: World Health Organization.

World Health Organization (1988). *Learning together to work together for health.* [Technical Report] Geneva: Author.

World Health Organization (2010). *Framework of action on interprofessional education and collaborative practice.* [Technical Report]. Geneva: Author.

WEBSITES

Australasian Interprofessional Practice & Education Network: http://www.aippen.net

Centre for Advancement of Interprofessional Education: http://www.caipe.org.uk/news

Canadian Interprofessional Health Collaborative: http://www.cihc.ca

CHAPTER 33

RESEARCH IN INTERPROFESSIONAL PRACTICE

DAWN FORMAN AND SUE FYFE

CHAPTER OVERVIEW

This chapter covers the following topics:

- Research in interprofessional education and collaborative practice
- Gathering evidence
- Evidence for interprofessional practice

KEY TERMS

Collaborative practice
Interprofessional care (IPC)
Interprofessional education
Interprofessional practice (IPP)
Practitioner

Health policy-makers internationally are seeking to find ways in which future health-care systems can be equipped to cope with needed changes in the way health professionals deliver health care. In developed countries the trend for the last three decades has been to move towards a more primary care focus with an emphasis on health **practitioners** working more effectively as a team (WHO, 2010). **Interprofessional care (IPC)** and **collaborative practice** models are now acknowledged as critical to ensuring a workforce that can optimise health services, strengthen health systems, and improve health outcomes (WHO, 2010; Goldberg, Koontz, Rogers, & Brickell, 2012).

There is a need to be clear about what the terms mean. **Interprofessional practice (IPP)**, or interprofessional care (IPC), is a process in which the practitioners from two or more professions work together with patients, families, and their communities to provide care and support (WHO, 2010). It encompasses the process of developing and maintaining effective interprofessional working relationships (Canadian Interprofessional Health Collaborative, 2012). Orchard, Curran and Kabene (2009) emphasise the importance of the health professional team being in a partnership with the patient/client in a 'participatory, collaborative and coordinated approach to shared decision making around health issues' (p. 4). **Interprofessional education** occurs when 'students from two or more professions learn about, from and with each other to enable effective collaboration and improve health outcomes' (WHO, 2010, p. 7).

RESEARCH IN INTERPROFESSIONAL EDUCATION AND COLLABORATIVE PRACTICE

Over the last 15 years, research into interprofessional practice has developed, but more is needed to show whether and how this new way of working can improve health outcomes and make a difference to the clients' experiences of health care.

RESEARCH ALIVE 33.1
SYSTEMATIC REVIEW

A systematic review investigating collaborative practice found only five studies that evaluated the effects of practice-based interprofessional collaborative interventions (Zwarenstein, Goldman & Reeves, 2009). Three of these studies found that collaborative interventions led to improvements in patient care, such as effective drug use, reduced length of hospital stay and fewer total hospital costs. One study showed no impact, and one study showed mixed outcomes. The studies indicate that practice-based IPC interventions can lead to positive

[continued next page]

Practitioner
A person recognised by a professional group.

Interprofessional care (IPC)
The provision of care, treatment and support for people based on the concept of interprofessional practice.

Collaborative practice
Practice involving many health workers from different professional backgrounds working together with patients, families, carers and communities to deliver the highest quality of care.

Interprofessional practice (IPP)
An approach to practice and service provision which incorporates interprofessional values.

Interprofessional education
Education in which students from various professions learn about, from and with each other.

changes in health care, but further studies are needed to better understand the range of possible interventions and their effectiveness, how they affect interprofessional collaboration and how they may be most useful. Examples of two interprofessional practice interventions where the collaborative care was evident were two randomised controlled trials of a collaborative care model. One involved nurses and psychiatrists in the United Kingdom treating severe mental illness (Bauer et al., 2006) and the second was the 'True Blue' study in Australia (Morgan et al., 2013), which involved practice nurses and general practitioners treating depression in patients with heart disease and/or diabetes. In both trials collaborative care interventions improved the outcomes for patients compared with traditional single profession treatment.

GATHERING EVIDENCE

Since the 1990s there have been many research reports, consultation papers and policy statements aimed at providing evidence for best practice. A review of background policies and articles which provide a rationale to the history in the United Kingdom between 1960 and 1998 can be found in Forman and Nyatanga (1999).

Every day, accidents, like the one outlined in Case Study 33.1, occur. While it may be generally expected that those involved in an adverse health event will be seen as people who have meaningful relationships and connections with others and not merely as individuals with a series of conditions, sadly that is not always the case, not just in Aotearoa New Zealand, but internationally.

CASE STUDY 33.1

WHAT HAPPENED?

On the news: A heavily pregnant woman and her daughter, aged 4, were today rescued from the scene of an accident outside Bunnings on Maple Road, Howick. Both mother and daughter were in a great deal of distress and the mother was bleeding heavily from a badly damaged left leg. The paramedics who arrived were concerned for the welfare of the unborn baby as well as for the mother. The daughter seemed shocked but to have received only cuts and bruises. We hope to bring you more news of their progress in the 4 o'clock news. Police would like to hear from anyone who witnessed the accident near ...

On arrival at Auckland City Hospital
Accident and Emergency report
Ms Renee C, aged 34, address:...
Arrived 2:38 p.m.

Nursing notes: triage category 1, heavily pregnant, compound fracture of the leg, bone visible, considerable blood loss and in pain

Doctor's actions: call for obstetrician and orthopaedic surgeon, emergency assessment needed for welfare of mother and baby and treatment of left leg

Bloods taken, BP 80/50, tachycardia 96 b/min, heavy smoker—30 per day

No further injuries apparent

Child: Clare C, 4.5 years of age of same address, triage category 5, low priority, distressed with minor cuts and bruises to face, dislodged front tooth

Aunt (Renee's sister) called at 3:00 p.m. waiting in waiting room with hospital volunteer

Depending on how the story unfolds for the mother, the unborn child and the daughter, more than 15 health and social care professionals could be involved in their care over a four-week period: paramedics, accident and emergency doctor, accident and emergency nurse, radiographer, obstetrician, orthopaedic surgeon, medical scientist, dentist, midwife, podiatrist, physiotherapist, occupational therapist, social worker, and health promotion professional.
   Some of the research questions from this situation could be:

- How might collaborative care make a difference to the treatment for Renee, her unborn child and Clare? How would we know?
- How might all these professionals communicate well to ensure the care of all three clients?
- How can the effectiveness of interprofessional care be measured?
  A number of outcomes could be chosen to explore this, such as research to measure:
  - performance of health professionals involved in the care;
  - satisfaction of the patients and clients receiving the care;
  - patient length of stay;
  - incidence rates of secondary complications;
  - re-admission with problems after discharge from hospital.

EVIDENCE FOR INTERPROFESSIONAL PRACTICE

International research has provided an evidence base from which to develop a model of interprofessional practice appropriate for individual countries and cultural contexts. The model focuses on both the community and the individual, and helps identify, at a local level, how interprofessional or collaborative practice could be a way to improve health outcomes. Local needs are identified and guidance given as to how interprofessional or collaborative practice is a route to improving health outcomes.

RESEARCH ALIVE 33.2
WORLD HEALTH ORGANIZATION

Researchers across mainly the UK, US, Canada and Australasia started researching IPP in the 1980s. Their work was collected into a World Health Organization Framework for Action on Interprofessional Education and Collaborative Practice (WHO, 2010). The framework used published research but also undertook two years of original research involving almost 400 health professionals, educators, administrators and researchers in 42 countries. These respondents answered questionnaires and took part in interviews to explain how interprofessional education is undertaken in their country. The report is rich with comments that individuals and groups have made about interprofessional education and collaborative care.

RESEARCH ALIVE 33.3
SHIFTING PARADIGMS

Research using a psychological and sociological approach has been conducted to investigate and explain why health professionals may be concerned about IPE affecting their professional distinctiveness. Beattie (1995) found that tribalism in health care originates and is reinforced in every cohort of student professionals. Each discipline or profession has a specific culture, as does an organisation. Culture in this way incorporates the shared values, beliefs, expectations, language, attitudes, assumptions and norms that underpin a specific group, discipline, team or organisation. This culture has been termed 'ethnocentrism'.

It is argued that a paradigm shift is needed for health professionals to move from one culture to another and that shift involves changing those understandings, values and attitudes in order to accept the other culture (Thistlethwaite, 2012). In this shift of culture, professional identity can be re-categorised in a way that sees all members of the re-categorised group as a single 'in group' (Tajfel, Flament, Billig, & Bundy, 1971). Where health professionals such as speech pathologists or occupational therapists could have seen themselves as separate and perhaps even competing groups, a re-categorised group working as an interprofessional team will see a new group and culture. In this new 'in group', the occupational therapists and speech pathologists, for example, recognise their own roles, each other's strengths and how they can best work together for the benefit of the client and the team. This new 'in group' will have a different set of values, attitudes and beliefs where collaboration will not be seen as a threat to any one professional role. Thistlethwaite and Nisbet (2011) see this as students moving first into their own profession, gradually increasing their understanding of their own role, observing their role within an IP team and then taking their place in the team, with an understanding of their own identity and their IP team role.

WHO (2010) has identified interprofessional and collaborative working as a critically important way of working. As a result, many tools have been developed to monitor the attitudes of students who are learning interprofessionally.

CASE STUDY 33.2

RESEARCH TOOLS

A report from the Canadian Interprofessional Health Collaborative (2012) lists all the research tools developed for interprofessional practice and collaborative research. They measure six main factors: attitudes, knowledge skills and abilities, behaviours, organisation practice, patient satisfaction and organisational satisfaction.

Most measures of change evaluate attitudes because, for cultural change to occur, attitudes must also change. Hylin, Nyholm, Mattiasson, and Ponzer (2007) evaluated the effect of a two-week IPP placement in an interprofessional training ward two years later. Just over half of the 633 students, now working

[continued next page]

in practice, responded. They had very positive impressions of the course, their own professional role development, patient care and teamwork during the placement. As importantly, 92% of them reported encouraging teamwork in their current workplaces. Similarly in Queensland, Jackson, Nicholson, Davidson, and McGuire (2006) found that IPE workshops for undergraduate nursing, medicine and allied health disciplines significantly improved students' reported knowledge and decreased their interprofessional boundaries. However, there was no evidence of changes in attitudes to patient care.

Really making a difference to patient/client care and improved health outcomes requires an evidence base demonstrating changes in patient satisfaction with care and improvement in outcomes. Showing that interprofessional practice has made a difference to the client or patient is difficult as people may experience a number of interventions to support their health and well-being. Patient satisfaction with interprofessional student placement is reportedly high (Arthur, 2012), but it is uncertain whether the interprofessional approach improved care. The effectiveness of IPP is more difficult to assess and quantify, but this is what must be investigated and measured to move towards the WHO goal of collaborative practice.

CASE STUDY 33.3

TEAMWORK IN ACTION

One UK study looked specifically at the effect of teamwork training in emergency department (ED) teams on the team behaviour, attitudes and opinions of staff and patients (Morey et al., 2002). The teams, consisting of doctors, nurses and technicians, received training and practice in 48 specific teamwork behaviours and roles, including the coordinating actions for effective ED teams such as good planning, reporting error, standing up for a position that a team member believes to be correct, and communicating and resolving conflict. The performance of the ED was evaluated using admission data and observed error. An example of error identified was that of a trauma patient who was brought in by ambulance, and had been receiving oxygen by mask in the ambulance. The mask was left in place when the patient was admitted, but not connected to the oxygen flow in the room.

The trained ED teams improved their quality of team behaviour and their attitudes to teamwork, and the clinical error rate in the trained groups significantly decreased from an average of 30.9% before the training to 4.4% afterwards. One point made by the authors of this study is that teamwork is not a natural product of working together and is more than team members getting along well.

Some IPP outcomes can be measured quantitatively, as was undertaken for emergency departments by Morey et al. (2002) (for example, error rates and team behaviour skills), and by Young et al. (2005) in treating mental health (measures of teamwork and overall competency). A qualitative approach may aim to elicit the thoughts and feelings of the patients or participants and their conceptions of participating in care from interprofessional teams (Kvarnstrom, Willumsen, & Anderson-Gare, 2012) and health professionals involved (Young et al., 2005), and explore the culture and processes of interprofessional practice (Drummond, Abbott, Williamson, & Somali, 2012; Schwartz, Wright, & Lavoie-Tremblay, 2011).

However, people and their health and disability experiences are as complex as the professional groups, teams and institutions providing care and support. This natural human complexity lends itself to research approaches that appreciate the many variables. The use of both qualitative and quantitative research methods is needed in the continuing investigations into collaborative and interprofessional care and education.

SUMMARY

To date, IPP research has focused on measuring health-care student and practitioner attitudinal changes in response to collaborative practice experiences. Further research is needed to examine the difference collaborative practice makes to the patient/client and the service provided.

REFLECTION POINTS

- Why should the client/patient always be at the centre of collaborative practice?
- From your own experience, what questions do you think IPP researchers should explore?

STUDY QUESTION

What research methods are appropriate in interprofessional education and practice?

ADDITIONAL READING

Arthur, N., Deutschlander, S., Law, R., Lait, J., McCarthy, P., Pallaveshi, L., et al. (2012). *An inventory of quantitative tools to measure interprofessional education and collaborative practice*. Retrieved from http://www.chd.ubc.ca/files/file/instructor-resources/CIHC_tools_report_Aug26%202012.pdf

Nichol, P. (2013). *Interprofessional education for health professionals in western Australia: perspectives and activity*. Sydney: Centre for Research in Learning and Change, Faculty of Arts and Social Sciences, University of Technology.

Reason, P., & Bradbury, H. (2001). *A handbook of action research participative inquiry and practice: groundings, practices, exemplars and skills*. London: Sage Publications.

World Health Organization. (2010). *Framework for action on interprofessional education and collaborative practice*. Geneva: Author.

REFERENCES

Arthur, N., Deutschlander, S., Law, R., Lait, J., McCarthy, P., Pallaveshi, L., et al. (2012). An inventory of quantitative tools to measure interprofessional education and collaborative practice. Retrieved from www.chd.ubc.ca/files/file/instructorresources/CIHC_tools_report_Aug26%202012.pdf

Bauer, M. S., McBride, L., Williford, W. O., Glick, H., Kinosian, B., Altshuler, L., et al. (2006). Collaborative care for bipolar disorder: Part II. Impact on clinical outcome, function, and costs. *Psychiatric Services, 57*(7), 937–45.

Beattie, A. (1995). *War and peace among the health tribes*. In K. Soothill, L. Mackay, & C. Webb. (Eds.), *Inter-professional relations in health care*. London: Edward Arnold.

Canadian Interprofessional Health Collaborative (CIHC) (2012). *An inventory of quantitative tools to measure interprofessional education and collaborative practice*.

Drummond, N., Abbott, K., Williamson, T., & Somali, B. (2012). Interprofessional primary care in academic family medicine clinics: implications for education and training. *Canadian Family Physician, 58*(8), 450–458.

Forman, D., & Nyatanga, L. (1999). The evolution of shared learning: some political and professional imperatives. *Medical Teacher, 21*(5), 489–96.

Goldberg, L. R., Koontz, J. S., Rogers, N., & Brickell, J. (2012). Considering accreditation in Gerontology: The importance of interprofessional collaborative competencies to ensure quality health care for older adults. *Gerontology & Geriatrics Education, 33*(1), 95–110.

Hylin, U., Nyholm, H., Mattiasson, A. C., & Ponzer, S. (2007). Interprofessional training in clinical practice on a training ward for healthcare students: a two-year follow-up. *Journal of Interprofessional Care, 21*(3), 277–288.

Jackson, C. L., Nicholson, C., Davidson, B., & McGuire, T. (2006). Training the primary care team; a successful interprofessional education initiative. *Australian Family Physician, 35*(10), 829–832.

Kvarnstrom, S., Willumsen, E., & Anderson-Gare, B.(2012). How service users perceive the concept of participation, specifically in interprofessional care. *British Journal of Social Work, 42*(1), 129–146.

Morey, J. C., Simon, R., Jay, G. D., Wears, R. L., Salisbury, M., Dukes, K. A., et al. (2002). Error reduction and performance improvement in the emergency department through formal teamwork training: Evaluation results of the MedTeams Project. *Health Services Research, 37*, 1553–1581.

Morgan, M. A. C., Coates, M. J., Dunbar, J. A., Reddy, P., Schlicht, K, & Fuller, J. (2013). The TrueBlue model of collaborative care using practice nurses as case managers for depression alongside diabetes or heart disease: a randomised trial. *British Medical Journal Open 2013, 3*, e002171.

Orchard, C., Curran, V., & Kabene, S. (2009). Creating a culture for interdisciplinary collaborative professional practice. *Medical Education Online, 10*(11), 1–13. Retrieved from http://med-ed-online.net/index.php/meo/article/view/4387.

Schwartz, L., Wright, D., & Lavoie-Tremblay, M. (2011). New nurses' experience of their role within interprofessional health care teams in mental health. *Archives of Psychiatric Nursing, 25*(3), 153–63.

Tajfel, H., Flament, C., Billig, M. G., & Bundy, R. P. (1971). Social categorisation and inter-group behaviour. *European Journal of Social Psychology, 1*, 149–178.

Thistlethwaite, J. E. (2012). Interprofessional education: A review of context, learning and the research agenda. *Medical Education, 46*, 58–70.

Thistlethwaite, J. E., & Nisbet, G. (2011). Preparing educators for interprofessional learning: rationale, educational theory and delivery. In S. Kitto, J. Chesters, J. Thistlethwaite, & S. Reeves (Eds.), Sociology of interprofessional health care practice: Critical reflections and concrete solutions (pp. 169–184). Hauppauge, NY: Nova Science Publishers.

World Health Organization (WHO). (2010). *Framework for action on interprofessional education and collaborative practice.* Geneva: Author.

Young, A. S., Chinman, M., Forquer, S. L., Knight, E. L., Vogel, H., Miller, A., et al. (2005). Use of a consumer-led intervention to improve provider competencies. *Psychiatric Services, 56*(8), 967–975.

Zwarenstein, M., Goldman, J., & Reeves, S. (2009). *Interprofessional collaboration: Effects of practice-based interventions on professional practice and healthcare outcomes. Cochrane Database of Systematic Reviews, 2009*(3). Art. No.: CD000072.

WEBSITES

Centre for the Advancement of Interprofessional Education:
http://www.caipe.org.uk

World Health Organization:
http://www.who.int/en

Canadian Interprofessional Health Collaborative:
http://www.cihc.ca

The Network Towards Unity for Health:
http://www.the-networktufh.org

GLOSSARY

Applied
Put to practical use.

Average
A measure that represents the middle point in a set of data (mean, median or mode are all types of average).

Behaviour
The response of a living thing (including people) to stimulation.

Best practice
An approach to practice that has been investigated and has been acknowledged as enabling optimum outcomes.

Bias
The preference of one particular response over another one.

Biological
Pertaining to biology—the science of life.

Biomedical
Relating to a way of thinking about health and illness with a focus on diseases as physical entities that affect physical bodies. This is the dominant Western model of health care.

Blinding
A research process that maintains anonymity, such as preventing research participants and/or researchers from identifying key details.

Capacity-building
The process of developing knowledge and skills within a group.

Cariogenic
Relating to a process or element that promotes tooth decay.

Case control trial
A study design that compares two groups of similar people, where the members of one group have a condition that members of the other group do not.

Clinical trial
A formally structured approach to research which includes standards and processes for identifying the problem and investigating it.

Cochrane Collaboration
An organisation which acts as a repository for evidence-based practice in health-care practice.

Cochrane Reviews
Reviews produced by the Cochrane Collaboration.

Collaborative practice
Practice involving many health workers from different professional backgrounds working together with patients, families, carers and communities to deliver the highest quality of care.

Community
A group of people with defined commonality. This may include geographical location, belief systems or any other social construct.

Complexity
The result of interaction between entities that results in effects whose sum is greater than the effects produced by the component parts.

Conditioning
A process of using reinforcement to develop a behavioural response.

Confidence interval
A range of values within which a parameter is expected to lie.

Consensus
A general agreement on any given issue.

Constructivist
A view that learning is not passively received, but actively constructed by individuals or groups.

Contested
Open to debate.

Control
A research cohort not treated in an active way to provide a point of comparison.

Critical
Of significance or a deliberate attempt to bring about social change.

Critical appraisal
A process of considering information from a perspective of critique.

Critical theory
An approach that examines hidden imbalances of power and knowledge in society and involves an in-depth analysis of social constructs in order to effect change.

Critical thinking
The application of sceptical inquiry to examine knowledge claims and taken-for-granted assumptions.

Cross-cultural research
Research that takes place across more than one cultural context.

Cultural
Relating to beliefs, traditions, practices and rituals originating within the family and community into which a person is born and raised, and transmitted from one generation to the next through a common language.

Data
Information that is gathered for the purpose of analysis and research.

Deductive reasoning
An approach to thinking that involves identifying common principles from which specific conclusions can be drawn.

Delphi
A process for gathering data that involves layers of collection.

Design
The process of planning and creating a solution to a problem.

Determinants
Factors that lead to a particular outcome.

Disease susceptibility
The tendency or likelihood of acquiring a disease.

Drug responsiveness
How a person responds to medication.

Editing
Selecting and preparing information in a variety of media for publication or presentation through a process of review and crafting. It involves, correction, condensation and other modifications of the original text or medium.

Empirical
Relating to a scientific approach to defining knowledge based on objective information and processes.

Empowerment
Giving or receiving the power in a particular situation.

Engagement
Meaningful interaction.

Epistemology
The study of the basis of knowledge.

Equity
Equal rights for all people in any situation.

Ethics
Moral values that are identified by any group of people, such as health professionals.

Ethnography
The process of recording and describing human behaviour.

Evaluation
The process of determining value.

Evidence-based practice
Practice that is informed by the careful consideration and evaluation of relevant information, and client/patient and practitioner experience and preference.

Experimentation
A process of testing hypotheses.

Expertise
Expert skills and knowledge.

Filter
Sort elements into categories.

Fluoride
A mineral associated with prevention of tooth decay in humans.

Fringe science
Knowledge or information considered not to be mainstream.

Genotype
The genetic make-up of an organism or cell; also refers to the specific set of alleles inherited for one gene.

Grey literature
Published information which is not peer reviewed.

Guidelines
Information providing advice on how to interpret policy or procedure.

Haplotype
A set of alleles (one of the possible alternative forms of a gene) from genes that are closely linked on a chromosome and inherited together.

Hapū
A subtribe.

Hauora
Philosophy of health.

Hermeneutic
A set of principles or a method of interpretation.

Hierarchy of evidence
A tool for evaluating research findings according to the degree of scientific rigour.

Hinengaro
Mental well-being.

Holistic
An emphasis on the whole, rather than separate parts.

Humanism
The belief that people are fundamentally good and that reasoning can prevail to address problems.

Hypothesis
A speculative explanation for a problem that can be tested by further research.

Inductive reasoning
An approach to thinking that involves developing general propositions from particular examples.

Information literacy
Competence to access and understand information from appropriate sources.

Informed consent
The process where research participants, having been fully informed, agree to engage in the study; also used in clinical settings to ensure patients are informed and agree to procedures or treatments.

Internet
The electronic means (and protocols) to connect computer users to information from a vast array of sources.

Interpretation
Adapting or explaining information in a meaningful and relevant way.

Interpretative
Interpreting in order to explain or make sense.

Interprofessional
Relating to the interaction between two or more professionals.

Interprofessional care (IPC)

The provision of care, treatment and support for people based on the concept of interprofessional practice.

Interprofessional collaboration

The process of practitioners from different professions working together in a meaningful way.

Interprofessional education

Education in which students from various professions learn about, from and with each other.

Interprofessional learning

Learning that involves students engaging (learning with and about) their professional groups.

Interprofessional practice (IPP)

An approach to practice and service provision which incorporates interprofessional values.

Interviews

Conversations held for the purpose of gathering information.

Intuition

The process of knowing something as a result of personal and/or professional insight.

Iwi

Main tribe.

Kaumātua

Esteemed, wise members of the Māori community.

Kaupapa Māori

Philosophy or agenda of the Māori community.

Knowing

Understanding, through being informed and aware.

Library databases

Tools for cataloguing information that enable many sources to be searched.

Limitations

Restrictions on applicability or consequences.

Mana

Pride or sense of esteem.

Māori-centred

Focused on Māori (by, for and about the indigenous people of Aotearoa New Zealand).

Mātauranga Māori

Māori knowledge and wisdom.

Mean

A particular type of average value calculated by the addition of all values in a data set, divided by the number of data points.

Measurement

The process of measuring the size or amount of something; also, the size or amount itself.

Medical model

An approach to health care that privileges biological, mechanistic and reductive understandings of bodily structures and functions.

Mental

Relating to the mind.

Meta-analysis

The process of undertaking a quantitative analysis of similar research studies.

Methods

Systematic procedures for undertaking an inquiry.

Methodology

Particular principles, rules and processes for undertaking research.

Mind

That which thinks, reasons and perceives.

Mixed methods

An approach to research that encompasses multiple elements—commonly both qualitative and quantitative approaches.

Model

A framework for describing concepts.

Naturalistic

An approach that emphasises viewing and exploring things in their natural environment.

Noa

Normal (not sacred).

Normal distribution

A statistical concept that describes the expected symmetrical distribution of a set of data around the mean.

Normative

Relating to the norms that form expectations about how people should behave, individually and as a society.

Null hypothesis

The position that states there is no relationship between defined variables.

Objective

An approach that implies a completely external or detached view of an object or phenomenon.

Occupation

An activity that people engage in.

Ontology

The view a person holds of the nature of being or existence.

Oral therapists

Practitioners utilising the skills of dental therapy and dental hygiene.

Pacific world view

A philosophical view that incorporates elements of Pacific culture and history.

Paradigm shift

A change in the theoretical framework or perspective from which information and knowledge has been viewed.

Participants

People who choose to take part in research.

Participation

The process of being involved.

Partnership

Genuine and respectful relationship between people.

Peer-review

The process of appropriately qualified individuals evaluating work for the purpose of maintaining quality.

Personalised medicine

Prevention, diagnosis and treatment of disease based on an individual's genetic profile.

Pharmacogenetics

The study of variation between individuals within a single gene that causes different responses to drug treatment.

Pharmacogenomics

The study of how all the genes within the genome function and interact to bring about a drug response.

Phenomenology

The study of human experience and consciousness.

Philosophy

The study of thought, meaning and existence.

PICO

An acronym for developing research questions: Problem/Population; Intervention; Comparison/Control; Outcome.

Placebo

An apparently inert intervention used in research as a control to test the effectiveness of an active intervention.

Positivist

An approach that emphasises natural phenomena, objectivity and empirical scientific approaches to knowledge.

Power

The exercise of strength or control, or a judgment about the importance or weight of a statistic.

Practitioner

A person recognised by a professional group.

Pragmatism

The demonstration of logical and practical responses to problems.

Presenting

The process of sharing information.

Primary sources

Acknowledged research findings traceable to their original sources.

Probability

The likelihood of a particular outcome.

Professional cultures

The ways of thinking, talking and interacting that develop within defined groups of practitioners.

Professionalisation

The process of a group of practitioners becoming recognised as a profession.

Protection
The act of looking after or taking care of.

Pseudo-scientific
Relating to information which purports to be scientific but is not based on sound principles or analysis.

Publishing
The process of having research scrutinised and promulgated to an audience in a particular medium.

Purpose
The intended outcome, reason or goal.

P-value
The statistical probability that the result is arrived at by chance.

Qualitative
Relating to analysis based on quality rather than the quantity of information and the value of human experience.

Qualitative evidence
Information collected through a rigorous research process that emphasised the quality and richness of data.

Qualitative research
Research carried out in a qualitative manner.

Quantitative
Relating to analysis based on quantity of information.

Quantitative evidence
Information collected through rigorously conducted research processes with an emphasis on the quantity of data.

Quantitative research
Research carried out in a quantitative manner.

Random
Without plan or pattern.

Randomisation
The process of allocating research participants or elements to different parts of an experiment (such as control group or active treatment group).

Randomised clinical trial
A highly specialised and prescriptive approach to research often used within the health sector. It isolates the trial population into active and control groups and investigates the outcomes for each group.

Reading

The process of engaging with published information.

Realism

A view that emphasises external sources of existence independent of human interpretation.

Reflection

The process of considering action.

Reflexivity

The process of using learning from a reflective process to inform development.

Relationships

The similarities and connections between people or variables in any given situation.

Relativist

A view that information must be considered according to its relationship with other known facts.

Reliability

The extent to which the same results are elicited when an investigation is repeated.

Replicate

The process of repeating an investigation.

Research

The purposeful collection and consideration of information to investigate a defined question.

Research proposal

A document that outlines the intention and design of a study.

Research utilisation

The process of using knowledge provided by research.

Researcher attributes

The characteristics of a researcher.

Research–practice gap

The gap between what is known about practice and when or how it changes to reflect that knowledge.

Rigour

The degree to which research process and findings stand up to challenge.

Sampling

The process of identifying participants for a study.

Scholarly

Relating to rigorously exploring, sharing and developing knowledge.

Science

The body of processes used to develop and extend knowledge (often with an emphasis on empiricism and positivism).

Scientist–practitioner

A professional who engages with science as they practice.

Secondary sources

References to publications or research that are found within another publication or source.

Social

Relating to people and the interactions between them.

Social media

Technological tools that enable communication to be interactive.

Standard deviation

A description of how widely data points are spread around a mean value.

Systematic review

A specific process for analysing similar studies for the purpose of informing practice and practitioners.

Tapu

A restricted or protected state, to be treated with the appropriate respect to ensure people are safe.

Te āo Māori

Māori world.

Te reo Māori

Māori language (voice).

Te Tiriti o Waitangi

An agreement (written in te reo Māori) between Māori and the Crown, sometimes referred to as the founding document of Aotearoa New Zealand. *Also see* Treaty of Waitangi and note that the English translation of Te Tiriti o Waitangi is not identical to the Treaty of Waitangi.

Theoretical

Relating to theory.

Theory

An explanation of a phenomenon.

Theory–practice gap

See research–practice gap.

Tikanga

Māori way of doing things; Māori protocol.

Tinana

Physical well-being.

Treatment

The act of carrying out an intervention for the purpose of alleviating or curing a problem.

Treaty of Waitangi

An agreement (written in English) between Māori and the Crown, sometimes referred to as the founding document of Aotearoa New Zealand. *See* Te Tiriti o Waitangi and note that there is also an English translation of Te Tiriti o Waitangi.

Trial and error

The process of developing practice by trying various approaches and deciding what seems to be most effective.

Triangulation

The process of linking more than two pieces of information to improve the trustworthiness of findings.

Unconscious

The part of the human mind that the individual is unaware of.

Validity

Fitness for purpose.

Variability

An indication of the spread of data values.

Variable

A factor that can be controlled or changed in an experiment.

Variance

A measure of how far each value in a data set is from the mean.

Wairua

Spiritual well-being.

Whānau

Family.

World view

A set of beliefs or concepts held by an individual informing how they interpret their environment and experience.

Writing

The process of developing a written piece of work.

INDEX

Printed in Australia
05 Mar 2019
701169